CANCER ETIOLOGY, DIAGNOSIS AND TREATMENTS

# THE SENTINEL LYMPH NODE

## DETECTION, PROCEDURES AND CLINICAL IMPLICATIONS

# CANCER ETIOLOGY, DIAGNOSIS AND TREATMENTS

Additional books and e-books in this series can be found on Nova's website under the Series tab.

CANCER ETIOLOGY, DIAGNOSIS AND TREATMENTS

# THE SENTINEL LYMPH NODE

## DETECTION, PROCEDURES AND CLINICAL IMPLICATIONS


AMBROGIO PIETRO LONDERO
SERENA BERTOZZI
AND
CARLA CEDOLINI
EDITORS



nova
Medicine & Health
New York

**Library of Congress Cataloging-in-Publication Data**

ISBN 978-1-53614-557-1
Library of Congress Control Number: 2018958577

*Published by Nova Science Publishers, Inc. † New York*

# CONTENTS

# PREFACE

Sentinel lymph node biopsy is a minimally invasive surgical procedure that consists in the intraoperative detection of the first lymph node draining a certain cancer. The purpose of this technique is to allow adequate lymph node staging while sparing patients from unnecessary complete lymph node dissections and the traditional harmful complications associated with them.

This book gathers an overview of the knowledge on the sentinel lymph node biopsy procedure in the staging and treatment of cancers such as melanoma, breast, thyroid, vulva, endometrium, cervix, colon, anus and liver cancers. In addition, it also provides information on other malignancies that represent a less common indication for sentinel lymph node biopsy but may also benefit from this procedure such as gastric, urological and ovarian cancers.

Furthermore, it outlines the rationale for sentinel lymph node biopsy, together with the technical aspects of the procedure, which are also accurately covered, from the various intraoperative sentinel node detection techniques to the subsequent sentinel lymph node analysis methods. Finally, the book provides information also on preoperative lymph node diagnostics and sentinel lymph node biopsy perioperative complications in different nodal districts.

In: The Sentinel Lymph Node
Editors: A. Londero, S. Bertozzi and C. Cedolini
ISBN: 978-1-53614-557-1


*Chapter 1*

# CANCER DISSEMINATION PATHWAYS, CONSERVATIVE SURGERY AND THE RATIONALE FOR SENTINEL LYMPH NODE BIOPSY

***Luca Seriau*[1], *Serena Bertozzi*[1,*], *Carla Cedolini*[1] and *Ambrogio P. Londero*[2]**
[1]Breast Unit, University Hospital of Udine, Italy
[2]Clinic of Obstetrics and Gynecology, University Hospital of Udine, Italy

**Abstract**

Cancer is known to be a multifactorial disease, which may somehow be influenced by many different factors that can trigger the process of carcinogenesis. Malignant tumors have a metastatic capacity that is often a function of their size and biology. In the case of breast cancer, it is estimated that about 10% of cancers of less than 1 cm have nodal metastases. In this regard, axillary lymphadenectomy fully meets all diagnostic and prognostic needs, but is a very invasive surgery, and therefore burdened with potential severe complications. Hence, sentinel lymph node biopsy has permanently entered the protocol of surgical management of many malignant tumors, obtaining a particular consensus in the field of breast surgery, where it arises as an adequate alternative to complete axillary lymphadenectomy in clinically node-negative patients, preventing the harmful complications of such radical intervention when not necessary. Sentinel lymph node biopsy has a high predictive capacity, which reaches values of approximately 96% in the case of negativity. Furthermore, the likelihood that the other lymph nodes of the chain are involved with cancer is about 4% and a possible local recurrence of the disease does not exceed 3% of cases. As a consequence, it seems rational to subordinate the potential lymphadenectomy to those cases in which sentinel lymph node biopsy ascertains the metastatic involvement of the lymph node. Alternatively, its negativity will serve to provide a valuable tool for the staging of the disease for prognostic and therapeutic purposes.

**Keywords:** carcinogenesis, lymphatic metastases, sentinel lymph node biopsy, conservative surgery

---

*Corresponding Author E-mail: dr.bertozzi@gmail.com.

## 1. Introduction

Cancer is known to be a multifactorial disease. Therefore, by definition, it can be influenced by many different factors that can trigger the process of carcinogenesis, including age, metabolic factors, such as obesity or hyperinsulinemia, sedimentary lifestyle, tobacco smoking habits and exposure to carcinogenic factors, such as ionizing radiation or chemical agents. However, the most important role in carcinogenesis seems to be played by the genetic heritability of mutations, which may increase cancer susceptibility and can now be tested in patients with a strong familial history and, consequently, at high risk of cancer.

Most of these mutations occur in genes that encode proteins involved in regulating the cell cycle, but, subsequently, cancer cells can acquire a large number of other mutations that affect the genes that encode proteins involved in cellular adhesion and neoangiogenesis, allowing cancer to gain the ability to spread to other parts of the body. There are two primary ways cancer cells can disseminate to distant organs: through the lymphatic system, where they are usually blocked by the filter function of lymph nodes until they succeed in evading the surveillance of lymphocytes, or through the bloodstream, from where they can theoretically reach any part of the body.

During the first half of the 20$^{th}$ century, the TNM classification was developed, which enhances the important role of both lymphatic and distant metastases in prognosis prediction. In particular, the TNM classification provides a description of the stage of a cancer based on tumor size, possible lymphatic involvement and possible presence of distant solid organ metastases [1]. For this reason, lymphatic surgery has become an integral part of oncologic surgery over the decades.

In this chapter, we will describe the aforementioned pathways of neoplastic cells diffusion, the rationale for lymph node evaluations in the case of neoplastic disease and the evolution of lymphatic surgery in favor of an increasingly more conservative surgery.

## 2. Lymphatic Diffusion

After the introduction of the lymphatic system concept in 1653, many authors devoted a lot of time and resources to the study of this complex system, which consists of an intricate network of vessels that is present throughout the body and some nodes that have a filtering function of a particulate matter called lymph [2].

The embryology, anatomy and physiology of the lymphatic system are necessary to understand the process of lymphatic metastasization of tumors [3]. In particular, the primary function of the lymphatic system is to deposit the interstitial fluid and intestinal nutrients into the circulation. Subsequently, during the evolutionary process, lymphocyte collections have developed in the lymph nodes, which interrupt the lymph flow and are supplemented by a system of analysis of antigens from the hostile external environment. This type of lymphocyte collections allows a multilayer defense, but also an adaptive immunologic response. The lymphocyte trafficking between blood, lymph, and lymph nodes is extremely complex and allows the body to defend itself against "foreign" substances or even against its own cells when transformed in neoplastic cells.

Since lymph is produced and drained by all parts of the body, it has been suspected that it may also drain substances from neoplastic lesions. Hence, the lymph nodes draining the particular region of the body where the tumor is located should filter the lymph from the tumor and, consequently, block and annihilate any diseased cells that move through the lymphatic system. However, despite the clear difference between normal and cancer cells, the latter are sometimes not "foreign" enough and, by acquiring the ability to circumvent the lymphatic system surveillance, can finally spread to the entire lymphatic pathway and bloodstream. A possible mechanism of immune escape may be cytokine interaction, which prevents lymphatic entrapment and antibody production.

Over the past century, there has been growing evidence that lymph flow is not a random event, but an anatomically defined, highly structured, reliable, rational and coherent phenomenon that leads the lymph from the organ or limb tumor site to the regional lymphatic basin, initially encountering one, or occasionally more, sentinel lymph nodes [4].

In the lymphatic diffusion process, diseased cells, after being detached from the tumor, invade the lymphatic capillaries and collectors and, by following the flow of the lymph, reach the lymph nodes, where they remain blocked, at least temporarily. In fact, they can then pass into the post-lymph node collectors moving to other lymph nodes, and so on, until they complete their path in the main lymphatic trunks and finally enter the bloodstream, from which they can colonize everywhere. However, metastatic cells can potentially spread into the bloodstream during each stage of the lymphatic pathway through lymphovascular shunts in more peripheral regions, as well as before entering the lymphatic system. This kind of hematogenous metastatic property will be discussed in the next section.

The lymphatic diffusion of metastases has some peculiar aspects in comparison with the hematogenous diffusion. Firstly, it is slower, since it must follow the entire lymphatic pathway, and also being braked, as mentioned, by the lymph nodes, before it reaches the bloodstream and becomes systemic. Secondly, it proceeds in sequence and is therefore very reliable and predictable, as the metastases, advancing along the lymphatic chain, invade the lymph nodes from the very first one they meet (i.e. the sentinel lymph node) proceeding gradually with all the remaining ones until the involvement of the entire lymph node basin.

For this reason, knowledge of the topography of the drainage pathways of viscera and single anatomic districts is of fundamental importance, as it allows the surgeon to subject the correct nodes to histological examination. For instance, if we consider tumors located in the upper or lower limb, it is very likely that the lymph coming from those regions will be drained by the axillary and groin lymph nodes, respectively (Figure 1). However, in case of tumors of the trunk, it is very difficult to predict which nodal station will first drain the neoplastic lesion.

With regard to intra-thoracic or intra-abdominal cancer, a specific lymphatic drainage has been described for every organ, but also many variants have been observed. Then, also in this case, the lymph node stations to be dissected are not always so intuitive.

Lymphatic dissemination of tumor cells is not a passive process, and the metastastic spread to the lymph nodes may occur even in the absence of tumor lymphangiogenesis in some animal models [5]. However, some animal models using lymphangiogenetic growth factors and histochemical markers that discriminate between blood and lymphatic vessels show that lymphangiogenesis actively promotes the metastasization process [6, 7].

Both experimental models and clinicopathological data indicate that lymphatic vessel growth in the vicinity of solid tumors not only modifies the adhesive properties of the lymphatic endothelium, but also promotes lymph node metastases [8]. There are several factors, secreted by the tumor, responsible for lymphangiogenesis and lymphatic diffusion of the tumor, which have been shown to induce lymphangiogenesis both near the tumor site and within adjacent lymph nodes even before the arrival of metastatic tumor cells.

These lymphangiogenetic factors include the tumor-secreted vascular endothelial growth factors C (VEGF-C) and D (VEGF-D). They act through their cognate receptor tyrosine kinase (VEGFR-3), which is located on the lymphatic endothelial cells. Other additional signaling molecules reported to have a key role in both lymphangiogenesis and lymphatic metastasization are VEGF-A, platelet-derived growth factor BB (PDGF-BB), hepatocyte growth factor, and chemokines. All these factors involved in the molecular signaling pathways that control lymphangiogenesis can be targeted by biological drugs with the aim of counteracting lymphatic metastasization.

The most studied lymphangiogenetic molecular pathway consists of the tumor-secreted glycoproteins VEGF-C and VEGF-D, which activate the MAPK/AKT signaling cascade through the surface receptor tyrosin kinase VEGFR-3, resulting in the prevention of apoptosis and subsequent induction of cell proliferation and migration [9, 10].

Lymph node metastases are not usually considered to be a life-threatening manifestation of neoplastic disease [11], as regional lymph nodes do not play an essential life-sustaining function. Exceptions are extremely rare, but may occur in the lymphatic vessels in the case of lethal lymphangitic pulmonary carcinoma or in the lymphatic collectors by secondary compression or narrowing of an adjacent hollow lumen. Since nodal disease does not appear to significantly increase cancer-related mortality, over time nodal excision has acquired a prognostic rather than a curative function, providing useful information for clinicians in choosing adjuvant therapy.

The prognostic significance of lymphatic metastasization is still a subject of debate. In particular, some authors observed that the inhibition of lymph node metastases is associated with reduced metastases of distant organs in animal cancer models, suggesting that there may be a pathway that facilitates distant organ metastases via lymph nodes [12, 13]. However, in other studies there was no evidence of a correlation between lymphatic and hematogenous metastases.

A large number of factors influence whether the primary tumor metastasizes to the lymphatic pathway or the blood vessels, and consequently how tumor cells will reach the systemic circulation [14]. Morphological differences between blood and lymphatic vessels affect the initial diffusion path. In fact, peritumoral lymphatics may be considered a default pathway for tumors unable to cross blood endothelial boundaries. However, innate differentiation programs, together with additional genetic and epigenetic changes, determine the metastatic phenotype and the consequent ability of tumor cells to intravasate. For example, there are some subtypes of tumors, such as luminal A breast cancers, which are very likely to metastasize to lymph nodes but not to distant organs, and other subtypes, such as basal-like breast cancers, which are more likely to metastasize to distant viscera than to regional nodes.

## 3. Hematogenous Diffusion and Metatasization Cascade

Cancer progression through the process of metastasization comprises a series of sequential steps (Figure 2) [15]. The so-called metastasization cascade begins with tumor cells locally

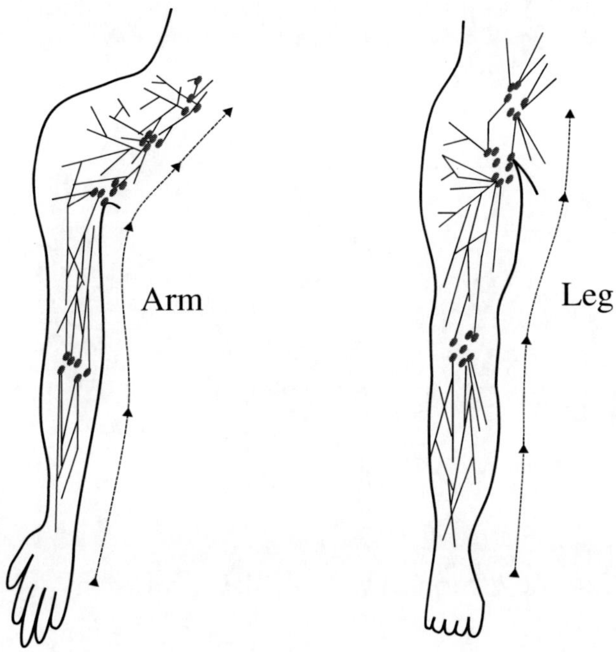


Figure 1. Lymphatic drainage of the limbs: on the left side arm and on the rigth side leg (drawing by SB and APL).

invading the surrounding host tissue, intravasating into the bloodstream or the lymphatic vessels and disseminating to distant organs. As a result, tumor cells undergo cell cycle arrest and adhere to capillary beds within the target organ before extravasating into the organ parenchyma, proliferating and promoting angiogenesis [16, 17]. During these numerous steps, tumor cells must evade the host immune response and apoptotic signals in order to survive, and failing to complete any of these steps will arrest the process [16, 18].

The local invasion step is favored by the progressive alteration of the adhesion of tumor cells to other cells or to the extracellular matrix (ECM), often due to an alteration of the cadherin family function [19]. In particular, E-cadherin down-regulation plays a key role in the outgrowth of metastatic cancer cells and has been associated with poor prognosis [20, 21, 22, 23]. On the other hand, N-Cadherin is closely associated with mesenchymal cells and related to epithelial-to-mesenchymal transition (EMT), which plays a major role in tumor progression by facilitating invasion and intravasation into the bloodstream and inducing proteases involved in the degradation of the ECM [24, 25, 26, 27, 28, 29, 30].

The adhesion of tumor cells to the ECM is usually mediated by integrins, which are transmembrane receptors found on ECM components such as fibronectin, laminin, collagen, fibrinogen and vitronectin [31, 19]. Integrins are known to participate in the modulation of tumor motility by promoting the ECM degradation, primarily through the activity of metalloproteinases (MMPs) and the urokinase plasminogen activator system, and to promote

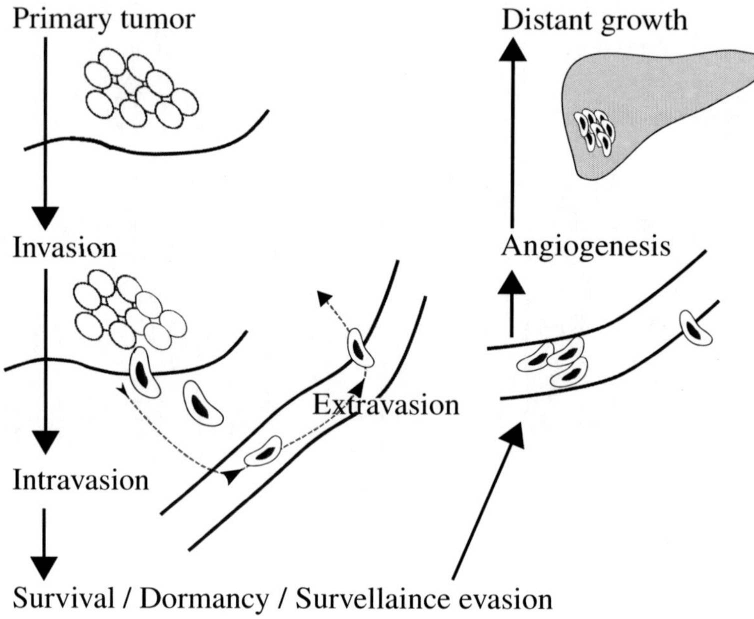


Figure 2. Metastatization cascade (drawing by SB and APL).

local invasion by enabling the penetration of tissue boundaries [32, 33].

To achieve an invasive phenotype, tumor cells are then able to migrate from the confined primary site, either individually or coordinately [34, 35]. Single tumor cells migrate in two ways, mainly by protease-dependent mesenchymal movement or protease-independent amoeboid movement [29, 34, 31]. Cell polarity is altered from apical-basal polarity to front-rear polarity to initiate cell migration through changes in actin fibers that induce cytoskeleton remodeling, and proteolytic enzymes such as MMPs are activated to modify cell matrix adhesion and produce channels in the ECM, so that tumor cells can move through the paths of least resistance [36]. Due to the presence of intercellular junctions, clusters of cells circulate commonly in the form of emboli in the blood or the lymphatic vessels, creating tube-like microtracks by cleaving and orientating collagen fibers using the membrane type 1 MMP for the subsequent collective mass migration of tumor cells through the ECM [37, 38, 39, 40].

Based on Paget's 'seed and soil' theory for metastases, the 'seed' (tumor cell) is postulated to grow only when it finds a suitable 'soil' (environment) [41]. Therefore, the microenvironment of metastatic tumor cells is crucial for establishing both tumor growth and malignant progression, consisting of many different specialized blood and lymph vessel cells, including fibroblasts, immune cells, endothelial cells and mural cells, together with the ECM [42, 43, 44, 45, 46, 47, 48, 49, 50, 51, 52]. For instance, the recruitment of macrophages by non-invasive breast tumor cells induces angiogenesis and promotes malignant transformation and metastatic spread [53, 54, 55, 56, 57, 58].

Another hallmark of the metastasization cascade is the establishment of tumor angiogenesis, which plays a significant role in the generation and growth of metastases, disrupting the balance between pro-angiogenic and anti-angiogenic factors with a slant towards the pro-angiogenic side [59, 60, 61, 62, 63]. Genetic mutations, mechanical stresses, inflammatory processes, tumor expression of angiogenic proteins and, above all, hypoxia are considered causes of the "angiogenic switch", favouring the production of more pro-angiogenic factors and creating an abnormal vasculature [64, 65, 66, 67].

Metastasization is regarded as a highly inefficient process, as the sheer number of tumor cells daily entering the bloodstream is estimated to be about 4 x 10[6] tumor cells released per gram of primary tumor [68, 69]. However, distant metastases constitute the major cause of cancer-related death rather than the insufficiency of the organ of origin of the primary tumor. Therefore, it is of extreme importance to understand every detail of the metastasization process in order to be successful in the future in blocking this mechanism before the tumor completes its first steps of metastasization.

## 4. Conservative Surgery Evolution

By taking on the filter role of lymph nodes, regional lymph node excision has become a key part of oncological surgery. The number and degree of involvement of the lymph nodes examined provide useful information on tumor aggressiveness and locoregional extent, and allow accurate staging, with the aim of best predicting both the response to adjuvant treatments and the patients' overall and disease-free survival. Moreover, this information also helps guide the clinician toward the type of intervention that best guarantees the necessary surgical radicality.

The initial concept of radicality was born at the end of the $19^{th}$ century from the hypothesis that tumors are a local disease, therefore initially circumscribed and capable of metastasizing only in its most advanced phases. As a result, there were no significant differences in the surgical approach to early or advanced cancers, although the aim was different: to prevent the risk of future metastatic dissemination in the first case or to try to save the lives of patients in the latter.

Lymph node dissection must include a variable number of regional nodes depending on the site involved. Many techniques have been developed in order to correctly detect and quantify the potential lymph nodes involvement.

As expected, complete lymph node dissection is correlated with different complications depending on the site involved. Although the locoregional failure of the lymphatic system is unlikely to have life-threatening consequences, it can have a very severe impact on patients' quality of life. In fact, lymphedema may result in acute onset of pain and significantly reduce both sensitivity and motility of the affected part of the body. In order to avoid lymphatic complications and reduce evident overtreatment in the case of clinically node-negative patients, we have witnessed an evolution of lymphatic surgery from radical toward conservative therapy.

The acquisition over time of new knowledge in the field of the tumor biology [70] and, in particular, the discovery that malignant neoplasms are to be regarded as systemic diseases, as they are capable of spreading metastatic cells already at their onset, has led to a revision over the years of the concept of radicality. This process has had significant effects on the surgical approach to early-stage tumors, particularly.

Through the introduction of organized screening programs (i.e. mammographic screening for breast cancer, PAP-test for cervical cancer and occult fecal blood test for colon cancer), we have witnessed a progressive reduction in locally advanced cancers in favor of an increase in early stage cancers, which currently represent the majority of neoplastic diseases [71, 72, 73]. Limited excisions are the gold standard surgical procedure for this type of tumors, as it is sufficient to eradicate the diseased tissue, leaving it to adjuvant therapy to combat any systemic dissemination.

The same principle applies to the role of lymphadenectomy. In particular, the removal of lymph nodes invaded by tumor cells is appropriate, while the removal of disease-free lymph nodes appears to be useless and even harmful. Furthermore, the curative intent of lymphadenectomy has been completely replaced by its staging intent. For this reason the removal of an adequate number of lymph nodes is mainly aimed at post-surgical treatments rather than at curing nodal disease.

In addition to contain the surgical extension, the tendency to reduce the surgical impact has led to a decrease in both the number of surgeries and the duration of the operation. As for the number of interventions, many techniques have been developed to intraoperatively analyze the sentinel lymph node with an accuracy comparable to a definitive histological examination and, consequently, to decide promptly whether complete lymph node dissection is necessary [74, 75, 76, 77, 78, 79, 80, 73, 81, 72].

Previously, there were two potentially viable routes to evaluate the sentinel node. In the first case, sentinel lymph node biopsy (SLNB) was performed a few days before the excision of the primary cancer in order to find out the lymph node status and, if necessary, perform complete lymph node dissection. However, this option was clearly limited to the types of cancers that usually metastasize to the groin or the axillary nodes, which are easier to excise. In the second case, SLNB was performed immediately before or after the excision of the cancer, with the risk of a subsequent second intervention to completely remove the remaining regional lymph nodes. This risk was found to vary depending on the location of the primary cancer site. For example, it is about 25% in the case of breast cancer.

In particular, the immediate intraoperative SLNB evaluation resulted to be superior to the scheduled delayed after surgery evaluation, as in about 14-38% it has allowed the prevention of a second operation in patients candidates for complete lymphadenectomy for sentinel node positivity, together with a few obvious consequential advantages, such as cost-effectiveness, a favorable impact on the psychosomatic well-being of patients and the prevention of potential surgical difficulties during the reoperation of recent surgically injured axillary tissues [74, 77, 82].

As for the duration of anaesthesia and surgery, many efforts have been made to reduce the time of analysis of the sentinel node, and different intraoperative techniques have been tested in order to reduce anesthesiological time as much as possible. In the case of breast cancer, for example, we have witnessed a great technical evolution, from the use of histological (frozen section analysis) or cytological (touch imprinting) techniques to the application of biomolecular technologies (OSNA), with a successful reduction in the time of analysis of the sentinel node.

In conclusion, if we take a look at breast cancer, for instance, we have an exemplary picture of the evolution of treatments in an increasingly conservative direction. Over time, in fact, there has been a clear tendency to quantitatively and qualitatively reduce the impact of surgical and non-surgical breast treatments on breast cancer patients. In the mid-1990s, we witnessed the introduction of quadrantectomy, which succeeded in substituting mastectomy for early breast cancers, achieving optimal aesthetic results while maintaining adequate oncological outcomes [83, 84]. Thereafter, axillary lymph nodes were systematically spared in patients with early breast cancer by introducing the SLNB procedure [74]. Moreover, the spread of partial breast irradiation techniques to spare most of the mammary gland from radiotherapy was remarkable, further reducing local aesthetic complications [85]. Finally, there was an interesting development of tailored biological therapies that can only act on targeted tissues and kill tumor cells while sparing healthy cells.

## 5. Rationale for the Sentinel Lymph Node Biopsy

SLNB was originally designed in the 1970s for penile and testicular cancers, but only in 1989 was initially performed for the treatment of malignant melanoma, and in 1995 for the treatment of breast cancer [86, 87, 88]. Subsequently, the technique was applied to many other primary tumors, including cancers of the gynecological organs (endometrium, vulva, cervix), the digestive tract (stomach, liver, colon, anus) and other specific organs (thyroid).

The rationale for the sentinel lymph node biopsy is to avoid unnecessary lymphadenectomy in node-negative patients and simultaneously provide the necessary indications, given its high predictive value.

The success of this technique, which today is an integral part of the surgical treatment of malignant tumors, is linked to the importance of the responses that histological examination can provide. In particular, the finding of metastases in the sentinel node attests that a local spread of the tumor is underway. While it does not allow to establish the degree of involvement of the lymphatic chain, once the pathological status is ascertained, it provides a precise indication for the excision of other regional nodes, known as radical lymphadenectomy.

On the other hand, the failure to detect neoplastic cells in the sentinel node suggests that the spreading of the disease is to be excluded at least at the lymphatic level, and, in certain types of tumors, it is a contraindication for complete lymph node dissection [75, 76, 77, 78].

However, some objections can be raised. Firstly, the result may be negative because the sentinel lymph node is not detected due to technical errors or insufficient preparation. Secondly, it could be a false-negative node. Thirdly, it is also possible to assume that the metastases have skipped, for some reason, the sentinel node directly reaching the following ones.

These doubts, which to some extent undermine the reliability of the examination, have found convincing answers over the years in numerous scientific studies on the subject. Most of these studies are breast pathology researches, a field in which SLNB has rapidly established itself as a viable alternative to the lymphatic emptying of the axillary cavity.

This technique involves the detection, excision and evaluation of only the first lymph node draining a specific neoplastic lesion. The first experiments were carried out using the vital staining method, which consists in injecting patent blue dye around the tumor site a few minutes before surgery. Then, the dye spreads rapidly into the lymphatic network and reaches the sentinel lymph node, which can be then easily identified by its blue color.

The rather high failure percentage has led to the testing of alternative methods based on the use of radioactive tracers, which have given better results. These new techniques are certainly much more expensive, compared with the previous one, since they require protected environments and specialized physicians (i.e. the specialist in nuclear medicine, the radiologist in the case of non-palpable lesions). Nevertheless, they are the most practiced techniques in cancer centers. If desired, after a few hours, a lymphoscintiscan can be performed to fix the image of the tracer diffusion into the lymphatic network and allow the identification of the sentinel node at its cutaneous projection [72, 89, 81].

More recently, to avoid the necessity of many specialists once again, another experimental method is being studied, based on the use of indocyanine green, which highlights the sentinel lymph node in the axillary cavity, without resorting to radioactive tracers. In the case of breast cancer, it is injected subcutaneously into the quadrant affected by the neoplasm, in the operating room, immediately after the induction of general anaesthesia. At this point, stimulated by an infrared lamp, the dye becomes fluorescent and its path can be visualized and followed subcutaneously, until it reaches the sentinel node [90, 91].

The detection rate of the sentinel lymph node in expert hands reaches very high values, of about 95-99%, when the vital dye and the radioactive tracer are used together, and surgical treatment of the neoplasia can be exhausted in a single session [92, 83]. With regard to cancer staging, SLNB represents a valid alternative to radical dissection. In fact, its accuracy in detecting breast cancer metastases is over 95% [93, 84, 74, 85].

## Conclusion

Malignant tumors have a metastatic capacity that is often, but not always, a function of their size. In particular, in the case of breast cancer, it is estimated that about 10% of cancers of less than 1 cm and about 5% of those of less than 0.5 cm have nodal metastases. Therefore, the decision to abstain from lymph node excision in the presence of smaller tumors is not acceptable.

Axillary lymphadenectomy fully meets all diagnostic and prognostic needs, but is a very invasive surgery, therefore burdened with potential severe complications. In addition, it requires more recovery time and, thereby, leads to an increase in hospitalization times and healthcare costs. Therefore, SLNB has permanently entered the protocol of surgical treatment of many malignant tumors, obtaining particular consensus in the field of breast surgery, where it arises as an adequate alternative to complete axillary lymphadenectomy in clinically node-negative patients and prevents the harmful complications of such radical intervention when not necessary.

SLNB has a high predictive capacity, which reaches values of around 96% in the case of negativity. Furthermore, the likelihood that the other lymph nodes of the chain are involved with cancer is about 4%, and a local recurrence of the disease does not exceed 3% of cases. As a consequence, it seems rational to subordinate the potential lymphadenectomy to those cases in which SLNB ascertains the metastatic involvement of the lymph node. Alternatively, its negativity will serve to provide a valuable tool for the staging of the disease for prognostic and therapeutic purposes.

## References


[1] American College of Surgeons. *AJCC Cancer Staging Manual (Eighth Edition)*. Springer. 2017.

[2] Halsted W. S. I. The Results of Operations for the Cure of Cancer of the Breast Performed at the Johns Hopkins Hospital from June, 1889, to January, 1894. *Ann Surg. 1894*;20:497–555.

[3] Cady B. Regional lymph node metastases, a singular manifestation of the process of clinical metastases in cancer: contemporary animal research and clinical reports suggest unifying concepts. *Cancer Treat Res. 2007*;135:185–201.

[4] Cabanas RM. An approach for the treatment of penile carcinoma. *Cancer. 1977*; 39:456–466.

[5] Wong S. Y., Haack H., Crowley D., Barry M., Bronson R. T., Hynes R. O., Tumor-secreted vascular endothelial growth factor-C is necessary for prostate cancer lymphangiogenesis, but lymphangiogenesis is unnecessary for lymph node metastasis. *Cancer Res. 2005*;65:9789–9798. doi:10.1158/0008-5472.CAN-05-0901.

[6] Saharinen P., Tammela T., Karkkainen M. J., Alitalo K., Lymphatic vasculature: development, molecular regulation and role in tumor metastasis and inflammation. *Trends Immunol. 2004*;25:387–395. doi:10.1016/j.it.2004.05.003.

[7] Stacker S. A., Achen M. G., Jussila L., Baldwin M. E., Alitalo K., Lymphangiogenesis and cancer metastasis. *Nat Rev Cancer. 2002*;2:573–583. doi:10.1038/nrc863.

[8] Achen M. G., Stacker S. A., Molecular control of lymphatic metastasis. *Ann N Y Acad Sci. 2008*;1131:225–234. doi:10.1196/annals.1413.020.

[9] Joukov V., Pajusola K., Kaipainen A., Chilov D., Lahtinen I., Kukk E. et al., A novel vascular endothelial growth factor, VEGF-C, is a ligand for the Flt4 (VEGFR-3) and KDR (VEGFR-2) receptor tyrosine kinases. *EMBO J. 1996*;15:290–298.

[10] Achen M. G., Jeltsch M., Kukk E., Mkinen T., Vitali A., Wilks A. F. et al., Vascular endothelial growth factor D (VEGF-D) is a ligand for the tyrosine kinases VEGF receptor 2 (Flk1) and VEGF receptor 3 (Flt4). *Proc Natl Acad Sci U S A. 1998*; 95:548–553.

[11] Taneja C., Cady B., Decreasing role of lymphatic system surgery in surgical oncology. *J Surg Oncol. 2005*;89:61–66. doi:10.1002/jso.20198.

[12] Krishnan J., Kirkin V., Steffen A., Hegen M., Weih D., Tomarev S. et al., Differential in vivo and in vitro expression of vascular endothelial growth factor (VEGF)-C and VEGF-D in tumors and its relationship to lymphatic metastasis in immunocompetent rats. *Cancer Res. 2003*;63:713–722.

[13] Hirakawa S., Brown L. F., Kodama S., Paavonen K., Alitalo K., Detmar M., VEGF-C-induced lymphangiogenesis in sentinel lymph nodes promotes tumor metastasis to distant sites. *Blood. 2007*;109:1010–1017. doi:10.1182/blood-2006-05-021758.

[14] Wong S. Y., Hynes R. O., Lymphatic or hematogenous dissemination: how does a metastatic tumor cell decide? *Cell Cycle. 2006*;5:812–817. doi:10.4161/cc.5.8.2646.

[15] Poste G., Fidler I. J., The pathogenesis of cancer metastasis. *Nature. 1980*;283:139–146.

[16] Hunter K. W., Crawford N. P. S., Alsarraj J., Mechanisms of metastasis. *Breast Cancer Res. 2008*;10 Suppl 1:S2. doi:10.1186/bcr1988.

[17] Talmadge J. E., Fidler I. J., AACR centennial series: the biology of cancer metastasis: historical perspective. *Cancer Res. 2010*;70:5649–5669. doi:10.1158/0008-5472.CAN-10-1040.

[18] Fidler I. J., Gersten D. M., Hart I. R., The biology of cancer invasion and metastasis. *Adv Cancer Res. 1978*;28:149–250.

[19] Li D. M., Feng Y. M., Signaling mechanism of cell adhesion molecules in breast cancer metastasis: potential therapeutic targets. *Breast Cancer Res Treat. 2011*;128:7–21. doi:10.1007/s10549-011-1499-x.

[20] Wendt M. K., Taylor M. A., Schiemann B. J., Schiemann W. P., Down-regulation of epithelial cadherin is required to initiate metastatic outgrowth of breast cancer. *Mol Biol Cell. 2011*;22:2423–2435. doi:10.1091/mbc.E11-04-0306.

[21] Gould Rothberg B. E., Bracken M. B., E-cadherin immunohistochemical expression as a prognostic factor in infiltrating ductal carcinoma of the breast: a systematic review and meta-analysis. *Breast Cancer Res Treat. 2006*;100:139–148. doi:10.1007/s10549-006-9248-2.

[22] Kowalski P. J., Rubin M. A., Kleer C. G., E-cadherin expression in primary carcinomas of the breast and its distant metastases. *Breast Cancer Res. 2003*;5:R217–R222. doi:10.1186/bcr651.

[23] Berx G., Cleton-Jansen A. M., Nollet F., de Leeuw W. J., van de Vijver M., Cornelisse C., et al., E-cadherin is a tumour/invasion suppressor gene mutated in human lobular breast cancers. *EMBO J. 1995*;14:6107–6115.

[24] Kotb A. M., Hierholzer A., Kemler R., Replacement of E-cadherin by N-cadherin in the mammary gland leads to fibrocystic changes and tumor formation. *Breast Cancer Res. 2011*;13:R104. doi:10.1186/bcr3046.

[25] Thiery J. P., Epithelial-mesenchymal transitions in tumour progression. *Nat Rev Cancer. 2002*;2:442–454. doi:10.1038/nrc822.

[26] Guarino M., Rubino B., Ballabio G., The role of epithelial-mesenchymal transition in cancer pathology. *Pathology. 2007*;39:305–318. doi:10.1080/00313020701329914.

[27] Bonnomet A., Brysse A., Tachsidis A., Waltham M., Thompson E. W., Polette M. et al., Epithelial-to-mesenchymal transitions and circulating tumor cells. *J Mammary Gland Biol Neoplasia. 2010*;15:261–273. doi:10.1007/s10911-010-9174-0.

[28] Ota I., Li X. Y., Hu Y., Weiss S. J., Induction of a MT1-MMP and MT2-MMP-dependent basement membrane transmigration program in cancer cells by Snail1. *Proc Natl Acad Sci U S A. 2009*;106:20318–20323. doi:10.1073/pnas.0910962106.

[29] Yilmaz M., Christofori G., Mechanisms of motility in metastasizing cells. *Mol Cancer Res. 2010*;8:629–642. doi:10.1158/1541-7786.MCR-10-0139.

[30] Cavallaro U., Christofori G., Cell adhesion and signalling by cadherins and Ig-CAMs in cancer. *Nat Rev Cancer. 2004*;4:118–132. doi:10.1038/nrc1276.

[31] Mego M., Mani S. A., Cristofanilli M., Molecular mechanisms of metastasis in breast cancer–clinical applications. *Nat Rev Clin Oncol. 2010*;7:693–701. doi: 10.1038/nrclinonc.2010.171.

[32] Dan K., Behrendt N., Hyer-Hansen G., Johnsen M., Lund L. R., Ploug M. et al., Plasminogen activation and cancer. *Thromb Haemost. 2005*;93:676–681. doi: 10.1160/TH05-01-0054.

[33] Egeblad M., Werb Z., New functions for the matrix metalloproteinases in cancer progression. *Nat Rev Cancer. 2002*;2:161–174. doi:10.1038/nrc745.

[34] McSherry E. A., Donatello S., Hopkins A. M., McDonnell S., Molecular basis of invasion in breast cancer. *Cell Mol Life Sci. 2007*;64:3201–3218. doi:10.1007/s00018-007-7388-0.

[35] Bell C. D., Waizbard E., Variability of cell size in primary and metastatic human breast carcinoma. *Invasion Metastasis. 1986*;6:11–20.

[36] Sahai E., Marshall C. J., Differing modes of tumour cell invasion have distinct requirements for Rho/ROCK signalling and extracellular proteolysis. *Nat Cell Biol. 2003*;5:711–719. doi:10.1038/ncb1019.

[37] Fidler I. J., Metastasis: quantitative analysis of distribution and fate of tumor emboli labeled with 125 I-5-iodo-2'-deoxyuridine. *J Natl Cancer Inst. 1970*;45:773–782.

[38] Fidler I. J., The relationship of embolic homogeneity, number, size and viability to the incidence of experimental metastasis. *Eur J Cancer. 1973*;9:223–227.

[39] Friedl P., Wolf K., Tube travel: the role of proteases in individual and collective cancer cell invasion. *Cancer Res. 2008*;68:7247–7249. doi:10.1158/0008-5472.CAN-08-0784.

[40] Wolf K., Wu Y. I , Liu Y., Geiger J., Tam E., Overall C. et al., Multi-step pericellular proteolysis controls the transition from individual to collective cancer cell invasion. *Nat Cell Biol. 2007*;9:893–904. doi:10.1038/ncb1616.

[41] Lin E. Y., Pollard J. W., Tumor-associated macrophages press the angiogenic switch in breast cancer. *Cancer Res. 2007*;67:5064–5066. doi:10.1158/0008-5472.CAN-07-0912.

[42] Mantovani A., Allavena P., Sica A., Balkwill F., Cancer-related inflammation. *Nature. 2008*;454:436–444. doi:10.1038/nature07205.

[43] Wu Y., Deng J., Rychahou P. G., Qiu S., Evers B. M., Zhou B. P., Stabilization of snail by NF-kappaB is required for inflammation-induced cell migration and invasion. *Cancer Cell. 2009*;15:416–428. doi:10.1016/j.ccr.2009.03.016.

[44] Robinson B. D., Sica G. L., Liu Y. F., Rohan T. E., Gertler F. B., Condeelis J. S. et al., Tumor microenvironment of metastasis in human breast carcinoma: a potential prognostic marker linked to hematogenous dissemination. *Clin Cancer Res. 2009*; 15:2433–2441. doi:10.1158/1078-0432.CCR-08-2179.

[45] Mundy G. R., Metastasis to bone: causes, consequences and therapeutic opportunities. *Nat Rev Cancer. 2002*; 2:584–593. doi:10.1038/nrc867.

[46] Parker B., Sukumar S., Distant metastasis in breast cancer: molecular mechanisms and therapeutic targets. *Cancer Biol Ther. 2003*; 2:14–21.

[47] Hiratsuka S., Nakamura K., Iwai S., Murakami M., Itoh T., Kijima H. et al., MMP9 induction by vascular endothelial growth factor receptor-1 is involved in lung-specific metastasis. *Cancer Cell. 2002*;2:289–300.

[48] Minn A. J., Kang Y., Serganova I., Gupta G. P., Giri D. D., Doubrovin M. et al., Distinct organ-specific metastatic potential of individual breast cancer cells and primary tumors. *J Clin Invest. 2005*;115:44–55. doi:10.1172/JCI22320.

[49] Minn A. J., Gupta G. P., Siegel P. M., Bos P. D., Shu W., Giri D. D. et al., Genes that mediate breast cancer metastasis to lung. *Nature. 2005*;436:518–524. doi: 10.1038/nature03799.

[50] Kang Y., Siegel P. M., Shu W., Drobnjak M., Kakonen S. M., Cordn-Cardo C. et al., A multigenic program mediating breast cancer metastasis to bone. *Cancer Cell. 2003*; 3:537–549.

[51] Mller A., Homey B., Soto H., Ge N., Catron D., Buchanan M. E. et al., Involvement of chemokine receptors in breast cancer metastasis. *Nature. 2001*;410:50–56. doi: 10.1038/35065016.

[52] Bruce J., Carter D. C., Fraser J., Patterns of recurrent disease in breast cancer. *Lancet. 1970*;1:433–435.

[53] De Castro Junior G., Puglisi F., De Azambuja E., El Saghir N. S., Awada A., Angiogenesis and cancer: A cross-talk between basic science and clinical trials (the “do ut des” paradigm). *Crit Rev Oncol Hematol. 2006*;59:40–50. doi: 10.1016/j.critrevonc.2006.02.007.

[54] Hanahan D., Weinberg R. A., Hallmarks of cancer: the next generation. *Cell. 2011*; 144:646–674. doi:10.1016/j.cell.2011.02.013.

[55] Hanahan D., Weinberg R. A., The hallmarks of cancer. *Cell. 2000*;100:57–70.

[56] Bergers G., Benjamin L. E., Tumorigenesis and the angiogenic switch. *Nat Rev Cancer. 2003*;3:401–410. doi:10.1038/nrc1093.

[57] Carmeliet P., Jain R. K., Angiogenesis in cancer and other diseases. *Nature. 2000*; 407:249–257. doi:10.1038/35025220.

[58] Fan F., Schimming A., Jaeger D., Podar K., Targeting the tumor microenvironment: focus on angiogenesis. *Journal of oncology. 2012*;2012:281261. doi: 10.1155/2012/281261.

[59] Ferrara N., Houck K., Jakeman L., Leung D. W., Molecular and biological properties of the vascular endothelial growth factor family of proteins. *Endocr Rev. 1992*;13:18–32. doi:10.1210/edrv-13-1-18.

[60] Mareel M., Oliveira M. J., Madani I., Cancer invasion and metastasis: interacting ecosystems. *Virchows Arch. 2009*;454:599–622. doi:10.1007/s00428-009-0784-0.

[61] Chia S. K., Speers C. H., D'yachkova Y., Kang A., Malfair-Taylor S., Barnett J. et al., The impact of new chemotherapeutic and hormone agents on survival in a population-based cohort of women with metastatic breast cancer. *Cancer. 2007*;110:973–979. doi:10.1002/cncr.22867.

[62] Luu T., Chung C., Somlo G., Combining emerging agents in advanced breast cancer. *Oncologist. 2011*;16:760–771. doi:10.1634/theoncologist.2010-0345.

[63] Von Hoff D. D., Layard M. W., Basa P., Davis H. L., Von Hoff A. L., Rozencweig M. et al., Risk factors for doxorubicin-induced congestive heart failure. *Ann Intern Med. 1979*;91:710–717.

[64] Alvarez R. H., Present and future evolution of advanced breast cancer therapy. *Breast Cancer Res. 2010*;12 Suppl 2:S1. doi:10.1186/bcr2572.

[65] Jaiyesimi I. A., Buzdar A. U., Decker D. A., Hortobagyi G. N., Use of tamoxifen for breast cancer: twenty-eight years later. *J Clin Oncol. 1995*;13:513–529. doi: 10.1200/JCO.1995.13.2.513.

[66] Mouridsen H., Sun Y., Gershanovich M., Perez-Carrion R., Becquart D., Chaudri-Ross H. A. et al., Superiority of letrozole to tamoxifen in the first-line treatment of advanced breast cancer: evidence from metastatic subgroups and a test of functional ability. *Oncologist. 2004*;9:489–496. doi:10.1634/theoncologist.9-5-489.

[67] Thrlimann B., Hess D., Kberle D., Senn I., Ballabeni P., Pagani O. et al., Anastrozole ('Arimidex') versus tamoxifen as first-line therapy in postmenopausal women with advanced breast cancer: results of the double-blind cross-over SAKK trial 21/95–a sub-study of the TARGET (Tamoxifen or 'Arimidex' Randomized Group

Efficacy and Tolerability) trial. *Breast Cancer Res Treat. 2004*;85:247–254. doi:10.1023/B:BREA.0000025420.78346.f9.

[68] Hamilton G., Rath B., Insights into mechanisms of tumor dissemination from circulating tumor cell lines of small cell lung cancer. *Journal of Cancer Metastasis and Treatment. 2016*;2:446. doi:10.20517/2394-4722.2016.57.

[69] Bockhorn M., Jain R. K., Munn L. L., Active versus passive mechanisms in metastasis: do cancer cells crawl into vessels, or are they pushed? *Lancet Oncol. 2007*; 8:444–448. doi:10.1016/S1470-2045(07)70140-7.

[70] Fisher B., Redmond C., Fisher E. R., The contribution of recent NSABP clinical trials of primary breast cancer therapy to an understanding of tumor biology–an overview of findings. *Cancer. 1980*;46:1009–1025.

[71] Cedolini C., Bertozzi S., Londero A. P., Bernardi S., Seriau L., Concina S. et al., Type of breast cancer diagnosis, screening, and survival. *Clin Breast Cancer. 2014*; 14:235–240. doi:10.1016/j.clbc.2014.02.004.

[72] Cedolini C., Bertozzi S., Seriau L., Londero A. P., Concina S., Cattin F. et al., Eight-year experience with the intraoperative frozen section examination of sentinel lymph node biopsy for breast cancer in a North-Italian university center. *Int J Clin Exp Path. 2014*;7:364–371.

[73] Driul L., Bernardi S., Bertozzi S., Schiavon M., Londero A. P., Petri R., New surgical trends in breast cancer treatment: conservative interventions and oncoplastic breast surgery. *Minerva Ginecol. 2013*;65:289–296.

[74] Nwariaku F. E., Euhus D. M., Beitsch P. D., Clifford E., Erdman W., Mathews D. et al., Sentinel lymph node biopsy, an alternative to elective axillary dissection for breast cancer. *Am J Surg. 1998*;176:529–531.

[75] Travagli J. P., Atallah D., Mathieu M. C., Rochard F., Camatte S., Lumbroso J. et al., Sentinel lymphadenectomy without systematic axillary dissection in breast cancer patients: predictors of non-sentinel lymph node metastasis. *Eur J Surg Oncol. 2003*; 29:403–406.

[76] Gipponi M., Clinical applications of sentinel lymph-node biopsy for the staging and treatment of solid neoplasms. *Minerva Chir. 2005*;60:217–233.

[77] Veronesi U., Galimberti V., Paganelli G., Maisonneuve P., Viale G., Orecchia R. et al., Axillary metastases in breast cancer patients with negative sentinel nodes: a follow-up of 3548 cases. *Eur J Cancer. 2009*;45:1381–1388. doi:10.1016/j.ejca.2008.11.041.

[78] Gentilini O., Veronesi P., Gatti G., Intra M., Mazzarol G., Trifir G. et al., [Conservative approach for breast cancer. The experience of the European Institute of Oncology]. *Minerva Chir. 2007*;62:447–458.

[79] Bertozzi S., Londero A. P., The sentinel lymph node biopsy for breast cancer over the years. *Eur J Gynaecol Oncol. 2016*;37:13–16.

[80] Bertozzi S., Londero A. P., Giacomuzzi F., Angione V., Carbone A., Petri R. et al., Applicability of two different validated models to predict axillary non-sentinel lymph node status by sentinel node biopsy in a single Italian center. *Breast Cancer. 2015*; 22:350–355. doi:10.1007/s12282-013-0485-z.

[81] Bernardi S., Bertozzi S., Londero A. P., Giacomuzzi F., Angione V., Dri C. et al., Nine years of experience with the sentinel lymph node biopsy in a single Italian center: a retrospective analysis of 1,050 cases. *World J Surg. 2012*;36:714–722. doi: 10.1007/s00268-011-1420-0.

[82] Veronesi U., Paganelli G., Galimberti V., Viale G., Zurrida S., Bedoni M. et al., Sentinel-node biopsy to avoid axillary dissection in breast cancer with clinically negative lymph-nodes. *Lancet. 1997*;349:1864–1867. doi:10.1016/S0140-6736(97)01004-0.

[83] Cody H. S., *Sentinel lymph node mapping in breast cancer*. Oncology (Williston Park). 1999;13:25–34; discussion 35–6, 39, 43.

[84] Giuliano A. E., Sentinel lymphadenectomy in primary breast carcinoma: an alternative to routine axillary dissection. *J Surg Oncol. 1996*;62:75–77. doi: 10.1002/(SICI)1096-9098(199606)62:2¡75::AID-JSO1¿3.0.CO;2-N.

[85] Feldman S. M., Krag D. N., McNally R. K., Moor B. B., Weaver D. L., Klein P., Limitation in gamma probe localization of the sentinel node in breast cancer patients with large excisional biopsy. *J Am Coll Surg. 1999*;188:248–254.

[86] Tanis P. J., Nieweg O. E., Valdes Olmos R. A., Th Rutgers E. J., Kroon B. B., History of sentinel node and validation of the technique. *Breast Cancer Res. 2001*;3:109–112.

[87] Giuliano A. E., Dale P. S., Turner R. R., Morton D. L., Evans S. W., Krasne D. L., Improved axillary staging of breast cancer with sentinel lymphadenectomy. *Ann Surg. 1995*;222:394–9; discussion 399–401.

[88] Veronesi, Zurrida., Optimal Surgical Treatment of Breast Cancer. *Oncologist. 1996*; 1:340–346.

[89] Bernardi S., Bertozzi S., Londero A. P., Angione V., Petri R., Giacomuzzi F., Prevalence and risk factors of intraoperative identification failure of sentinel lymph nodes in patients affected by breast cancer. *Nucl Med Commun. 2013*;34:664–673. doi: 10.1097/MNM.0b013e328361cd84.

[90] Foster D., Choy N., Porter C., Ahmed S., Wapnir I., Axillary reverse mapping with indocyanine green or isosulfan blue demonstrate similar crossover rates to radiotracer identified sentinel nodes. *J Surg Oncol. 2017*;doi:10.1002/jso.24859.

[91] Hokimoto N., Sugimoto T., Namikawa T., Funakoshi T., Oki T., Ogawa M. et al., A Novel Color Fluorescence Navigation System for Intraoperative Transcutaneous Lymphatic Mapping and Resection of Sentinel Lymph Nodes in Breast Cancer: Comparison with the Combination of Gamma Probe Scanning and Visible Dye Methods. *Oncology. 2017*;doi:10.1159/000484050.

[92] O'Hea B. J., Hill A. D., El-Shirbiny A. M., Yeh S. D., Rosen P. P., Coit D. G. et al., Sentinel lymph node biopsy in breast cancer: initial experience at Memorial Sloan-Kettering Cancer Center. *J Am Coll Surg. 1998*;186:423–427.

[93] Giuliano A. E., Barth A. M., Spivack B., Beitsch P. D., Evans S. W., Incidence and predictors of axillary metastasis in T1 carcinoma of the breast. *J Am Coll Surg. 1996*; 183:185–189.

In: The Sentinel Lymph Node
Editors: A. Londero, S. Bertozzi and C. Cedolini
ISBN: 978-1-53614-557-1


*Chapter 2*

# Sentinel Lymph Node Detection Technique

***Michela Andretta***[1,*]***, Serena Bertozzi***[1]***, Roberta Di Vora***[1]***,***
***Carla Cedolini***[1] ***and Ambrogio P. Londero***[2]
[1]Breast Unit, DAME, University of Udine,
University Hospital of Udine, Italy
[2]Clinic of Obstetrics and Gynecology,
University Hospital of Udine, Italy

**Abstract**

The feasibility and safety of intraoperative sentinel node identification was first assessed in 1991, with the injection of isosulfan blue vital dye into breast cancer to obtain a vital dye-directed lymphatic mapping. Then, with a well-defined technique and experience, an accuracy of almost 100% in the prediction of axillary nodal status was achieved. Subsequently, other technical approaches for sentinel node identification in breast cancer were developed in order to improve the accuracy and reduce the operative time of the procedure without any impact on surgical outcomes. The technique currently most used involves the use of a radiotracer, technetium-99 nanocolloid, which is injected preoperatively near the tumour site, and its subsequent preoperative and intraoperative localization by lymphoscintigraphy and by the use of a gamma camera, respectively. Other techniques include the use of indocyanine green with its near-infrared fluorescence properties and of superparamagnetic iron oxide particles detected by a magneto-metric probe. Despite the high detection rate of each of these techniques, the highest detection rates are achieved by the combination of at least two of them.

**Keywords:** radiotracer, vital staining, near-infrared fluorescence, superparamagnetic iron oxide, sentinel lymph node detection failure

## 1. Introduction

Sentinel lymph node biopsy (SLNB) has become the most widely used procedure for determining lymph node involvement in clinically node-negative primary tumors such as melanoma, breast, gynecological and gastroenterological cancers.

*Corresponding Author E-mail: andretta.michela@gmail.com.

The introduction of SLNB has been one of the greatest advances in the surgical treatment of breast cancer in order to reduce surgical complications, while achieving adequate axillary staging, not inferior to that achieved with complete axillary lymph node dissection. This procedure is particularly suitable for patients with invasive breast cancer with clinically and radiologically negative lymph nodes. However, SLNB can also be performed in selective patients in the presence of ductal carcinoma in situ, in the case of suspected infiltrations, predictive factors of lymph node involvement or mastectomy [1]. In the latter case, for example, SLNB is performed mainly because, if necessary, the procedure is no longer reliable after complete excision of the breast gland and consistent excision of all breast lymphatic drainage ducts.

Although sentinel node detection is now a standard technique for axillary staging in breast cancer patients, there are many options to implement it, which may be used differently in the various settings worldwide. With regard to the tracer used to identify the sentinel node, the most commonly used are a radioisotope or a vital dye, which may be applied alone or in combination. Moreover, they may be injected into different sites, such as periareolar or perilesional, with comparable success rates. [2]. In conclusion, the choice of the sentinel node detection technique depends not only on the scientifically proven oncological safety described in the literature, but also on the disposable resources of the local setting, such as the presence of a nuclear medicine specialist, the surgeon's experience and sustainable costs.

Due to the different contraindications and complications of the tracers currently used for lymph node detection, other techniques, such as fluorescent dyes, are emerging in the literature and in the clinical practice, always bearing in mind that the guidelines are being developed with the aim of conserving axillary lymph nodes as much as possible.

## 2. Vital Staining

The feasibility and safety of intraoperative sentinel node identification was first assessed in 1991, with the injection of isosulfan blue vital dye in breast cancer to obtain a vital dye-directed lymphatic mapping [3]. Then, with a well-defined technique and experience, an accuracy of almost 100% in the prediction of axillary nodal status was achieved [3, 4]. Subsequently, other technical approaches for sentinel node identification in breast cancer were developed in order to improve the accuracy and reduce the operative time of the procedure, without any impact on surgical outcomes.

Blue dye administration is usually performed by the injection of 3-5 ml of isosulfan blue vital dye into the subcutaneous tissue of the breast lesion area or the nipple areola complex. This procedure is performed 5-10 minutes prior to the incision and is accompanied by an accurate massage of the injected area to facilitate lymphatic drainage to the axilla [5]. All blue lymph nodes and any lymph nodes at the end of a blue lymphatic channel are removed as sentinel lymph nodes. The surgeon must carefully identify the proximal blue nodes because dye transit is rapid and may stain also secondary nodes, leading to overtreatment in the case of excision of secondary non-sentinel lymph nodes. [6].

In clinical practice, in addition to isosulfan blue other vital dyes have been used, such as patent blue and methylene blue. Methylene blue appears to be cheaper than other dyes and more readily available. Some authors reported similar detection rates between patent and methylene blue dyes [7, 8], with a lower risk of anaphylaxis compared with the other vital dyes and the possibility of using them in pregnant patients. The methylene blue method alone has gained popularity especially in developing countries because of its affordability and the fact that it does not have the restrictions of isosulfan and patent blue dyes. However, some authors claim that the use of blue dye alone leads to a lower sentinel node identification rate [9]. On the other hand, Giuliano and colleagues reported an increase from 66% to 94% in the detection rate with patent blue alone on account of the surgeon's achievement of the learning curve [4].

Complications due to blue dye injection are very rare and include allergic reactions up to anaphylactic shock, local skin reactions, transient drop in saturation and the persistence of a blue tattoo. A case of pulmonary edema has also been reported in the literature [10, 11, 12, 13, 14, 15]. Furthermore, since deeply located blue lymph vessels can be difficult to find, this technique requires considerable experience from the surgeon. Finally, with regard to the surgical technique, with blue dye the surgeon needs a larger skin incision in order to identify the blue lymphatic view without cutting it.

The standard sentinel node identification method suggested by the current literature is the combined one, performed with the injection of both radiotracer and blue dye in order to obtain the lowest possible false-negative rate. In order to avoid blue dye complications, several studies have been conducted to demonstrate the non-superiority between the combined technique and the radiotracer alone in terms of false-negative rate, overall survival and local recurrence rate [2, 16, 17]. On the other hand, other studies compared the use of blue dye alone with the combined use of blue dye and indocyanine green in order to avoid the radiotracer implications, determining the superiority, in terms of detection rate, of the fluorescence and dye combination compared with the blue dye alone, being thus comparable to the combination of radioisotope and blue dye. [18].

## 3. Radiotracer

Nowadays, the most commonly used technique worldwide for the sentinel node identification is radio-guided surgery with preoperative lymphoscintigraphy. The most frequently used radioisotope is filtered technetium-99 sulfur colloid, which is usually injected into the intradermal, subdermal, or peritumoral region, in a single dose of 0.3-1.0 mCi, between 3 and 24 hours prior to surgery. Lymphoscintigraphy is commonly performed after the injection to track the migration of the radioisotope and identify the location of the most radioactive nodes, also referred to as hot nodes [19] (Figure 1).

In the case of a difficult preoperative identification of the sentinel node or even of a completely negative lymphoscintigraphy, a single photon emission computed tomography (SPECT) can be performed to better evaluate the axillary status. This technique is a tomographic medical imaging of nuclear medicine that uses ionizing radiations called gamma rays. It is very similar to the planar imaging of conventional nuclear medicine in that it uses a gamma camera (Figure 2), but is also able to provide real biotopological data in three dimensions. This information is typically presented as axial slices of the patient, but the powerful processing of computer images can easily reformat them into sagittal or coronal sections, or depending on the needs, manipulate them with techniques of subtraction of selected structures or with the perfectly rotatory reconstruction of the isolated structure to be studied. Therefore, SPECT is able to precisely define the location of hot nodes to better guide the surgeon in performing SLNB.

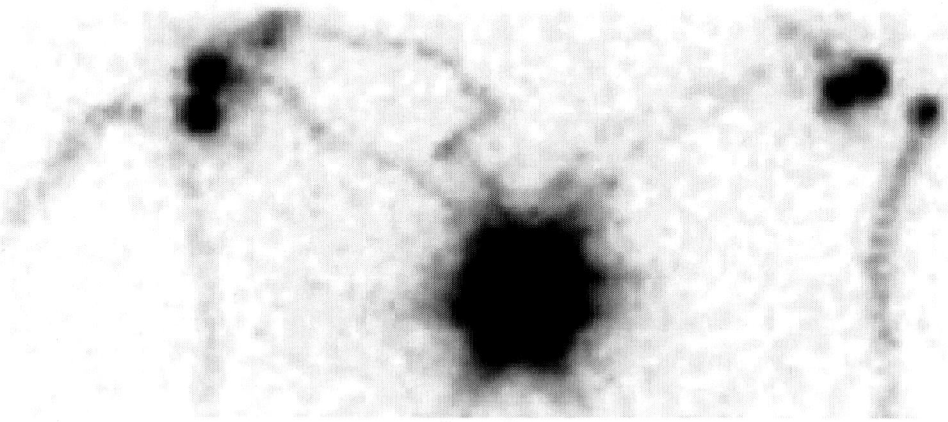

Figure 1. Lymphoscintigraphy.

A radioactive node has been defined as a node with a cumulative 10-second count greater than 25, the hottest node in absolute counts, a 10:1 sentinel to background ratio, or a four-fold reduction in counts after the removal of the sentinel node [20]. Verification is performed by comparing ex vivo sentinel node counts with residual in vivo background counts and removing additional radioactive nodes until the background is less than one-tenth of the value of the hottest node. Although the radioactive uptake is usually related to the tumor burden in metastatic lymph nodes, the nodes replaced by the tumor can sometimes present a lymphatic obstruction with a consequent reduction in radioactive uptake, supporting the removal also of nodes with low count rate [21].

Radiocolloid preparation drainage intuitively depends on the size of injected particles. In particular, preparations with large particles tend to remain at the injection site, while preparations with a small particle size tend to migrate to the axillary lymph nodes, causing diffuse nodal uptake and consequently overtreatment [22]. Three types of preparations are widely used: technetium-99 sulfur colloid with a wide variation in particle size, resulting in a variable daily performance; technetium-99 albumin nanocolloid with a more consistent particle size and less variable performance; and technetium-99 antimony trisulfide, which has the most consistent particle size of them all. Moreover, this interesting property of radiocolloid particles has led to the development of other radio-guided techniques for the localization of non-palpable structures. For example, the radio-guided occult lesion localization (ROLL) allows the intraoperative identification of non-palpable breast lesions by preoperative injection of large radioactive colloids that consequently do not move from the injection site [23].

The combined technique (radiotracer and blue dye) for the identification of the sentinel node should continue to be preferred in terms of detection rate. In particular, a detection rate of 96%-97% was achieved in the AMAROS [24]and the ALMANAC trials [25]. Despite this fact, many centers have started using the radiotracer alone method to avoid blue

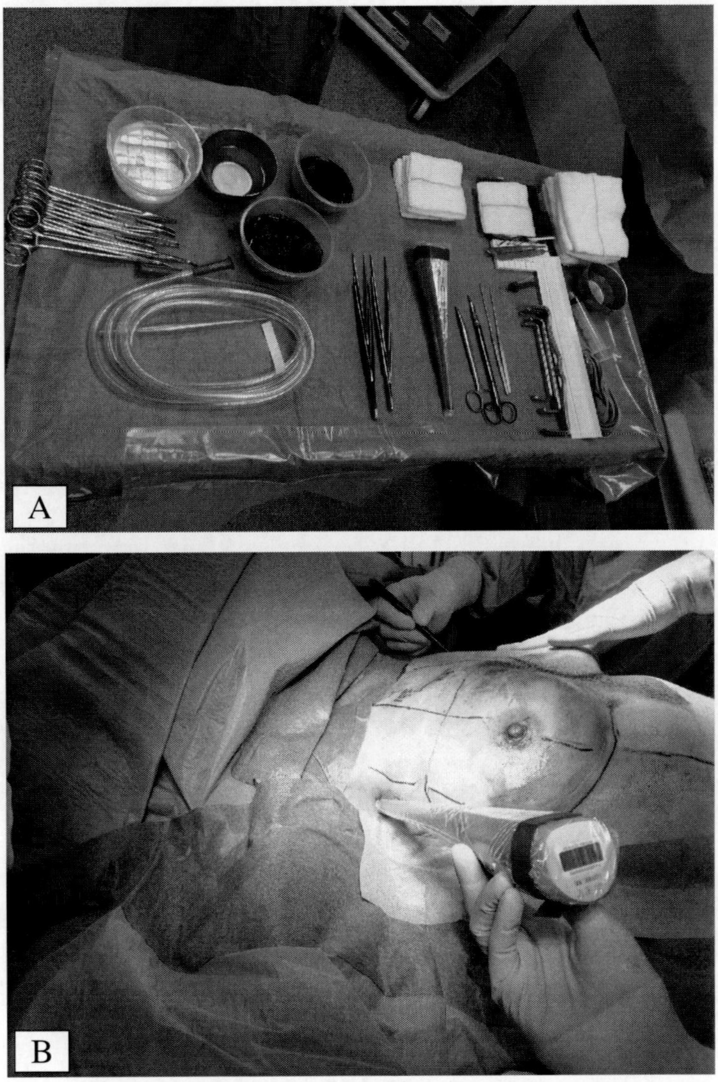


Figure 2. Panel A) Surgical instruments and the gamma camera in the operative room. Panel B) The gamma camera used to find the sentinel lymph node.

dye complications, such as anaphylaxis and chronic skin coloration. Moreover, in the literature it has been shown that, in the hands of experts, the radiotracer alone method is not inferior to the combined technique in terms of false-negative rates [26]. Therefore, several authors have argued that the added value of the blue dye over the radiotracer alone technique is minimal and that the marginal benefit of the dye decreases with increased surgical experience [27]. In addition, the superiority of the dual tracer may be limited in the case of negative lymphoscintigraphy or in patients who have undergone neoadjuvant chemotherapy [17]. Furthermore, a recent review of the combined technique (radiotracer and blue dye) [28] did not help lower false-negative rates, although it showed a higher success rate of sentinel node identification. For this reason, the conversion from the combined technique to the single tracer technique with the radioisotope alone would help facilitate the biopsy procedure and reduce complications and costs.

The major problems with the radioactive tracer technique are its high costs and the technological complexity it involes, only found in hospitals with a nuclear medicine department. [1]. If nuclear medicine is not present in the hospital, the costs of transporting patients to perform the injection for the sentinel lymph node identification in another hospital will obviously increase.

## 4. Near-Infrared Fluorescence

Multiple techniques use dye or radioisotope or a combination of both for the sentinel node identification. In fact, indocyanine green has been introduced in the clinical practice with the aim of developing always increasingly efficient methods for the implementation of SLNB.

Indocyanine green is an interesting radiation-free substance that can potentially be used for the sentinel node detection [29, 30]. Approved for medical use in 1956, it is commonly used nowadays for the diagnosis of liver function, in ophthalmology, cardiology and microcirculation diagnostics. Within the body it bonds to proteins and other macromolecules that change the intensity of its fluorescence and its emission spectrum to near-infrared, which is invisible to the naked eye but detectable through special devices with photodynamic cameras [31].

In the case of breast cancer, indocyanine green is injected near the tumor site and passes through the lymphatic ducts to the sentinel lymph node in about 1-3 minutes. The lymphatic pathway is individualized using an excitation illumination system combined with a high-sensitivity camera that detects the emitted fluorescence. Since indocyanine green is a fluorophore displaying fluorescence in incident light, along with its green color on visual inspection, its emitted radiation permeates through tissues allowing the visualization of deeply located structure, unlike common dyes.

A study showed that the sensitivity of indocyanine green may be related to the size of the particles of the tracer. This means that smaller particles are transported more quickly, and therefore early and dynamic observation of the fluorescence is important to exclude secondary nodes from sentinel nodes in case smaller particles spill into them [32].

Although indocyanine green has several advantages in clinical practice, it also has some limitations. In fact, studies have shown the difficulty of detecting the sentinel lymph node in obese patients (defined as patients with BMI $> 40$ kg/m$^2$) [33] because of the lower capacity of tissue penetration of near-infrared fluorescence compared to gamma rays. As with the blue dye, skin staining or permanent tattooing and subcutaneous nodules may occur also in the case of indocyanine green injection.

However, reducing fluorescence emission and its concentration can be a challenge for the routine use of indocyanine green. For this reason, there are some studies in the literature on its injection dose and volume, which have been standardized between 0.625 and 15 mg in 1 or 15 ml [34]. In any case, there is no consensus yet on the optimal dose of indocyanine green. Since SLNB is a difficult procedure, as with the other potential tracers, the use of indocyanine green requires an adequate learning curve. Avoiding damage to the lymphatic vessels is important because it can cause a highlighted fluorescence in the surgical field resulting in difficulties in the localization of sentinel lymph nodes.

## 5. Superparamagnetic Iron Oxide

Some experimentations have been published using superparamagnetic iron oxide particles detected by a magneto-metric probe (Sentimag®) (Figure 3). Sentimag is a handheld probe used to identify the sentinel node like a gamma probe with a detection and false-negative rates similar to those of the radioisotope [35, 36]. The Sienna+® is a dextran-coated superparamagnetic iron oxide nanoparticle with a size of 59 nm that drains to the lymphatics and accumulates in the sentinel lymph node.

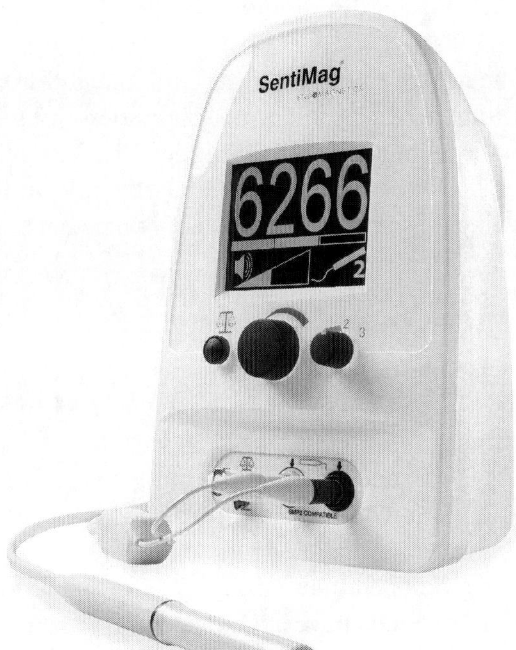


Figure 3. The Sentimag instrument.

The Sentimag method offers several advantages. The surgeon can inject the magnetic tracer by himself directly in the operating room, regardless of the complex time scheduling with the department of nuclear medicine, and there is no risk of tracer unavailability [37]. As reported by the manufacturer, the subareolar injection of the tracer can be performed at least 20 minutes prior to the incision and the tracer can be detected within seven days of injection.

The improved timing between the tracer injection and SLNB offers at least three beneficial effects: a short preparation time, the possibility of performing a higher number of procedures per day and improved patient comfort. Sienna has a great ease of use, is not associated with any special precautions, has a long half-life and the expiration date is negligible [38].

The published data verifies that its detection rates do not differ from those of radiotracers and that the presence of metastases does not affect the effectiveness of the method. Constantly, high concordance rates between the different sentinel node identification methods also suggest that superparamagnetic iron oxide correctly identifies the sentinel node [39]. In fact, when using Sentimag the mean number of sentinel nodes removed is 1.9, and thus even lower than the mean number of nodes removed with indocyanine green which is about 3.4 [37].

However, magnetic detection has also some disadvantages, such as the large volume of the detection substance that needs to be applied and the risk of skin discoloration at the injection site. Some studies reported discoloration in 19% of cases, which progressively faded after 6 months, while others reported an incidence of 40% at 6 months, which was transient in 91% of pigmented cases [39]. In any case, pigmentation was usually very light in color and did not constitute a real problem for the patient. As soon as the surgeons became more familiar with the technique, this side effect was controlled by performing the injection slightly deeper [38]. On the other hand, the dark color of the solution allows the nodes to become dark as well, and sometimes helps surgeon detect the sentinel lymph node more easily [39].

The Sentimag method appears to be easier than the conventional technetium-99 techniques, as it does not have the limitations of isotope manipulation. However, with this method there is the need to use plastic surgical instruments (which to date do not render at the level of metal tools) and to reset the magnetic baseline level to avoid incorrect use of the probe, resulting in brief interruptions during SLNB that must be taken into account.

A theoretical disadvantage of superparamagnetic iron oxide is the inability to obtain a simple and inexpensive preoperative localization scan, which is of great importance for example for the localization of the sentinel node in melanoma patients. On the other hand, it is not necessary to perform a preoperative scintigraphy for the sentinel node detection in breast cancer patients, and most centers have abandoned this practice [39].

In conclusion, this new method has none of the disadvantages of the standard technique and represents a promising, safe and effective alternative, especially in the absence of nuclear medicine facilities [39].

## 6. Other Techniques

In addition to the economical and logistical aspects, considering that the surgical conservation of the axillary lymph nodes in breast cancer patients is a current challenge, new techniques have been developed in order to limit the surgical impact on the axilla, while ensuring adequate staging. For example, the percutaneous biopsy of the sentinel lymph node identified by contrast-enhanced ultrasound is a developing technique to find an alternative and less invasive method to achieve axillary staging [40].

In particular, a new technique has been introduced by Omoto and colleagues [41] and consists in an intradermal injection of 1 ml of an ultrasound contrast agent into the periareolar area, whose the microbubbles are followed during their drainage through the lymphatic pathway to the axillary lymph nodes. The most used contrast agents are SonoVue and Sonozoid. The first lymph node to mantain contrast after a time ranging between 45 seconds and 5 minutes is supposed to be the sentinel node. Once the sentinel node is detected, a biopsy is performed and a clip is left inside the node.

In order to determine the sensitivity of this technique, the surgical biopsy of the sentinel node was conducted by detecting the node through wire hook localization, skin marking or radioactive iodine seed placement. The sensitivity of this sentinel node identification technique was about 50% [40]. The negative predictive value was also high, as assessed by Verheuvel and colleagues [42], and showed a difference in the overall survival between women with ultrasound-detected lymph nodes and surgically biopsied metastatic lymph nodes.

As already mentioned, the most accurate technique is usually a combination of the disposable techniques. In general, the best combination is technetium-99 with a blue dye, although this last substances can cause hypersensitivity reactions. Therefore, the identification of substances with fewer sides effects became a challenge, while trying not to reduce the sensitivity of the combined technique. For this reason, Pinheiro and colleagues [43] demonstrated in an experimental research on animals the efficacy of hemosiderin (a protein obtained from the degradation of hemoglobin) as an autologous dye in association with technetium-99. The same technique was then reported in 14 patients using hemosiderin obtained from autologous blood. In the study, this technique was safer than the one with blue dye, without any adverse reaction and was oncologically equivalent to thechnetium-99 in terms of detection rate.

## 7. Sentinel Lymph Node Detection Failure

The prevalence of intraoperative sentinel node identification failure varies in the literature between 1% and 10%, mostly depending on advanced age, high BMI, large breast size, tumor location other than the upper-outer quadrant, tumor size, previous breast surgery or recent breast biopsy, regional lymph node metastases, number of positive lymph nodes, type of injected radiocolloid, site of injection, injected radiocolloid volume and dose, time between injection of radiocolloid and surgery, lack of captation at the preoperative lymphoscintiscan, late lack of captation at the intraoperative sentinel node research and low institutional experience [44, 45, 46, 25, 47, 48, 49, 50, 51, 24]. As a consequence, we have witnessed a progressive evolution of the SLNB technique to optimize the sentinel node identification, both with regard to the tracers used (radioisotope, blue dye, indocyanine green or combinations) [52] and their injection site (peri-tumoral, intra-tumoral, or peri-areolar) [53].

According to the literature, failure to demonstrate axillary uptake by preoperative lymphoscintiscan can predict the consequent failure of intraoperative sentinel node identification, depending on patient's characteristics affecting breast lymphatic drainage, as well as technical factors [54]. In particular, assuming that the learning curve for sentinel node lymphoscintiscan requires at least 30 procedures to be performed [55, 56], the limited experience of the nuclear medicine specialist may compromise the success of SLNB [57]. In any case, even with the presence of expert operators, the necessity of routinely performing a preoperative lymphoscintiscan for the sentinel node identification remains subject of debate [48, 58, 59, 60, 61].

There is also strong disagreement regarding other risk factors for sentinel node detection failure. For example, in many studies, advanced age did not significantly influence SLNB failure; a low breast radiological density did not influence SLNB failure either, reflecting the progressive, physiological, adipose replacement of the breast and then correlating with the patient's age [44, 55, 62]. Subsequently, advanced age not only does not represent an absolute contraindication for SLNB, but can also be very useful to reduce surgical complications in patients with many comorbidities by limiting the surgical extension in node-negative patients [47, 63, 64, 65].

Another individual characteristic that represents a current subject of debate among SLNB indications is overweight, which can compromise the lymphoscintigraphic mapping by altering the lymphatic drainage of the breast and make intraoperative sentinel node detection more technically challenging due to the increased difficulty of identifying a hot spot in a large fatty axilla [65, 66]. Although other studies do not include the patient's BMI, no correlation was found between SLNB failure and a low breast density, which is sensitive indicator of breast adiposity [44].

The instrumental guidance of the radiotracer injection (by stereotactic mammography or ultrasonography), which reflects the non-palpability of the lesion and then correlates with smaller-sized lesions, does not appear to significantly influence SLNB failure [47]. Also the characteristics of the tumor did not seem to play any fundamental role in the intraoperative identification of the sentinel node. Considering the site of injection, there appear to be no differecens in terms of sentinel node detection failure rates. Nowadays, the peri-areolar injection is preferred, especially in the case of mastectomy, being more comfortable for patients who do not require any preoperative radiological localization of the lesion, as happens, on the contrary, in the case of quadrantectomy.

Some authors found that the failure to detect the sentinel node is influenced by the sentinel node location. In particular, in the case of melanoma of the head or neck, they showed a higher incidence of failed sentinel node mapping and a higher recurrence rate following SLNB compared to truncal or extremity localizations [67].

In conclusion, the low prevalence of SLNB failure confirms the accuracy of the procedure when performed by specialized operators. Also, when compared to other radio-guided surgical techniques, such as the breast ROLL, radio-guided SLNB appears to have a significantly lower failure rate [23]. A possible explanation may be that ROLL is more dependent on the operator's experience, while SLNB depends mainly on the patient's lymphatic pathways, which are very reliable regardless of the injection site and the operator's experience.

Finally, the impact of SLNB failure on patient's diagnostic and therapeutic management is minimal, considering the low invasiveness and complications of the procedure and the possibility of staging the cancer through a lymph node sampling if necessary. In fact, in the literature the lack of sentinel node captation required the procedure to be repeated in very few patients, while in some cases the sentinel node was found intraoperatively and in other cases patients directly underwent a lymph node sampling or complete axillary lymph node dissection [44].

## 8. Axillary Reverse Mapping

Axillary reverse mapping was originally introduced in 2007 to allow the distinction between the lymphatic drainage of the breast and the upper arm [11, 14]. The upper extremity is usually drained by nodes most commonly located in the upper outer part of the axilla, just caudal to the axillary vein and lateral to the ascending lateral thoracic vein, which is a tributary vein of the axillary vein, while the breast is most frequently drained by nodes located in the lower basin of the axilla [15]. Although it is assumed that the breast and the upper arm have their own lymphatic drainage pathways, there may be an overlap between the two [68].

The rationale of this technique is that the discrimination of the two different pathways, in the case of a positive sentinel node can allow the surgeon to selectively dissect only the nodes draining the breast and spare those draining exclusively the arm, in order to prevent as much as possible the potential complications of complete axillary lymph node dissection, such as lymphedema.

This technique involves the use of two different methods of nodal identification. Initially, the arm lymphatic drainage is mapped by using blue dye, while the breast lymph nodes are classically identified with a radiotracer [11, 14]. The identification rates are very variable in the literature, ranging between 20% and 90%, probably due to the type of axillary surgery, the type of "successful identification" definition, and the surgeon's experience and technique.

From an oncological point of view, there is still disagreement on the safety of this procedure, as some authors found a metastatic involvement of the nodes that apparently drained the arm exclusively in about 14% of breast cancer node-positive patients who underwent complete axillary lymph node dissection [69]. Therefore, complete axillary lymph node dissection remains the only recommended technique in the case of intraoperative presence of a positive sentinel node or preoperative detection of a positive lymph node.

## Conclusion

Since the introduction of SLNB for routine use, physicians have tried to find a safe method to detect sentinel nodes with adequate accuracy and a low false-negative rate [70]. Sentinel node identification in breast cancer is technically feasible, safe and represents an accurate predictor of the status of the axilla using a variety of technical approaches. Studies comparing blue dye alone with the combined use of radioisotope and blue dye showed no differences between the identification rates of the two groups [71], as well as studies comparing indocyanine green with blue dye [72, 73, 74, 75, 76] or radioisotope [77, 78, 79, 80]. On the other hand, studies showed that only the surgeon experience can have a significant impact on sentinel node identification and false-negative rates.

The literature describes various lymph node detection techniques with different pros and cons in terms of complications, contraindications, detection rate, false-negative rate and costs. For this reason, there are many differences in the choice of the SLNB technique worldwide. However, the literature highlights the combined use of different sentinel node detection techniques, with the benefit that the identification rate can be improved and the false-negative rate minimized, particularly in the case of patients with a high BMI, prior axillary or breast surgery or preoperative neoadjuvant therapies. In these selected cases, misidentification and false-negative rates are known to be higher. In addition, in these particular cases, misidentification and false-negative rates are known to be higher and preoperative lymphoscintigraphy may be very useful [6].

Furthermore, the palpation of the axillary space for any suspicious nodes will avoid missing a metastatic node with a lymphatic obstruction, which may not be blue or radioactive. All suspicious palpable nodes must be removed at the time of the SLNB, regardless of the chosen technique.

Finally, different new techniques are emerging as a result of the tendency to conserve axillary lymph nodes as much as possible, while obtaining a reliable staging of the axillary tumor. For this reason, each surgeon has to find the method that best suits his/her practice and the local setting in which he/she is working, also taking into account the costs and the availability of the structures needed.

## References

[1] Paulinelli R. R., Freitas-Junior R., Rahal RMdS, Oliveira LFdP, Vilela M. H. T., Moreira MAR et al., A prospective randomized trial comparing patent blue and methylene blue for the detection of the sentinel lymph node in breast cancer patients. *Rev Assoc Med Bras. 2017*;63:118–123. doi:10.1590/1806-9282.63.02.118.

[2] Garbay J. R., Skalli-Chrisostome D., Leymarie N., Sarfati B., Rimareix F., Mazouni C., The Role of Blue Dye in Sentinel Node Detection for Breast Cancer: A Retrospective Study of 203 Patients. *Breast care (Basel, Switzerland). 2016*;11:128–132. doi:10.1159/000445368.

[3] Giuliano A. E., Kirgan D. M., Guenther J. M., Morton D. L., Lymphatic mapping and sentinel lymphadenectomy for breast cancer. *Ann Surg. 1994*;220:391–8; discussion 398–401.

[4] Giuliano A. E., Jones R. C., Brennan M., Statman R., Sentinel lymphadenectomy in breast cancer. *J Clin Oncol. 1997*;15:2345–2350. doi:10.1200/JCO.1997.15.6.2345.

[5] Bass S. S., Cox C. E., Salud C. J., Lyman G. H., McCann C., Dupont E. et al., The effects of postinjection massage on the sensitivity of lymphatic mapping in breast cancer. *J Am Coll Surg. 2001*;192:9–16.

[6] James T. A., Coffman A. R., Chagpar A. B., Boughey J. C., Klimberg V. S., Morrow M. et al., Troubleshooting Sentinel Lymph Node Biopsy in Breast Cancer Surgery. *Ann Surg Oncol. 2016*;23:3459–3466. doi:10.1245/s10434-016-5432-8.

[7] Varghese P., Abdel-Rahman A. T., Akberali S., Mostafa A., Gattuso J. M., Carpenter R., Methylene blue dye–a safe and effective alternative for sentinel lymph node localization. *Breast J. 2008*;14:61–67. doi:10.1111/j.1524-4741.2007.00519.x.

[8] Aydogan F., Celik V., Uras C., Salihoglu Z., Topuz U., A comparison of the adverse reactions associated with isosulfan blue versus methylene blue dye in sen-

tinel lymph node biopsy for breast cancer. *Am J Surg. 2008*;195:277–278. doi:10.1016/j.amjsurg.2007.03.008.

[9] Hung W. K., Chan C. M., Ying M., Chong S. F., Mak K. L., Yip A. W. C., Randomized clinical trial comparing blue dye with combined dye and isotope for sentinel lymph node biopsy in breast cancer. *Br J Surg. 2005*;92:1494–1497. doi:10.1002/bjs.5211.

[10] Tausch C., Baege A., Dietrich D., Vergin I., Heuer H., Heusler R. H. et al., Can axillary reverse mapping avoid lymphedema in node positive breast cancer patients? *Eur J Surg Oncol. 2013*;39:880–886. doi:10.1016/j.ejso.2013.05.009.

[11] Thompson M., Korourian S., Henry-Tillman R., Adkins L., Mumford S., Westbrook K. C., et al., Axillary reverse mapping (ARM): a new concept to identify and enhance lymphatic preservation. *Ann Surg Oncol. 2007*;14:1890–1895. doi:10.1245/s10434-007-9412-x.

[12] Khandelwal R., Poovamma C. U., Shilpy C., Prema M., Anthony P., Axillary reverse mapping: Is it feasible in locally advanced breast cancer patients? *Breast Dis. 2014*; 34:151–155. doi:10.3233/BD-140371.

[13] Rubio I. T., Cebrecos I., Peg V., Esgueva A., Mendoza C., Cortadellas T. et al., Extensive nodal involvement increases the positivity of blue nodes in the axillary reverse mapping procedure in patients with breast cancer. *J Surg Oncol. 2012*;106:89–93. doi:10.1002/jso.23048.

[14] Nos C., Lesieur B., Clough K. B., Lecuru F., Blue dye injection in the arm in order to conserve the lymphatic drainage of the arm in breast cancer patients requiring an axillary dissection. *Ann Surg Oncol. 2007*;14:2490–2496. doi:10.1245/s10434-007-9450-4.

[15] Casabona F., Bogliolo S., Valenzano Menada M., Sala P., Villa G., Ferrero S., Feasibility of axillary reverse mapping during sentinel lymph node biopsy in breast cancer patients. *Ann Surg Oncol. 2009*;16:2459–2463. doi:10.1245/s10434-009-0554-x.

[16] Kang T., Yi M., Hunt K. K., Mittendorf E. A., Babiera G. V., Kuerer H. et al., Does blue dye contribute to success of sentinel node mapping for breast cancer? *Ann Surg Oncol. 2010*;17 Suppl 3:280–285. doi:10.1245/s10434-010-1235-5.

[17] O'Reilly E. A., Prichard R. S., Al Azawi D., Aucharaz N., Kelly G., Evoy D. et al., The Value of Isosulfan Blue Dye in Addition to Isotope Scanning in the Identification of the Sentinel Lymph Node in Breast Cancer Patients With a Positive Lymphoscintigraphy: A Randomized Controlled Trial (ISRCTN98849733). *Annals of surgery. 2015*; 262:243–248. doi:10.1097/SLA.0000000000001213.

[18] Guo J., Yang H., Wang S., Cao Y., Liu M., Xie F. et al., Comparison of sentinel lymph node biopsy guided by indocyanine green, blue dye, and their combination in breast cancer patients: a prospective cohort study. *World J Surg Oncol. 2017*;15:196. doi:10.1186/s12957-017-1264-7.

[19] Johnson C. B., Boneti C., Korourian S., Adkins L., Klimberg V. S., Intraoperative injection of subareolar or dermal radioisotope results in predictable identification of sentinel lymph nodes in breast cancer. *Ann Surg. 2011*;254:612–618. doi: 10.1097/SLA.0b013e31823005bf.

[20] Hill A. D., Tran K. N., Akhurst T., Yeung H., Yeh S. D., Rosen P. P. et al., Lessons learned from 500 cases of lymphatic mapping for breast cancer. *Ann Surg. 1999*; 229:528–535.

[21] Tafra L., Lannin D. R., Swanson M. S., JJ VE, Verbanac K. M., Chua A. N. et al., Multicenter trial of sentinel node biopsy for breast cancer using both technetium sulfur colloid and isosulfan blue dye. *Ann Surg. 2001*;233:51–59.

[22] Goyal A., Sentinel lymph node biopsy in breast cancer: the node to recovery. *Indian J Surg Oncol. 2010*;1:10–13. doi:10.1007/s13193-010-0005-y.

[23] Bernardi S., Bertozzi S., Londero A. P., Gentile G., Giacomuzzi F., Carbone A., Incidence and risk factors of the intraoperative localization failure of nonpalpable breast lesions by radio-guided occult lesion localization: a retrospective analysis of 579 cases. *World J Surg. 2012*;36:1915–1921. doi:10.1007/s00268-012-1577-1.

[24] Straver M. E., Meijnen P., van Tienhoven G., van de Velde C. J. H., Mansel R. E., Bogaerts J. et al., Sentinel node identification rate and nodal involvement in the EORTC 10981-22023 AMAROS trial. *Ann Surg Oncol. 2010*;17:1854–1861. doi: 10.1245/s10434-010-0945-z.

[25] Goyal A., Newcombe R. G., Chhabra A., Mansel R. E., Group A. T., Factors affecting failed localisation and false-negative rates of sentinel node biopsy in breast cancer–results of the ALMANAC validation phase. *Breast Cancer Res Treat. 2006*;99:203–208. doi:10.1007/s10549-006-9192-1.

[26] Peek M. C., Kovacs T., Baker R., Hamed H., Kothari A., Douek M., Is blue dye still required during sentinel lymph node biopsy for breast cancer? *Ecancermedicalscience. 2016*;10:674. doi:10.3332/ecancer.2016.674.

[27] Bines S., Kopkash K., Ali A., Fogg L., Wool N., The use of radioisotope combined with isosulfan Blue dye is not superior to radioisotope alone for the identification of sentinel lymph nodes in patients with breast cancer. *Surgery. 2008*;144:606–9; discussion 609–10. doi:10.1016/j.surg.2008.06.023.

[28] He P. S., Li F., Li G. H., Guo C., Chen T. J., The combination of blue dye and radioisotope versus radioisotope alone during sentinel lymph node biopsy for breast cancer: a systematic review. *BMC Cancer. 2016*;16:107. doi:10.1186/s12885-016-2137-0.

[29] Niebling M. G., Pleijhuis R. G., Bastiaannet E., Brouwers A. H., van Dam G. M., Hoekstra H. J., A systematic review and meta-analyses of sentinel lymph node identification in breast cancer and melanoma, a plea for tracer mapping. *Eur J Surg Oncol. 2016*;42:466–473. doi:10.1016/j.ejso.2015.12.007.

[30] Reinhart M. B., Huntington C. R., Blair L. J., Heniford B. T., Augenstein V. A., Indocyanine Green: Historical Context, Current Applications, and Future Considerations. *Surg Innov. 2016*;23:166–175. doi:10.1177/1553350615604053.

[31] Owens E. A., Lee S., Choi J., Henary M., Choi H. S., NIR fluorescent small molecules for intraoperative imaging. *Wiley Interdiscip Rev Nanomed Nanobiotechnol. 2015*; 7:828–838. doi:10.1002/wnan.1337.

[32] Fujisawa Y., Nakamura Y., Kawachi Y., Otsuka F., Indocyanine green fluorescence-navigated sentinel node biopsy showed higher sensitivity than the radioisotope or blue dye method, which may help to reduce false-negative cases in skin cancer. *J Surg Oncol. 2012*;106:41–45. doi:10.1002/jso.23045.

[33] Grischke E. M., Rhm C., Hahn M., Helms G., Brucker S., Wallwiener D., ICG Fluorescence Technique for the Detection of Sentinel Lymph Nodes in Breast Cancer: Results of a Prospective Open-label Clinical Trial. *Geburtshilfe Frauenheilkd. 2015*; 75:935–940. doi:10.1055/s-0035-1557905.

[34] Ahmed M., Purushotham A. D., Douek M., Novel techniques for sentinel lymph node biopsy in breast cancer: a systematic review. *Lancet Oncol. 2014*;15:e351–e362. doi: 10.1016/S1470-2045(13)70590-4.

[35] Coufal O., Fait V., Liaov E., Chrenko V., aloudk J., [SentiMag–the magnetic detection system of sentinel lymph nodes in breast cancer]. *Rozhl Chir. 2015*;94:283–288.

[36] Teshome M., Wei C., Hunt K. K., Thompson A., Rodriguez K., Mittendorf E. A., Use of a Magnetic Tracer for Sentinel Lymph Node Detection in Early-Stage Breast Cancer Patients: A Meta-analysis. *Ann Surg Oncol. 2016*;23:1508–1514. doi: 10.1245/s10434-016-5135-1.

[37] Thill M., Kurylcio A., Welter R., van Haasteren V., Grosse B., Berclaz G. et al., The Central-European SentiMag study: sentinel lymph node biopsy with superparamagnetic iron oxide (SPIO) vs. radioisotope. *Breast. 2014*;23:175–179. doi: 10.1016/j.breast.2014.01.004.

[38] Ghilli M., Carretta E., Di Filippo F., Battaglia C., Fustaino L., Galanou I. et al., The superparamagnetic iron oxide tracer: a valid alternative in sentinel node biopsy for breast cancer treatment. *Eur J Cancer Care (Engl). 2017*;26. doi:10.1111/ecc.12385.

[39] Karakatsanis A., Christiansen P. M., Fischer L., Hedin C., Pistioli L., Sund M. et al., The Nordic SentiMag trial: a comparison of super paramagnetic iron oxide (SPIO) nanoparticles versus Tc(99) and patent blue in the detection of sentinel node (SN) in patients with breast cancer and a meta-analysis of earlier studies. *Breast Cancer Res Treat. 2016*;157:281–294. doi:10.1007/s10549-016-3809-9.

[40] Sharma N., Cox K., Axillary Nodal Staging with Contrast-Enhanced Ultrasound. *Curr Breast Cancer Rep. 2017*;9:259–263. doi:10.1007/s12609-017-0258-3.

[41] Omoto K., Hozumi Y., Omoto Y., Taniguchi N., Itoh K., Fujii Y. et al., Sentinel node detection in breast cancer using contrast-enhanced sonography with 25 *J Clin Ultrasound. 2006*;34:317–326. doi:10.1002/jcu.20241.

[42] Verheuvel N. C., van den Hoven I., Ooms H. W. A., Voogd A. C., Roumen R. M. H., The role of ultrasound-guided lymph node biopsy in axillary staging of invasive breast cancer in the post-ACOSOG Z0011 trial era. *Ann Surg Oncol. 2015*;22:409–415. doi: 10.1245/s10434-014-4071-1.

[43] Pinheiro L. G. P., Oliveira Filho R. S. D., Vasques P. H. D., Filgueira P. H. D. O., Aragão D. H. P., Barbosa P. M. E. et al., Hemosiderin: a new marker for sentinel lymph node identification. *Acta Cir Bras. 2009*;24:432–436.

[44] Bernardi S., Bertozzi S., Londero A. P., Angione V., Petri R., Giacomuzzi F., Prevalence and risk factors of intraoperative identification failure of sentinel lymph nodes in patients affected by breast cancer. *Nucl Med Commun. 2013*;34:664–673. doi: 10.1097/MNM.0b013e328361cd84.

[45] Rescigno J., Zampell J. C., Axelrod D., Patterns of axillary surgical care for breast cancer in the era of sentinel lymph node biopsy. *Ann Surg Oncol. 2009*;16:687–696. doi:10.1245/s10434-008-0195-5.

[46] Johnson M. T., Guidroz J. A., Smith B. J., Graham M. M., Scott-Conner C. E. H., Sugg S. L. et al., A single institutional experience of factors affecting successful identification of sentinel lymph node in breast cancer patients. *Surgery. 2009*;146:671–6; discussion 676–7. doi:10.1016/j.surg.2009.06.025.

[47] Straalman K., Kristoffersen U. S., Galatius H., Lanng C., Factors influencing sentinel lymph node identification failure in breast cancer surgery. *Breast. 2008*;17:167–171. doi:10.1016/j.breast.2007.08.008.

[48] Wang L., Yu Jm., Wang Ys., Zuo Ws., Gao Y., Fan J. et al., Preoperative lymphoscintigraphy predicts the successful identification but is not necessary in sentinel lymph nodes biopsy in breast cancer. *Ann Surg Oncol. 2007*;14:2215–2220. doi: 10.1245/s10434-007-9418-4.

[49] Pritsivelis C., Garcia Mendona C. A., Pinheiro Pessoa M. C., Coelho-Oliveira A., Gutfilen B., Barbosa Da Fonseca L. M., Failure predictors of the sentinel lymph node in patients with breast cancer using Tc-99m sulfur colloid and periareolar injection. *Q J Nucl Med Mol Imaging. 2007*;51:189–193.

[50] Chagpar A. B., Martin R. C., Scoggins C. R., Carlson D. J., Laidley A. L., El-Eid S. E. et al., Factors predicting failure to identify a sentinel lymph node in breast cancer. *Surgery. 2005*;138:56–63. doi:10.1016/j.surg.2005.03.003.

[51] Kern K. A., Concordance and validation study of sentinel lymph node biopsy for breast cancer using subareolar injection of blue dye and technetium 99m sulfur colloid. *J Am Coll Surg. 2002*;195:467–475.

[52] Gauthier T., Mollard J., Fermeaux V., Kapella M., Aubard Y., Axillary recurrence after negative sentinel lymph node biopsy under local anesthesia in breast cancer. *Eur J Surg Oncol. 2009*;35:464–468. doi:10.1016/j.ejso.2008.09.008.

[53] Visnjić M., Kovacević P., Dordević G., [Sentinel lymph node biopsy in breast neoplasms]. *Vojnosanit Pregl. 2009*;66:228–232.

[54] Soran A., Falk J., Bonaventura M., Keenan D., Ahrendt G., Johnson R., Does failure to visualize a sentinel node on preoperative lymphoscintigraphy predict a greater likelihood of axillary lymph node positivity? *J Am Coll Surg. 2007*;205:66–71. doi: 10.1016/j.jamcollsurg.2007.01.064.

[55] Krag D. N., Ashikaga T., Harlow S. P., Skelly J. M., Julian T. B., Brown A. M. et al., Surgeon training, protocol compliance, and technical outcomes from breast cancer sentinel lymph node randomized trial. *J Natl Cancer Inst. 2009*;101:1356–1362. doi: 10.1093/jnci/djp281.

[56] Davis K. G., Schriver J. P., Prevalence of teaching sentinel lymph node biopsy for breast cancer in general surgery residency programs. *Curr Surg. 2002*;59:420–422.

[57] Clarke D., Newcombe R. G., Mansel R. E., Group A. T., The learning curve in sentinel node biopsy: the ALMANAC experience. *Ann Surg Oncol. 2004*;11:211S–215S.

[58] Abdollahi A., Jangjoo A., Dabbagh Kakhki V. R., Rasoul Zakavi S., Memar B., Naser Forghani M. et al., Factors affecting sentinel lymph node detection failure in breast cancer patients using intradermal injection of the tracer. *Rev Esp Med Nucl. 2010*;29:73–77. doi:10.1016/j.remn.2009.10.001.

[59] McMasters K. M., Wong S. L., Tuttle T. M., Carlson D. J., Brown C. M., Dirk Noyes R. et al., Preoperative lymphoscintigraphy for breast cancer does not improve the ability to identify axillary sentinel lymph nodes. *Ann Surg. 2000*;231:724–731.

[60] Shoher A., Diwan A., Teh B. S., Lu H. H., Fisher R., Lucci A., Lymphoscintigraphy does not enhance sentinel node identification or alter management of patients with early breast cancer. *Curr Surg. 2006*;63:207–212. doi:10.1016/j.cursur.2006.02.008.

[61] Marchal F., Rauch P., Morel O., Mayer J. C., Olivier P., Leroux A. et al., Results of preoperative lymphoscintigraphy for breast cancer are predictive of identification of axillary sentinel lymph nodes. *World J Surg. 2006*;30:55–62. doi:10.1007/s00268-005-0145-3.

[62] Sato K., Tamaki K., Shigekawa T., Tsuda H., Kosuda S., Kusano S. et al., Clinicopathologic and technical factors associated with the uptake of radiocolloid by sentinel nodes in patients with breast cancer. *Surg Today. 2003*;33:403–407. doi: 10.1007/s10595-002-2525-9.

[63] Jinno H., Ikeda T., Asaga S., Muto T., Kitagawa Y., Fujii H. et al., Increasing age does not affect efficacy of sentinel lymph node biopsy using smaller-sized technetium-99m tin colloids for breast cancer patients. *Am J Surg. 2005*;190:51–54. doi: 10.1016/j.amjsurg.2004.08.067.

[64] Derossis A. M., Fey J. V., Cody H. S., Borgen P. I., Obesity influences outcome of sentinel lymph node biopsy in early-stage breast cancer. *J Am Coll Surg. 2003*; 197:896–901. doi:10.1016/j.jamcollsurg.2003.08.005.

[65] Cox C. E., Dupont E., Whitehead G. F., Ebert M. D., Nguyen K., Peltz E. S. et al., Age and body mass index may increase the chance of failure in sentinel lymph node biopsy for women with breast cancer. *Breast J. 2002*;8:88–91.

[66] Hughes M., Goffman T. G., Perry R. R., Laronga C., Obesity and lymphatic mapping with sentinel lymph node biopsy in breast cancer. *Am J Surg. 2004*;187:52–57.

[67] Kelly J., Fogarty K., Redmond H. P., A definitive role for sentinel lymph node mapping with biopsy for cutaneous melanoma of the head and neck. *Surgeon. 2009*;7:336–339.

[68] Pavlista D., Eliska O., Analysis of direct oil contrast lymphography of upper limb lymphatics traversing the axilla – a lesson from the past – contribution to the concept of axillary reverse mapping. *Eur J Surg Oncol. 2012*;38:390–394. doi: 10.1016/j.ejso.2012.01.010.

[69] Nos C., Kaufmann G., Clough K. B., Collignon M. A., Zerbib E., Cusumano P. et al., Combined axillary reverse mapping (ARM) technique for breast cancer patients requiring axillary dissection. *Ann Surg Oncol. 2008*;15:2550–2555. doi: 10.1245/s10434-008-0030-z.

[70] Nowikiewicz T., Kurylcio A., Polkowski W., Zegarski W., Imaging methods for the local lymphatic system of the axilla in early breast cancer in patients qualified for sentinel lymph node biopsy. *Prz Menopauzalny. 2016*;15:52–55. doi: 10.5114/pm.2016.58775.

[71] Morrow M., Rademaker A. W., Bethke K. P., Talamonti M. S., Dawes L. G., Clauson J. et al., Learning sentinel node biopsy: results of a prospective randomized trial of two techniques. *Surgery. 1999*;126:714–20; discussion 720–2.

[72] Hirano A., Kamimura M., Ogura K., Kim N., Hattori A., Setoguchi Y. et al., A comparison of indocyanine green fluorescence imaging plus blue dye and blue dye alone for sentinel node navigation surgery in breast cancer patients. *Ann Surg Oncol. 2012*;19:4112–4116. doi:10.1245/s10434-012-2478-0.

[73] Tong M., Guo W., Gao W., Use of Fluorescence Imaging in Combination with Patent Blue Dye versus Patent Blue Dye Alone in Sentinel Lymph Node Biopsy in Breast Cancer. *J Breast Cancer. 2014*;17:250–255. doi:10.4048/jbc.2014.17.3.250.

[74] Guo W., Zhang L., Ji J., Gao W., Liu J., Tong M., Evaluation of the benefit of using blue dye in addition to indocyanine green fluorescence for sentinel lymph node biopsy in patients with breast cancer. *World J Surg Oncol. 2014*;12:290. doi:10.1186/1477-7819-12-290.

[75] Pitsinis V., Provenzano E., Kaklamanis L., Wishart G. C., Benson J. R., Indocyanine green fluorescence mapping for sentinel lymph node biopsy in early breast cancer. *Surg Oncol. 2015*;24:375–379. doi:10.1016/j.suronc.2015.10.002.

[76] Toh U., Iwakuma N., Mishima M., Okabe M., Nakagawa S., Akagi Y., Navigation surgery for intraoperative sentinel lymph node detection using Indocyanine green (ICG) fluorescence real-time imaging in breast cancer. *Breast Cancer Res Treat. 2015*; 153:337–344. doi:10.1007/s10549-015-3542-9.

[77] Ballardini B., Santoro L., Sangalli C., Gentilini O., Renne G., Lissidini G. et al., The indocyanine green method is equivalent to the mTc-labeled radiotracer method for identifying the sentinel node in breast cancer: a concordance and validation study. *Eur J Surg Oncol. 2013*;39:1332–1336. doi:10.1016/j.ejso.2013.10.004.

[78] Xiong L., Gazyakan E., Yang W., Engel H., Hnerbein M., Kneser U. et al., Indocyanine green fluorescence-guided sentinel node biopsy: a meta-analysis on detection rate and diagnostic performance. *Eur J Surg Oncol. 2014*;40:843–849. doi: 10.1016/j.ejso.2014.02.228.

[79] Samorani D., Fogacci T., Panzini I., Frisoni G., Accardi F. G., Ricci M. et al., The use of indocyanine green to detect sentinel nodes in breast cancer: a prospective study. *Eur J Surg Oncol. 2015*;41:64–70. doi:10.1016/j.ejso.2014.10.047.

[80] Sugie T., Kinoshita T., Masuda N., Sawada T., Yamauchi A., Kuroi K. et al., Evaluation of the Clinical Utility of the ICG Fluorescence Method Compared with the Radioisotope Method for Sentinel Lymph Node Biopsy in Breast Cancer. *Ann Surg Oncol. 2016*;23:44–50. doi:10.1245/s10434-015-4809-4.

In: The Sentinel Lymph Node
Editors: A. Londero, S. Bertozzi and C. Cedolini
ISBN: 978-1-53614-557-1


*Chapter 3*

# TECHNICAL ASPECTS OF THE SENTINEL LYMPH NODE EVALUATION

***Maria Orsaria*[1,*], *Serena Bertozzi*[2], *Stefania Marzinotto*[1], *Ambrogio P. Londero*[3] and *Laura Mariuzzi*[1]**
[1]Institute of Pathology, DAME,
University of Udine, University Hospital of Udine, Italy
[2]Breast Unit, University Hospital of Udine, Italy
[3]Clinic of Obstetrics and Gynecology,
University Hospital of Udine, Italy

**Abstract**

Sentinel lymph node biopsy has become a common procedure in breast and melanoma surgery and its popularity is growing among other cancer staging procedures thanks to its conservative approach, which enables a reduced postoperative morbidity. In recent decades we have witnessed a technical evolution in the preoperative, intraoperative and postoperative steps of this procedure. Many different techniques are currently used in the literature and in the clinical routine to assess the sentinel node status, from conventional histological and immunohistochemical analyses to cytology, bimolecular tests, or physical tests based on spectrometry. In this chapter, we will discuss the conventional techniques and some of the new techniques to assess the sentinel node status, including the intraoperative biomolecular examination of the nodes. In particular, we will discuss the molecular tests developed for detecting lymph node metastases, which theoretically allows a more accurate lymph node assessment than the conventional histology techniques, as biomolecular examination allows the analysis of the whole sentinel node specimen. Currently, there are two available methods for the intraoperative sentinel node assessment in breast cancer, the one-step nucleic acid amplification (OSNA) method and Metasin, both based on the specific mRNA quantification to define the amount of nodal involvement (micrometastases or macrometastases).

**Keywords:** sentinel lymph node biopsy, cytology, histology, OSNA, Metasin

*Corresponding Author E-mail: mariaorsaria@yahoo.it.

# 1. Introduction

As expected, over time we have seen a technical evolution in the preoperative, intraoperative and postoperative examination procedures for the sentinel lymph node biopsy (SLNB). First of all, we have observed an evolution toward reducing the number of interventions with the introduction of the intraoperative frozen section evaluation of the sentinel node. Secondly, immunohistochemical and molecular biology techniques have begun to replace traditional morphological examination in order to increase accuracy and reduce operative time.

Considering SLNB in breast cancer, which is the field in which there is most experience with this procedure, the sentinel node detection rate in routine breast surgery has achieved a high success rate. According to our experience, the sentinel node detection rate is about 99%, with a mean number of biopsied nodes of 1.64 (±0.67), and axillary localization is by far the most common case [1].

The prevalence of isolated tumor cells (ITCs), micrometastases and macrometastases in our population using frozen section were 0.6%, 4.9%, and 7.5%, respectively [1]. Yet, in our experience, in women who have recived complete axillary lymph node dissection (CALND) the mean number of cleaned nodes was 16.36 (±6.19) and the mean number of metastatic non-sentinel nodes was less than 1 in the case of micrometastases, 2.65 in the case of macrometastases and up to 9.88 in the case of lymph node pericapsular invasion [1].

In the literature, the prevalence of micrometastases and ITCs by SLNB varies between 2% and 23% [2, 3, 4, 5, 6, 7, 8] and between 8.9% and 10.6%, respectively [4, 9, 2]. In accordance with the current literature, in our experience intraoperative frozen section histological examination of the sentinel node has revealed a low prevalence of micrometastases and ITCs. In fact, frozen section histological examination is well-known for having a higher false-negative rate [10], with a sensitivity of 83.3% for macrometastases, 40% for micrometastases and only 18.2% for ITCs [11].

With regard to the clinical significance of ITCs and micrometastases, it has been shown that the size of lymph node metastases is directly correlated with the likelihood of non-sentinel lymph node involvement, which is 4-9% for ITCs [12, 9, 13, 14], 0-80% for micrometastases [13, 9, 14, 12], and 46-80% for macrometastases [9, 13]. Based on current available evidence, CALND is not indicated in the presence of ITCs [15, 12] or micrometastases [16].

The reason for introducing frozen section histological examination or touch imprint cytology was to improve breast cancer management, allowing single-session surgery with intraoperative SLNB assessment and, if necessary, immediate CALND. In this chapter, we will discuss the conventional techniques along with the new approaches to intraoperative nodal status assessment.

# 2. Postoperative Histological Examination

Routine processing of sentinel nodes consist of fixing the nodes in 10% neutral formalin and cutting the nodes, after or before fixation, into 2-mm-thick slices. This 2-mm-spaced evaluation of the node allows the detection of all macrometastases (larger than 2 mm) (Figure 1), as well as most large micrometastases (ranging between 0.2 mm and 2 mm) (Figure 2). Subsequently, the slices of each node are placed in one or more bio-cassettes according

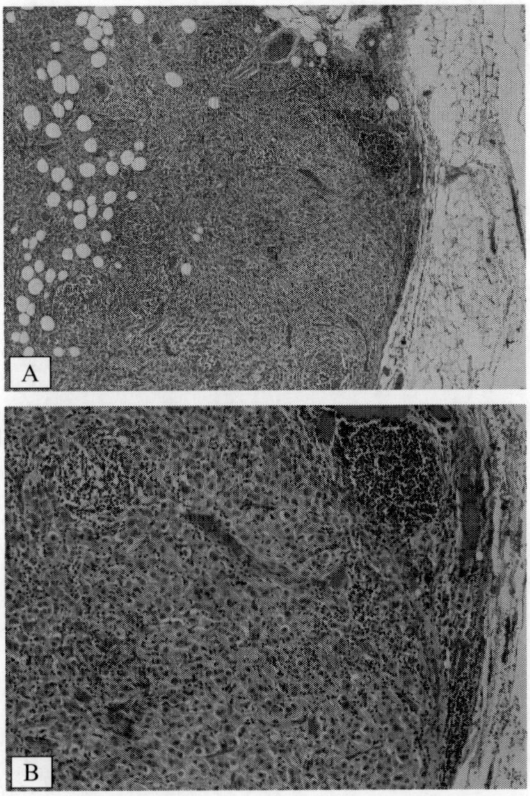


Figure 1. Hematoxylin-eosin stained sections showing macrometastatic disease. (Panel A) 4x magnification. (Panel B) 10x magnification.

to the node size and embedded in paraffin. Finally, 4 μm sections are cut and stained with hematoxylin-eosin.

In the literature there are several different practices. In some centers, only one slice is cut and stained per paraffin block, but it is also possible to process step sections (up to three from each block or until the lymph node tissue is exhausted). If the assessed lymph node is less than 5mm, it shall be fixed and embedded intact before the examination of the step sections.

In our setting, usually all biopsied lymph nodes undergo an accurate evaluation of 2-mm-spaced hematoxylin-eosin stained sections, followed by immunohistochemical evaluation of a random portion of the node to look for a potential positivity for cytokeratins [17, 2].

# 3. Postoperative Immunohistochemical Examination

Cytokeratin immunohistochemistry staining was introduced as part of the ultrastaging procedure to detect occult metastases. According to our experience, it is reasonable to stain at least one to three sections for pan-cytokeratin (AE1/AE3) if the hematoxylin-eosin-stained

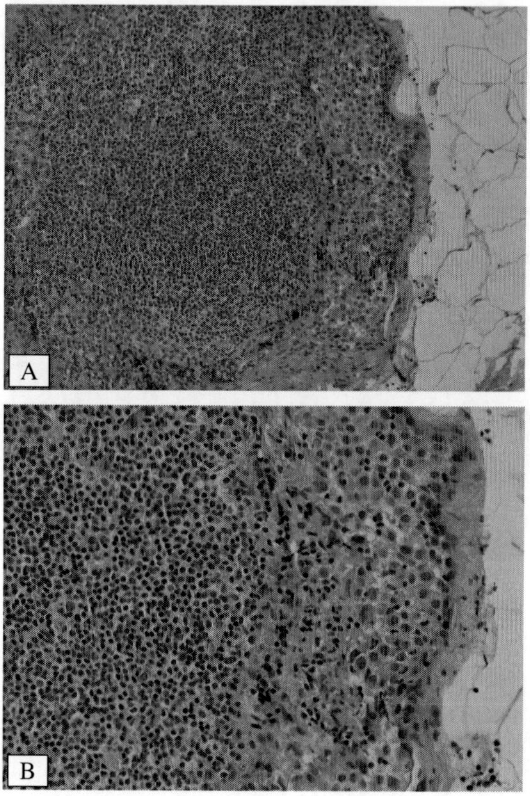


Figure 2. Hematoxylin-eosin stained sections showing micrometastatic disease. (Panel A) 10x magnification. (Panel B) 20x magnification.

sections do not show any presence of tumoral disease [18, 19].

This type of procedure helps identify small micrometastases and ITCs that are usually not found with the standard 2-mm-thick hematoxylin-eosin-stained slices [20]. In particular, the presence of micrometastases guides decision-making on adjuvant treatments [16]. Furthermore, cytokeratin immunohistochemistry staining is very useful in the case of invasive lobular carcinoma, since metastatic tumor cells are hardly identifiable in the sentinel lymph node with the standard hematoxylin-eosin-stained sections.

## 4. Intraoperative Histological Examination

In the case of intraoperative frozen section histological examination, the sentinel nodes are cut into 2-mm-thick parts, frozen-fixed and polyvinyl-alcohol-embedded before being submitted to intraoperative histological examination of 2-4 0.15-mm-spaced, hematoxylin-eosin-stained sections as well as to immunhistochemical evaluation of three random sections to look for a potential positivity for cytokeratins.

Subsequently, the remaining sentinel lymph nodes tissue is submitted to traditional definitive histological examination with evaluation of 0.15-mm-spaced, hematoxylin-eosin-stained sections [21, 1] and immunohistochemical evaluation of a random nodal portion [22, 1].

## 5. Intraoperative Touch Imprinting Cytology

Touch imprinting cytology represent one of the several methods proposed in the literature for the intraoperative assessment of the sentinel lymph node status [23, 24, 1, 25]. Although this technique is considered to be as accurate as frozen section histological examination for intraoperative nodal analysis [26, 27], the sensitivity of this method for intraoperative sentinel node assessment in breast cancer is not consistent among published studies [23, 24, 26, 28, 29, 30]. In fact, the sensitivity of touch imprinting cytology is found to be dependent on the size of the primary tumor and ranges from 54.4% (for 11-20 mm tumors) to 88.2% (for tumors over 50 mm) [27].

Furthermore, sentinel node metastases from invasive lobular carcinoma are reported to be more difficult to identify with touch imprinting cytology than those from ductal invasive carcinoma, because lobular invasive carcinoma has more often a low-grade cytomorphology and a propensity to infiltrate lymph nodes in a single-cell pattern, resembling lymphocytes [28, 29].

To perform touch imprinting cytology, the sentinel lymph node is cut into 2mm-thick sections (to detect macrometastases) and one or two imprints of the same surface are made for each section by touching the cut surface of the node on a glass slide. One imprint is tested by immunocytochemical cytokeratin staining, while the second imprinting glass is stained by the May-Grnwald-Giemsa method. Finally, the lymph node is formalin-fixed and paraffin-embedded to be processed with conventional postoperative histology or molecular techniques.

## 6. Intraoperative Biomolecular Examination

The aforementioned conventional techniques for intraoperative sentinel lymph node analysis, such as frozen section histological examination and touch imprint cytology, have a high specificity of up to 100%, but their sensitivity ranges between 60-70%, and is particularly low for micrometastases [31]. Therefore, molecular tests have been developed for the detection of lymph node metastases, which theoretically allow a more accurate and sensitive sentinel lymph node assessment than conventional formalin-fixed paraffin-embedded histology techniques, since biomolecular examination allows the analysis of the whole SLNB specimen [32].

There are currently two commercially available diagnostic methods for the intraoperative biomolecular evaluation of SLNB in breast cancer: the one-step nucleic acid amplification (OSNA) method (Gene Amplification Detector System RD-100i by Sysmex, Kobe, Japan) (Figure 3) [33, 34] and Metasin [35]. The Metasin system is similar to the GeneSearch BLN Assay (Veridex, Warren, New Jersey, USA), which is no longer available on the market [36, 37, 38, 39]. This system uses a real-time quantitative polymerase chain reaction (PCR) to detect the mRNA of two breast metastases markers: a breast-specific marker (mammaglobin) and an epithelial marker (cytokeratin 19). The porphobilinogen deaminase primer is used as an internal positive amplification control.

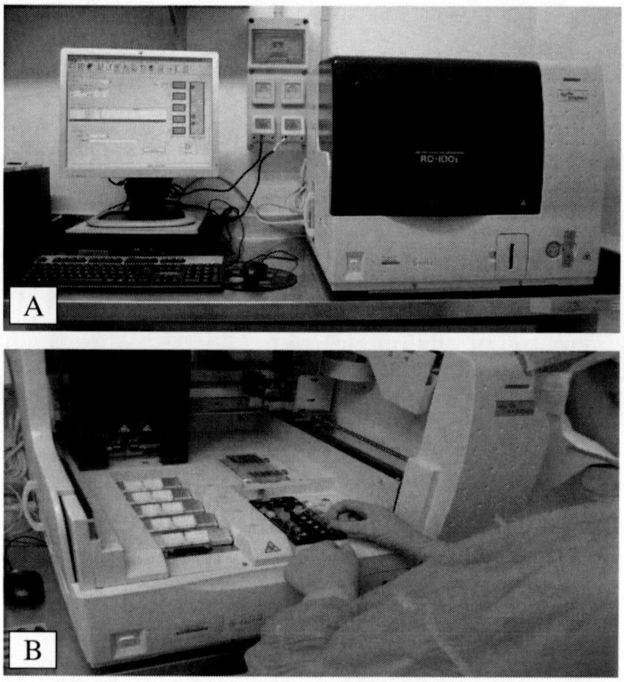

Figure 3. Gene Amplification Detector System RD-100i by Sysmex. (Panel A) The whole system. (Panel B) The system during the loading procedure.

Thanks to the publication of Metasin primer and probe sequences, in the scientific literature, any laboratory is now able to use commercially available reagents and real-time quantitative PCR platforms to validate this method for its own personal use [35]. In the original manuscript, Metasin was evaluated and tested against conventional histological techniques and GeneSearch [35]. The cut-off values of the real-time quantitative PCR quantification cycle to define macrometastases, micrometastases and negative status (including ITCs) were previously stated [40] (Table 1).

**Table 1. Cut-off values of RT-qPCR quantification cycle (Cq) to define SLNB status [40]**

| | CK19 | MGB |
|---|---|---|
| Negative/ITC | >32 | 32.3 |
| Micrometastases | >25 – <32 | >26 – <32.3 |
| Macrometastases | ≤25 | ≤26 |

In recent studies, a high concordance between Metasin and histology was found, ranging between 92-94% [40, 31]. In addition, a high sensitivity (89-92%) and specificity (93-97%) were found [40, 31].

The OSNA® method is a CE-IVD biomolecular quantitative system that significantly accelerates sentinel node analysis, resulting in reduced operative time and anesthesiological risk, cost-benefit gains, and a high accuracy of result [41, 42, 43]. The procedure begins with the homogenization of the collected sentinel nodes in a mRNA-stabilizing solution (LYNORHAG®, pH 3.5 Sysmex;), followed by an isothermal (65 C) CK19 amplification using the LYNOAMP® BC amplification kit (Sysmex;) through a reverse transcriptase amplification assay (RT-LAMP) in a gene amplification detector RD-100i (Sysmex;) [44, 45, 46, 47, 34]. A standard positive control sample and a negative control sample are always used for calibration in each assay, and the test results are automatically given in a semiquantitative way [46, 34, 48, 49]. In particular, the test is negative if the CK19 mRNA copy number/l lysate is less than 250/l; while it shows the presence of micrometastases for copy numbers between 250/l and 5000/l; and macrometastases for copy numbers equal to or greater than 5000/l (Table 2).

**Table 2. The results of OSNA are qualitatively illustrated in three categories (++, +, and -) and quantitatively expressed as the number of copies of CK19 mRNA present in the sample. The quantitative molecular result is therefore related to the volume of metastases**

| | Metastasis dimensions (mm) | CK19 mRNA (copies/l) | OSNA | TNM |
|---|---|---|---|---|
| Macrometastasis | $> 2$ | $> 5.000$ | ++ | pN1a |
| Micrometastasis | $0.2 < X < 2$ | $250 < X < 5.000$ | + | pN1mi |
| Negative or ITCs | $< 0.2$ | $< 250$ | - | pN0/pN0(i+) |

In the literature, the OSNA method is comparable with both postoperative histological examination and intraoperative frozen section evaluation in terms of overall and disease-free survival, and is able to significantly reduce surgical time from a mean operation length of 69.4 (±10.3) minutes in case of frozen section to a mean operation length of 41.9 (±4.9) minutes using OSNA [43, 50, 51]. Obviously, this result requires the accurate compliance with certain technical premises, such as a strong limitation of the number of excised nodes. As a consequence, both OSNA and frozen section are usually correlated with a smaller number of excised sentinel nodes than definitive histological examination. A new platform, RD210, is now available, allowing the simultaneous analysis of up to 14 lymph-nodes, and further reducing the time of analysis (11 minutes for 1 sample) [52].

In addition to a decrease in the use of frozen section analysis from 100% to 62% among more than 7,500 patients with clinically node-negative invasive breast cancer from 1997 to 2006, some authors also described the decrease in CALND after the detection of sentinel node metastases by serial sectioning or immunohistochemistry, likely due to the current trend toward sparing CALND for micrometastases [53].

Furthermore, the OSNA system allows a more efficient detection of micrometastases, consequently decreasing the number of false-negative histological examinations resulting from the small size of micrometastases, which may not be included in any microscopical section [54]. This may also explain the lower cumulative rate of local recurrences after evaluation with the OSNA method. However, it is not prudent to draw definitive conclusions about local recurrences, considering the quite recent introduction of the OSNA method and the observation of a peak of local recurrences after SLNB between the third and sixth year of follow-up [2].

Several publications provide evidence on the clinical utility of OSNA® and CK19 copy number for breast cancer patients. More recent data shows that CK19 also provides predictive and prognostic information beyond conventional pathology assessment. This helps to deliver less invasive interventions, more personalized treatments and improves patients' quality of life. The data confirms that using the CK19 mRNA concentration to determine the metastatic burden of the sentinel lymph node leads to increased predictive capabilities in terms of risk of further axillary node involvement [55, 56]. Recent studies also indicate a prognostic value that enables patients to be categorized into high- or low-risk groups based on 5-year disease-free survival [51].

## 7. Fourier-Transform Infrared Spectroscopy

With regard to the detection of metastatic lymph nodes, a new technique for detecting nodal metastases in thyroid cancer has been recently introduced [57], which applies a Fourier-transform infrared spectroscopy to the excised sentinel lymph node to predict the presence of cancer within the node [57]. This technique detects an absorption spectrum reflecting the vibrational characteristics of chemical functional groups in relation to composition and structure. Furthermore, it allows the identification of different chemical signatures following changes in the intracellular environment, thus providing important information at the molecular level [58].

Biological tissues are composed of water, proteins, RNA, DNA, carbohydrates and lipids. These components at Fourier-transform infrared spectroscopic analysis show distinct vibrational absorption features and in cancer cells most of these components change significantly. Therefore, differences between malignant and normal cells can be identified through a specific fingerprint in the Fourier-transform infrared spectroscopic analysis. This method is able to analyze the fresh sample after only a minimal preparation, preserving the sample for further conventional analysis [59]. Several researchers found Fourier-transform infrared spectroscopy to be a reliable method to detect cancer [60, 61, 62, 63, 64].

Analysis by Fourier-transform infrared spectroscopy shall be carried out as follows. After collecting the fresh sentinel lymph node, it is immediately washed in distilled water several times at room temperature to remove residual blood. As a second step, cool air is gently blown onto the tissue for about one minute to remove ambient moisture and reduce the effect of water on the spectra. Since Fourier-transform infrared spectroscopy can penetrate one centimeter of tissue, the whole node can be analyzed without tissue destruction. As final step, the samples are analyzed by a Fourier-transform infrared spectrometer. The background spectrum is recorded before each tissue sample is scanned [24], and the scanning procedure takes about 2-3 minutes [24].

A recent study found this method to be accurate for assessing breast cancer SLNB (94.7% sensitivity, 90.1% specificity, and 91.3% accuracy) [24]. Potentially, Fourier-transform infrared spectroscopy is a non-destructive, accurate and cost-effective method for intraoperative assessment of SLNB metastases.

# 8. Preoperative Fine Needle Aspiration Cytology

Fine needle aspiration cytology is a cost-effective technique with a high diagnostic accuracy to assess the status of a suspicious lymph node or the sentinel lymph node. It is a typical outpatient procedure that reduces the hospital ward workload, as it requires basic equipment and causes only minimal discomfort to the patient. Although fine needle aspiration cytology is a low-cost procedure, it requires an experienced operator for the sampling phase and a skilled pathologist for the interpretation of the results.

Fine needle aspiration cytology and core needle biopsy are part of routine assessment of breast lesions (clinical, radiological and histological assessment), and have an increasing clinical role in sentinel node evaluation before or during surgery. The cost of fine needle aspiration cytology is lower than the cost of core needle biopsy and significantly lower than open biopsy. Both techniques are outpatient procedures, but core needle biopsy showed a greater diagnostic accuracy, especially for small non-palpable lesions [65, 66, 67]. Moreover, although the specificity of both methods is documented to be 100%, the sensitivity was higher in core needle biopsy (88.2%) than in fine needle aspiration cytology (72.5%) [66]. In addition, despite its evident cost-effectiveness, fine needle aspiration cytology in many centers has been replaced by core needle biopsy, which allows also a more accurate determination of the cancer immunophenotype (Figure 4) [67].

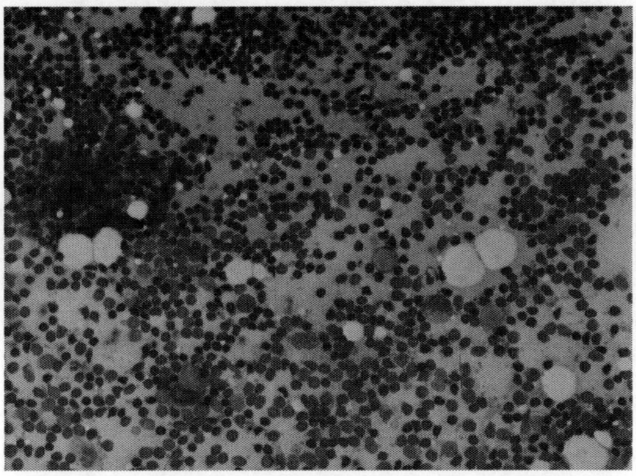

Figure 4. FNAC sample showing atypical cells.

However, there are some advantages of fine needle aspiration cytology over core needle biopsy, such as a greater mobility of the needle and the ability to feel the nature of the lesion and the texture of the tissue (soft low-resistance, rubbery, or firm texture, which are clues for final diagnosis), immediate assessment of the specimen adequacy, shorter processing time and and less time to final diagnosis. On the other hand, among the disadvantages of this procedure, we have a limited amount of tissue for further analysis, the presence of some lesions with a low cellular yield, inability to distinguish between in situ and invasive cancer, inaccurate determination of immunophenotypes and a high rate of insufficient sampling of microcalcifications or other non-palpable lesions due to the lack of epithelial tissue.

The fine need aspiration cytology equipment consist of local antisepsis material, potential local anesthesia, a needle, a syringe and a syringe holder (metal or plastic pistol-grip syringe) for the aspiration. In addition, a glass slide and liquid fixatives are needed. The needle diameter for this procedure is usually between 23 and 27 gauge (respectively 0.58-0.36mm). Most operators use a 10 ml syringe, but a 20 ml one can also be used. However, it should be noted that a good quality aspiration sample fills the needle hub and not the syringe and that a higher negative suction pressure could be associated with a higher risk of bleeding and therefore a lower-quality sample [68].

The breast lesion or the lymph node to be aspirated can be identified by palpation, with one hand used to immobilize the lesion and the other to perform the aspiration procedure. The lesion can be fixed along the axis of greatest mobility between the index and middle fingers [68]. The second option to localize the lesion and perform the procedure is the ultrasound-guided technique. Thanks to ultrasound it is possible to guide the needle into the lesion avoiding the vascular structures that might be in the way of the needle. For the aspiration procedure, the needle is inserted into the mass and the syringe plunger is pulled back creating a suction effect, while the needle is pushed forward and backward (30-40 excursions in 10-20 seconds).

The sample from the target mass is not obtained by suction, but through the cutting action of the needle. In fact, an alternative technique to perform fine needle aspiration cytology without the use of the syringe is the capillary method, which uses only the needle. At the end of the classical procedure, the suction is released while the needle is withdrawn and a pressure is applied at the needle insertion site to avoid bleeding [68].

Fine needle aspiration cytology, as well as core needle biopsy, can also be performed on the presumed sentinel node, identified by preoperative ultrasound examination with the aid of a microbubble contrast medium [69]. Therefore, preoperative microbubble contrast-enhanced axillary node core needle biopsy appears to be a valid option adopted in some breast units around the world [70]. In particular, microbubbles (usually 2-8 μm in diameter, mostly smaller than red blood cells) are ultrasound contrast agents that contain high molecular weight gases, which are less soluble and do not diffuse easily [71]. Microbubbles act as reflectors of the ultrasound beam and persist in the circulation for a few minutes, passing through the microcirculation [71].

In the case of breast cancer, microbubbles are injected intradermically allowing the identification of the sentinel nodes [69]. The sentinel nodes can then be assessed by ultrasound-guided fine needle aspiration or core needle biopsy [72]. Sever and colleagues found a detection rate of 93% in a population of 136 patients [72]. A positive SLNB was found among the negative nodes at the core biopsy in 8% of cases [72]. Furthermore, Cox and colleagues found a sensitivity of 61% and a specificity of 100% [73]. Due to the limited sensitivity of the technique, a negative biopsy requires a SLNB. In Figure 5 a possible algorithm including preoperative ultrasound-guided axillary node assessment is shown [70].

The following conditions are associated with an increased risk of sample inadequacy, in which case it is recommended to repeat the procedure to obtain a second sample [68]: fibrous lesions, small lesions due to their potential missing, specimen that clots immediately on the glass slide (diluted or hypocellular sample due to bleeding), sample that looks as smooth as a peripheral blood smear without visible particles and, finally, yellow or slightly oily aspirate in the case of adipose tissue sample.

After obtaining the sample, the smear is prepared either by a one-step procedure (pre-

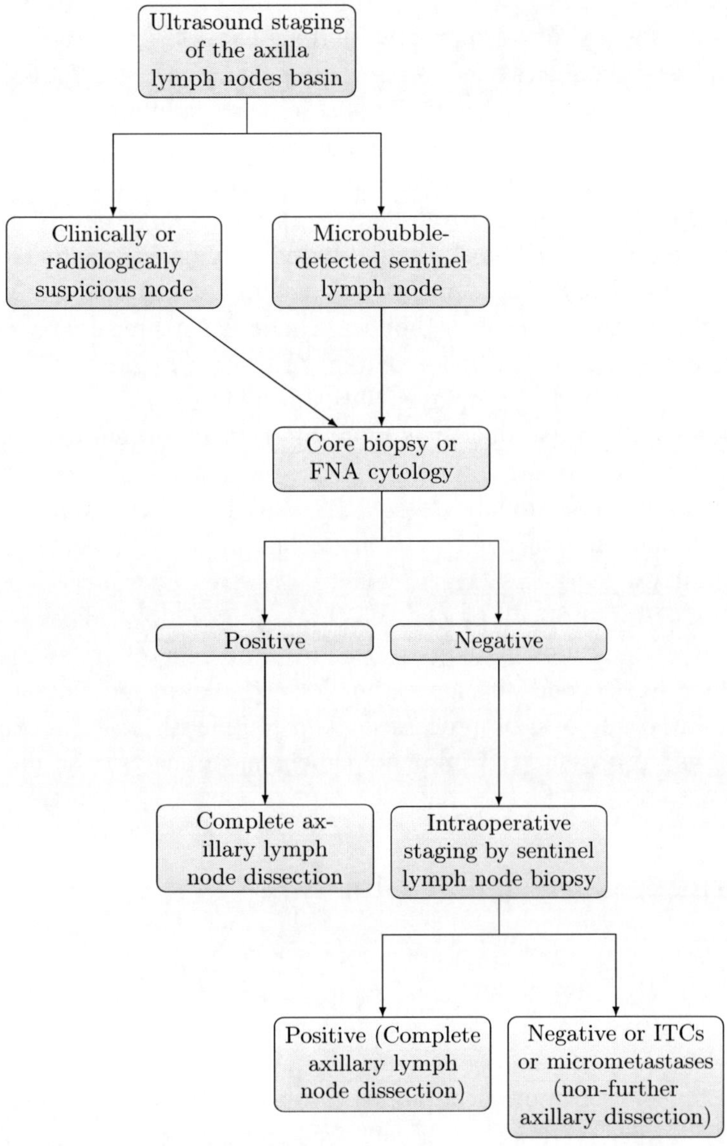


Figure 5. Sentinel lymph node algorithm with preoperative ultrasound staging modified from Shousha and colleagues [70].

ferred for low volume specimens) or a two-step procedure (preferred for liquid or hemorrhagic specimens) [68]. In the one-step method, the specimen is placed near the slide label, and a second spreader slide perpendicular to the first is used to gently touch and press the lower slide, allowing the specimen to be spread along the length of the lower slide (but not over the inferior limit of the spreader slide). In the two-step method, the fluid sample is placed first from the middle of the glass to the labeled edge, then the spreader slide is held at a 45 angle (using the short side) to the specimen bearing slide, advancing toward the label edge and returning back up to the center of the specimen. Finally, the spreader slide is used as in the one-step method.

Once the smear is ready, one can proceed with its fixation. In the case of Papanicolau (hematoxylin nuclear stain and two cytoplasmic stains, orange G and EA) or hematoxylin-eosin staining, the sample is fixed with 70-90% ethanol solution, while in the case of Romanowsky staining (Giemsa, May-Gruenwald-Giemsa, or Diff-Quik) the sample is air-dried before fixation, and treated with methanol after-fixation [68].

Recently, cytology has been improved with the introduction of new techniques such as the liquid-based cytology and cell block. Liquid-based cytology is a method implemented to reduce inadequacy rates in cytology screening by placing the material in a fixative solution and then filtering or centrifuging it to produce a monolayer preparation of cells on the slide glass. There are commercial methods (eg. ThinPrep or SurePath) and alternative manual methods to process the monolayer [74]. In addition, it has been found that the monolayer provides a definitive diagnosis more often than conventional cytology smear (73% vs 59%) [74]. Furthermore, immunohistochemical staining works better in liquid-based cytology than in conventional cytology [75, 76]. However, the loss of background and the epithelial fragmentation, typical of this technique, may hinder some diagnosis in breast cancer pathology.

Another options consist of cell blocks, which are prepared by embedding centrifuged cells from fine needle aspiration cytology procedures into agar, other gels, or directly into formalin to produce, as a second step, a paraffin block containing the cellular material. This procedure allows the sample to be processed as in routine histological examination and allows more staining processes and immunohistochemical analyses on the same sample [77].

## 9. Preoperative Core Needle Biopsy

Pathological assessment of the lymph node core needle biopsy is not different from the procedure used to analyze breast biopsies. Core needle biopsy is initially cut into three levels and every level is then analyzed with hematoxylin-eosin staining. This procedure allows accurate detections of tumor cells in the case of metastatic lymph nodes. In the case of a suspicious clinical or pathological picture (clinical history or suspicious cells in the original sections), further sections can be analyzed and eventually immunohistochemical examination can be performed (usually by testing pan-cytokeratin AE1/AE3). If core needle biopsy is composed only of tumor cells and no lymph node tissue is present, the biopsy should be considered as a second primary focus of breast cancer instead of a lymph node.

## 10. Notes on Radiation Safety

Given the use of radiotracers to identify the sentinel lymph node, there is concern that operators may be exposed to radioactive material when handling tissue samples. Already in the 2000s, the Surgical Pathology Committee of the College of American Pathologists and the Association of Directors of Anatomic and Surgical Pathology stated in their recommendations that apparently there are no reasons to delay the processing of the sentinel node [78]. However, it is good praxis to monitor the level of radiation in the working area and in the examined specimens because in some institutions an increased radioactivity level was found [79]. Therefore, specimens, envelopes and the area where the analyses are carried out must follow a radiation safety policy. These issues do not arise when using non-radioactive tracers (such as microbubble contrast, indocyanine green, or blue dye).

## References

[1] Cedolini C., Bertozzi S., Seriau L,, Londero A. P., Concina S., Cattin F., et al. Eight-year experience with the intraoperative frozen section examination of sentinel lymph node biopsy for breast cancer in a North-Italian university center. *Int J Clin Exp Path. 2014*;7:364–371.

[2] Bernardi S., Bertozzi S., Londero A. P., Giacomuzzi F., Angione V., Dri C., et al. Nine years of experience with the sentinel lymph node biopsy in a single Italian center: a retrospective analysis of 1,050 cases. *World J Surg. 2012*;36:714–722. doi: 10.1007/s00268-011-1420-0.

[3] Wasif N., Maggard M. A., Ko C. Y., Giuliano A. E., Underuse of axillary dissection for the management of sentinel node micrometastases in breast cancer. *Arch Surg. 2010*;145:161–166. doi:10.1001/archsurg.2009.269.

[4] Weaver D. L., Le U. P., Dupuis S. L., Weaver K. A. E., Harlow S. P., Ashikaga T., et al. Metastasis detection in sentinel lymph nodes: comparison of a limited widely spaced (NSABP protocol B-32) and a comprehensive narrowly spaced paraffin block sectioning strategy. *Am J Surg Pathol. 2009*;33:1583–1589. doi: 10.1097/PAS.0b013e3181b274e7.

[5] Gobardhan P. D., Elias S. G., Madsen E. V. E., Bongers V., Ruitenberg H. J. M., Perre C. I., et al. Prognostic value of micrometastases in sentinel lymph nodes of patients with breast carcinoma: a cohort study. *Ann Oncol. 2009*;20:41–48. doi: 10.1093/annonc/mdn535.

[6] Chen S. L., Hoehne F. M., Giuliano A. E., The prognostic significance of micrometastases in breast cancer: a SEER population-based analysis. *Ann Surg Oncol. 2007*; 14:3378–3384. doi:10.1245/s10434-007-9513-6.

[7] van der Heiden-van der Loo M., Bezemer P. D., Hennipman A., Siesling S., van Diest P. J., Bongers V., et al. Introduction of sentinel node biopsy and stage migration of breast cancer. *Eur J Surg Oncol. 2006*;32:710–714. doi:10.1016/j.ejso.2006.04.001.

[8] van Rijk M. C., Peterse J. L., Nieweg O. E., Oldenburg H. S. A., Rutgers E. J. T., Kroon B. B. R.. Additional axillary metastases and stage migration in breast cancer patients with micrometastases or submicrometastases in sentinel lymph nodes. *Cancer. 2006*;107:467–471. doi:10.1002/cncr.22069.

[9] Hansen N. M., Grube B., Ye X., Turner R. R., Brenner R. J., Sim M. S., et al. Impact of micrometastases in the sentinel node of patients with invasive breast cancer. *J Clin Oncol. 2009*;27:4679–4684. doi:10.1200/JCO.2008.19.0686.

[10] Tille J. C., Egger J. F., Devillaz M. C., Vlastos G., Pelte M. F., Frozen section in axillary sentinel lymph nodes for diagnosis of breast cancer micrometastasis. *Anticancer Res. 2009*;29:4711–4716.

[11] Khalifa K., Pereira B., Thomas V. A., Mokbel K. The accuracy of intraoperative frozen section analysis of the sentinel lymph nodes during breast cancer surgery. *Int J Fertil Womens Med. 2004*;49:208–211.

[12] Joseph K. A., El-Tamer M., Komenaka I., Troxel A., Ditkoff B. A., Schnabel F. Predictors of nonsentinel node metastasis in patients with breast cancer after sentinel node metastasis. *Arch Surg. 2004*;139:648–651. doi:10.1001/archsurg.139.6.648.

[13] Kim T., Giuliano A. E., Lyman G. H., Lymphatic mapping and sentinel lymph node biopsy in early-stage breast carcinoma: a metaanalysis. *Cancer. 2006*;106:4–16. doi: 10.1002/cncr.21568.

[14] Noguchi M. Avoidance of axillary lymph node dissection in selected patients with node-positive breast cancer. *Eur J Surg Oncol. 2008*;34:129–134. doi: 10.1016/j.ejso.2007.03.026.

[15] Lyman G. H., Giuliano A. E., Somerfield M. R., Benson A. B., Bodurka D. C., Burstein H. J., et al. American Society of Clinical Oncology guideline recommendations for sentinel lymph node biopsy in early-stage breast cancer. *J Clin Oncol. 2005*;23:7703–7720. doi:10.1200/JCO.2005.08.001.

[16] National Comprehensive Cancer Network (NCCN). *Breast Cancer (Version 1.2018).* Available at https://www.nccn.org/professionals/physician_gls/pdf/breast.pdf, accessed 27.05.2018.

[17] Bernardi S., Bertozzi S., Londero A. P., Angione V., Petri R, Giacomuzzi F., Prevalence and risk factors of intraoperative identification failure of sentinel lymph nodes in patients affected by breast cancer. *Nucl Med Commun. 2013*;34:664–673. doi: 10.1097/MNM.0b013e328361cd84.

[18] Yared M. A., Middleton L. P., Smith T. L., Kim H. W., Ross M. I., Hunt K. K., et al. Recommendations for sentinel lymph node processing in breast cancer. *Am J Surg Pathol. 2002*;26:377–382.

[19] Verma R., Sundara Rajan S., Verghese E. T., Horgan K., Hanby A. M., Lane S. Pathological evaluation of the staging axillary lymph nodes for breast cancer: a national survey in the United Kingdom. *Histopathology. 2014*;65:707–711. doi: 10.1111/his.12440.

[20] Turner R. R., Weaver D. L., Cserni G., Lester S. C., Hirsch K., Elashoff D. A., et al. Nodal stage classification for breast carcinoma: improving interobserver reproducibility through standardized histologic criteria and image-based training. *J Clin Oncol. 2008*;26:258–263. doi:10.1200/JCO.2007.13.0179.

[21] Viale G., Maiorano E., Mazzarol G., Zurrida S., Galimberti V., Luini A., et al. Histologic detection and clinical implications of micrometastases in axillary sentinel lymph nodes for patients with breast carcinoma. *Cancer. 2001*;92:1378–1384.

[22] Giobuin S. M., Kavanagh D. O., Myers E., Doherty A. O., Quinn C. M., Crotty T., et al. The significance of immunohistochemistry positivity in sentinel nodes which are negative on haematoxylin and eosin in breast cancer. *Eur J Surg Oncol. 2009*; 35:1257–1260. doi:10.1016/j.ejso.2009.04.004.

[23] Nowikiewicz T., Asrutek E., Zegarski W. Application of immunohistochemistry for detection of metastases in sentinel lymph nodes of non-advanced breast cancer patients. *Pol J Pathol. 2015*;66:22–29.

[24] Tian P., Zhang W., Zhao H., Lei Y., Cui L., Zhang Y., et al. Intraoperative detection of sentinel lymph node metastases in breast carcinoma by Fourier transform infrared spectroscopy. *Br J Surg. 2015*;102:1372–1379. doi:10.1002/bjs.9882.

[25] Cserni G., The potential value of intraoperative imprint cytology of axillary sentinel lymph nodes in breast cancer patients. *Am Surg. 2001*;67:86–91.

[26] Petropoulou T., Kapoula A., Mastoraki A., Politi A., Spanidou-Karvouni E., Psychogios I., et al. Imprint cytology versus frozen section analysis for intraoperative assessment of sentinel lymph node in breast cancer. *Breast cancer (Dove Medical Press). 2017*;9:325–330. doi:10.2147/BCTT.S130987.

[27] Patursson H. I., Kovacs A., Mattsson J., Olofsson Bagge R. Evaluation of intraoperative touch imprint cytology on axillary sentinel lymph nodes in invasive breast carcinomas, a retrospective study of 1227 patients comparing sensitivity in the different tumor subtypes. *PLoS ONE. 2018*;13:e0195560. doi:10.1371/journal.pone.0195560.

[28] Howard-McNatt M., Geisinger K. R., Stewart J. H., Shen P., Levine E. A. Is intraoperative imprint cytology evaluation still feasible for the evaluation of sentinel lymph nodes for lobular carcinoma of the breast? *Ann Surg Oncol. 2012*;19:929–934. doi: 10.1245/s10434-011-2038-z.

[29] Creager A. J., Geisinger K. R., Perrier N. D., Shen P., Shaw J. A., Young P. R., et al. Intraoperative imprint cytologic evaluation of sentinel lymph nodes for lobular carcinoma of the breast. *Ann Surg. 2004*;239:61–66. doi: 10.1097/01.sla.0000103072.34708.e3.

[30] Wang Y., Li L., Xu W., Zheng Z., Wu J., Yang W., et al. High sensitivity of touch imprint cytology in young patients with invasive lobular carcinoma of the breast. *Tumour Biol. 2014*;35:5741–5746. doi:10.1007/s13277-014-1761-z.

[31] Smith G. J., Hodges E., Markham H., Zhang S., Cutress R. I. Evaluation of the Metasin assay for intraoperative assessment of sentinel lymph node metastases in breast cancer. *J Clin Pathol. 2017*;70:134–139. doi:10.1136/jclinpath-2016-203728.

[32] Layfield D. M., Agrawal A., Roche H., Cutress R. I. Intraoperative assessment of sentinel lymph nodes in breast cancer. *Br J Surg. 2011*;98:4–17. doi:10.1002/bjs.7229.

[33] Visser M., Jiwa M., Horstman A., Brink A. A. T. P., Pol R. P., van Diest P., et al. Intra-operative rapid diagnostic method based on CK19 mRNA expression for the detection of lymph node metastases in breast cancer. *Int J Cancer. 2008*;122:2562–2567. doi: 10.1002/ijc.23451.

[34] Tsujimoto M., Nakabayashi K., Yoshidome K., Kaneko T., Iwase T., Akiyama F., et al. One-step nucleic acid amplification for intraoperative detection of lymph node metastasis in breast cancer patients. *Clin Cancer Res. 2007*;13:4807–4816. doi: 10.1158/1078-0432.CCR-06-2512.

[35] Al-Ramadhani S., Sai-Giridhar P., George D., Gopinath P., Arkoumani E., Jader S., et al. Metasin-an intra-operative RT-qPCR assay to detect metastatic breast cancer in sentinel lymph nodes. *Int J Mol Sci. 2013*;14:12931–12952. doi: 10.3390/ijms140712931. Original DateCompleted: 20130627.

[36] Martin Martinez M. D., Veys I., Majjaj S., Lespagnard L., Schobbens J. C., Rouas G., et al. Clinical validation of a molecular assay for intra-operative detection of metastases in breast sentinel lymph nodes. *Eur J Surg Oncol. 2009*;35:387–392. doi: 10.1016/j.ejso.2008.05.008.

[37] Mansel R. E., Goyal A., Douglas-Jones A., Woods V., Goyal S., Monypenny I., et al. Detection of breast cancer metastasis in sentinel lymph nodes using intra-operative real time GeneSearch BLN Assay in the operating room: results of the Cardiff study. *Breast Cancer Res Treat. 2009*;115:595–600. doi:10.1007/s10549-008-0155-6.

[38] Viale G., Dell'Orto P., Biasi M. O., Stufano V., De Brito Lima L. N., Paganelli G., et al. Comparative evaluation of an extensive histopathologic examination and a real-time reverse-transcription-polymerase chain reaction assay for mammaglobin and cytokeratin 19 on axillary sentinel lymph nodes of breast carcinoma patients. *Ann Surg. 2008*; 247:136–142. doi:10.1097/SLA.0b013e318157d22b.

[39] Blumencranz P., Whitworth P. W., Deck K., Rosenberg A., Reintgen D., Beitsch P., et al. Scientific Impact Recognition Award. Sentinel node staging for breast cancer: intraoperative molecular pathology overcomes conventional histologic sampling errors. *Am J Surg. 2007*;194:426–432. doi:10.1016/j.amjsurg.2007.07.008.

[40] Sai-Giridhar P., Al-Ramadhani S., George D., Gopinath P., Andrews W., Jader S., et al. A multicentre validation of Metasin: a molecular assay for the intraoperative assessment of sentinel lymph nodes from breast cancer patients. *Histopathology. 2016*; 68:875–887. doi:10.1111/his.12863.

[41] Huxley N., Jones-Hughes T., Coelho H., Snowsill T., Cooper C., Meng Y., et al. A systematic review and economic evaluation of intraoperative tests [RD-100i one-step nucleic acid amplification (OSNA) system and Metasin test] for detecting sentinel lymph node metastases in breast cancer. *Health Technol Assess. 2015*;19:v–xxv, 1–215. doi:10.3310/hta19020.

[42] Chaudhry A., Williams S., Cook J., Jenkins M., Sohail M., Calder C., et al. The real-time intra-operative evaluation of sentinel lymph nodes in breast cancer patients using

One Step Nucleic Acid Amplification (OSNA) and implications for clinical decision-making. *Eur J Surg Oncol. 2014*;40:150–157. doi:10.1016/j.ejso.2013.12.007.

[43] Cattin F., Castriotta L., Zumerle G., Scarpa E., Leo C. A., Semprini G., et al. The breast cancer: a comparison among different diagnostic and therapeutic protocols. *Breast J. 2013*;19:560–562. doi:10.1111/tbj.12171.

[44] Associazione Italiana di Oncologia Medica (AIOM). Linee guida: NEOPLASIE DELLA MAMMELLA. *Technical report, AIOM. 2016.*

[45] Schem C., Maass N., Bauerschlag D. O., Carstensen M. H., Lening T., Roder C., et al. One-step nucleic acid amplification-a molecular method for the detection of lymph node metastases in breast cancer patients; results of the German study group. *Virchows Arch. 2009*;454:203–210. doi:10.1007/s00428-008-0703-9.

[46] Pegolo E., Puppin C., Gerometta A., Damante G., Puglisi F., Di Loreto C. One-step nucleic acid amplification (OSNA) for intraoperative evaluation of sentinel lymph node status in breast cancer: a comparative study between CK19 protein expression and CK19 mRNA level in primary tumors and lymph node metastasis. *Virchows Arch. 2013*;463:7–15. doi:10.1007/s00428-013-1440-2.

[47] Tamaki Y., Akiyama F., Iwase T., Kaneko T., Tsuda H., Sato K., et al. Molecular detection of lymph node metastases in breast cancer patients: results of a multicenter trial using the one-step nucleic acid amplification assay. *Clin Cancer Res. 2009*; 15:2879–2884. doi:10.1158/1078-0432.CCR-08-1881.

[48] Feldman S., Krishnamurthy S., Gillanders W., Gittleman M., Beitsch P. D., Young P. R., et al. A novel automated assay for the rapid identification of metastatic breast carcinoma in sentinel lymph nodes. *Cancer. 2011*;117:2599–2607. doi: 10.1002/cncr.25822.

[49] Snook K. L., Layer G. T., Jackson P. A., de Vries C. S., Shousha S., Sinnett H. D., et al. Multicentre evaluation of intraoperative molecular analysis of sentinel lymph nodes in breast carcinoma. *Br J Surg. 2011*;98:527–535. doi:10.1002/bjs.7347.

[50] Ohi Y., Umekita Y., Sagara Y., Rai Y., Yotsumoto D., Matsukata A., et al. Whole sentinel lymph node analysis by a molecular assay predicts axillary node status in breast cancer. *British journal of cancer. 2012*;107:1239–1243. doi:10.1038/bjc.2012.387.

[51] Peg V., Sansano I., Vieites B., Bernet L., Cano R., Cordoba A., et al. Role of total tumour load of sentinel lymph node on survival in early breast cancer patients. *Breast (Edinburgh, Scotland). 2017*;33:8–13. doi:10.1016/j.breast.2017.02.011.

[52] Fanfani F., Monterossi G., Ghizzoni V., Rossi E. D., Dinoi G., Inzani F., et al. One-Step Nucleic Acid Amplification (OSNA): A fast molecular test based on CK19 mRNA concentration for assessment of lymph-nodes metastases in early stage endometrial cancer. *PloS one. 2018*;13:e0195877. doi:10.1371/journal.pone.0195877.

[53] Weber W. P., Barry M., Stempel M. M., Junqueira M. J., Eaton A. A., Patil S. M., et al. A 10-year trend analysis of sentinel lymph node frozen section and completion axillary dissection for breast cancer: are these procedures becoming obsolete? *Ann Surg Oncol. 2012*;19:225–232. doi:10.1245/s10434-011-1823-z.

[54] Tanis P. J., van Sandick J. W., Nieweg O. E., Valdes Olmos R. A., Rutgers E. J. T., Hoefnagel C. A., et al. The hidden sentinel node in breast cancer. *Eur J Nucl Med Mol Imaging. 2002*;29:305–311.

[55] Peg V., Espinosa-Bravo M., Vieites B., Vilardell F., Antenez J. R., de Salas M. S., et al. Intraoperative molecular analysis of total tumor load in sentinel lymph node: a new predictor of axillary status in early breast cancer patients. *Breast Cancer Res Treat. 2013*;139:87–93. doi:10.1007/s10549-013-2524-z.

[56] Di Filippo F., Di Filippo S., Ferrari A. M., Antonetti R., Battaglia A., Becherini F., et al. Elaboration of a nomogram to predict nonsentinel node status in breast cancer patients with positive sentinel node, intraoperatively assessed with one step nucleic amplification: Retrospective and validation phase. *Journal of experimental & clinical cancer research : CR. 2016*;35:193. doi:10.1186/s13046-016-0460-6.

[57] Liu Y., Xu Y., Liu Y., Zhang Y., Wang D., Xiu D., et al. Detection of cervical metastatic lymph nodes in papillary thyroid carcinoma by Fourier transform infrared spectroscopy. *Br J Surg. 2011*;98:380–384. doi:10.1002/bjs.7330.

[58] Mantsch H. H., Chapman D., editors. Infrared Spectroscopy of Biomolecules. *Wiley-Liss. 1996*.

[59] Wang L., Mizaikoff B. Application of multivariate data-analysis techniques to biomedical diagnostics based on mid-infrared spectroscopy. *Anal Bioanal Chem. 2008*;391:1641–1654. doi:10.1007/s00216-008-1989-9.

[60] Liu M. J., Wang Z., Wu R. C., Sun S. Q., Wu Q. Y. Monitoring all-trans-retinoic acid-induced differentiation of human acute promyelocytic leukemia NB4 cells by Fourier-transform infrared spectroscopy. *Leukemia. 2003*;17:1670–1674. doi: 10.1038/sj.leu.2403019.

[61] Li Q. B., Sun X. J., Xu Y. Z., Yang L. M., Zhang Y. F., Weng S. F., et al. Diagnosis of gastric inflammation and malignancy in endoscopic biopsies based on Fourier transform infrared spectroscopy. *Clin Chem. 2005*;51:346–350. doi: 10.1373/clinchem.2004.037986.

[62] Taylor S. E., Cheung K. T., Patel I. I., Trevisan J. , Stringfellow H. F., Ashton K. M., et al. Infrared spectroscopy with multivariate analysis to interrogate endometrial tissue: a novel and objective diagnostic approach. *Br J Cancer. 2011*;104:790–797. doi:10.1038/sj.bjc.6606094.

[63] Zwielly A. , Mordechai S., Brkic G., Bogomolny E., Pelly I. Z., Moreh R., et al. Grading of intrinsic and acquired cisplatin-resistant human melanoma cell lines: an

infrared ATR study. *Eur Biophys J. 2011*;40:795–804. doi:10.1007/s00249-011-0695-2.

[64] Zhang X., Xu Y., Zhang Y., Wang L., Hou C., Zhou X., et al. Intraoperative detection of thyroid carcinoma by fourier transform infrared spectrometry. *J Surg Res. 2011*; 171:650–656. doi:10.1016/j.jss.2010.05.031.

[65] Houssami N., Ciatto S., Turner R. M., Cody H. S., Macaskill P. Preoperative ultrasound-guided needle biopsy of axillary nodes in invasive breast cancer: meta-analysis of its accuracy and utility in staging the axilla. *Ann Surg. 2011*;254:243–251. doi:10.1097/SLA.0b013e31821f1564.

[66] Rautiainen S., Masarwah A., Sudah M., Sutela A., Pelkonen O., Joukainen S., et al. Axillary lymph node biopsy in newly diagnosed invasive breast cancer: comparative accuracy of fine-needle aspiration biopsy versus core-needle biopsy. *Radiology. 2013*; 269:54–60. doi:10.1148/radiol.13122637.

[67] Kocjan G., Bourgain C., Fassina A., Hagmar B., Herbert A., Kapila K., et al. The role of breast FNAC in diagnosis and clinical management: a survey of current practice. *Cytopathology. 2008*;19:271–278. doi:10.1111/j.1365-2303.2008.00610.x.

[68] Tse G., Tan P. H., Schmitt F. Fine Needle Aspiration Cytology of the Breast. *Springer Berlin Heidelberg. 2013*. doi:10.1007/978-3-642-35000-9.

[69] Sever A. R., Mills P., Jones S. E., Cox K., Weeks J., Fish D., et al. Preoperative sentinel node identification with ultrasound using microbubbles in patients with breast cancer. *AJR Am J Roentgenol. 2011*;196:251–256. doi:10.2214/AJR.10.4865.

[70] Shousha S. Axillary Lymph Node Biopsies. *In Breast Pathology, 175–187. Springer International Publishing. 2016*;doi:10.1007/978-3-319-28655-6_14.

[71] Goldberg B. B., Liu J. B., Forsberg F. Ultrasound contrast agents: a review. *Ultrasound Med Biol. 1994*;20:319–333.

[72] Sever A. R., Mills P., Weeks J., Jones S. E., Fish D., Jones P. A., et al. Preoperative needle biopsy of sentinel lymph nodes using intradermal microbubbles and contrast-enhanced ultrasound in patients with breast cancer. *AJR Am J Roentgenol. 2012*; 199:465–470. doi:10.2214/AJR.11.7702.

[73] Cox K., Sever A., Jones S., Weeks J., Mills P., Devalia H., et al. Validation of a technique using microbubbles and contrast enhanced ultrasound (CEUS) to biopsy sentinel lymph nodes (SLN) in pre-operative breast cancer patients with a normal grey-scale axillary ultrasound. *Eur J Surg Oncol. 2013*;39:760–765. doi: 10.1016/j.ejso.2013.03.026.

[74] Wauters C. A. P., Kooistra B., Strobbe L.J. A. The role of laboratory processing in determining diagnostic conclusiveness of breast fine needle aspirations: conventional smearing versus a monolayer preparation. *J Clin Pathol. 2009*;62:931–934. doi:10.1136/jcp.2009.066589.

[75] Leung S. W., Badard Y. C. Immunocytochemical staining on ThinPrep processed smears. *Mod Pathol. 1996*;9:304–306.

[76] Rossi E. D., Raffaelli M., Minimo C., Mule A., Lombardi C. P., Vecchio F. M., et al. Immunocytochemical evaluation of thyroid neoplasms on thin-layer smears from fine-needle aspiration biopsies. *Cancer. 2005*;105:87–95. doi:10.1002/cncr.21026.

[77] Al Jajeh I., Hok-Ling Chan N., Siok-Gek Hwang J., Tan P. H. A simple technique for augmenting recovery of cellular material from fine needle aspirates for adjunctive studies. *J Clin Pathol. 2012*;65:672–674. doi:10.1136/jclinpath-2012-200688.

[78] Fitzgibbons P. L., LiVolsi V. A. Recommendations for handling radioactive specimens obtained by sentinel lymphadenectomy. Surgical Pathology Committee of the College of American Pathologists, and the Association of Directors of Anatomic and Surgical Pathology. *Am J Surg Pathol. 2000*;24:1549–1551.

[79] Renshaw A. A., Kish R., Gould E. W. Increasing radiation from sentinel node specimens in pathology over time. *Am J Clin Pathol. 2010*;134:299–302. doi: 10.1309/AJCPWX3QAIBS2BTK.

In: The Sentinel Lymph Node
Editors: A. Londero, S. Bertozzi and C. Cedolini
ISBN: 978-1-53614-557-1


*Chapter 4*

# SENTINEL LYMPH NODE BIOPSY IN BREAST CANCER

***Serena Bertozzi*[1,*], *Carla Cedolini*[1] *and Ambrogio P. Londero*[2]**
[1]Breast Unit, DAME, University of Udine,
University Hospital of Udine, Italy
[2]Clinic of Obstetrics and Gynecology,
University Hospital of Udine, Italy

**Abstract**

Sentinel lymph node biopsy for breast cancer was originally introduced by Veronesi in the 1990s to spare clinically node-negative patients from unnecessary complete axillary dissection. The primary advantage of sentinel lymph node biopsy is its recognized accuracy in staging the axilla while preventing the high morbidity correlated with complete axillary lymph node dissection. This procedure, initially performed using blue vital dye, currently consists in the radio-guided identification of the first lymph node draining the primary tumor. However, the sentinel node can also be detected by using indocyanine green fluorescence. The subsequent evaluation of the sentinel node is usually carried out intraoperatively to reduce the number of interventions and immediately dissect the axilla in the case of macrometastases. Together with the traditional morphological evaluation by hematoxylin-eosin staining of the frozen section, a new method has been recently introduced, capable of amplifying the mRNA of cytokeratins within the lysate of the sentinel node, called the OSNA method. The latter, however, is not indicated in the case of neoadjuvant treatment, due to its controversial result in the case of partial response. Finally, it is important to remark the possibility of performing sentinel node biopsy in some special cases, such as pregnant women, patients who have undergone previous axillary surgery and patients affected by ductal carcinoma in situ. For the latter case, the sentinel lymph node biopsy is indicated in the presence of a suspected microinvasion or in the case of mastectomy.

**Keywords:** sentinel lymph node biopsy, breast cancer, OSNA, complete axillary lymph node dissection

*Corresponding Author E-mail: dr.bertozzi@gmail.com.

# 1. Introduction

Breast cancer was initially considered a local disease. Complete axillary lymph node dissection (CALND), in conjunction with mastectomy and excision of part of the ipsilateral chest wall, aimed at completely removing the cancer and controlling the disease with curative intent. During the first half of the 20$^{th}$ century, increased knowledge of cancer metastasization pathways gave importance to the axillary node evaluation with staging intent.

First introduced in 1948, the TNM classification is currently the most widely used system worldwide for breast cancer staging. The classification is generated through a combination of three variables taken into consideration: the tumor size, the lymph node status and the possible presence of distant localizations of the disease. The combination of these parameters is a highly predictive tool for determining patients' prognosis [1]. Axillary lymph node investigation later became an exclusive staging method to better tailor patients' treatment and follow-up.

In the 1990s, Veronesi and colleagues introduced a new technique in order to spare clinically node-negative patients from unnecessary CALND: the sentinel lymph node biopsy (SLNB). This new procedure consisted in the radio-guided identification of the first lymph node draining the primary tumor. The sentinel node is supposed to be the first lymph node affected by neoplastic cells in the case of tumor lymphatic dissemination [2]. The main advantage of SLNB is its proven accuracy in axillary staging, while preventing CALND-related high morbidity [2], such as ipsilateral arm lymphoedema or paresthesia, which were previously very frequent and disabling for several breast cancer survivors.

In 2009, Veronesi and colleagues subsequently introduced a new series of variables in order to improve the prognostic power of the TNM classification, such as the presence of lymph node micrometastases or isolated tumor cells (ITCs), the extracapsular invasion of lymphatic metastases and the presence of bunched lymph nodes [3]. These new histological variables taken into account have generated controversy in the field of axillary management, which is still a topic of debate. In particular, ITCs and micrometastases were initially identified as positive sentinel nodes, while currently no longer require axillary radicalization.

In the next sections we will discuss the rationale for SLNB, describe the techniques to intraoperatively identify and consequently analyze the sentinel node, and finally discuss some controversial issues about axillary management in particular situations, such as ductal carcinoma in situ (DCIS), pregnancy, neoadjuvant therapies, or previous surgery.

# 2. Sentinel Lymph Node Detection Technique

The feasibility and safety of intraoperative sentinel node identification was first evaluated in 1991, with the injection of isosulfan blue vital dye in breast cancer to obtain a vital dye-directed lymphatic mapping [4]. Blue dye administration is usually carried out by injecting from 3 to 5 ml of isosulfan blue vital dye into the subcutaneous tissue of the breast lesion area or the nipple-areola complex, from 5 to 10 minutes prior to incision, accompanied by a thorough massage of the injected area to facilitate the lymphatic drainage to the axilla [5].

Currently, the most commonly used technique for sentinel node identification worldwide is radio-guided surgery using filtered technetium-99 sulfur colloid, which is usually injected in either the intradermal, subdermal, or peritumoral region in a single dose from 0.3

to 1.0 mCi between 3 and 24 hours before surgery. Lymphoscintigraphy is generally performed after the injection to document the migration of the radioisotope, and in the case of difficult preoperative identification of the sentinel node, a single photon emission computed tomography (SPECT) can be performed to better evaluate the axillary status [6].

Approved for medicinal uses in 1956, indocyanine green is another valuable substance that can be used to detect the sentinel node [7, 8, 9]. Within the organism, it bonds to proteins and other macromolecules, and changes its fluorescence intensity and the emission spectrum to near-infrared, which is invisible to the human eye, but can be detected by using special devices with photodynamic cameras [10]. In addition, together with its green color at visual inspection, indocyanine green is a fluorophore that displays fluorescence in incident light and its emitted radiation permeates through tissues. Therefore, in contrast to common dyes, it can also visualize deeply located structures.

In conclusion, sentinel node identification in breast cancer is technically feasible, safe, and an accurate predictor of axillary status through a variety of technical approaches. Studies comparing blue dye alone with the combined use of radioisotope and blue dye, as well as studies comparing indocyanine green with blue dye [11, 12, 13, 14, 15] and indocyanine green with radioisotope [16, 17, 18, 19] showed no difference in the sentinel node identification rate between the two groups in comparison [20]. On the other hand, studies also showed that only the surgeon's experience has a significant impact on sentinel node identification and false-negative rates. In addition, palpation of the axillary space for any suspicious node can avoid missing a metastatic node, that may not be blue or radioactive due to lymphatic obstruction. Therefore, as a precaution, all suspicious palpable nodes must be removed during SLNB, regardless of the technique.

## 3. Sentinel Lymph Node Evaluation Technique

As expected, over the years, we have witnessed a technical evolution also with regard to intraoperative examination procedures for SLNB. First of all, the number of interventions has been reduced by introducing intraoperative frozen section evaluation of SLNB. Secondly, the traditional morphological examination has been replaced by molecular biology techniques in order to reduce the operative time.

In the case of intraoperative frozen section, the sentinel node is cut into parts 2-mm-thick, frozen-fixed and polyvinyl alcohol embedded before undergoing intraoperative histological examination of four hematoxylin-eosin-stained, 0.15-mm-spaced sections as well as immunohistochemical evaluation of three random sections to look for a potential positivity for cytokeratins. Subsequently, the residual sentinel lymph node tissue undergoes traditional definitive histological examination with evaluation of 0.15-mm-spaced, hematoxylin-eosin-stained sections and immunohistochemical evaluation of a random nodal portion.

The one-step nucleic acid amplification (OSNA) method is a biomolecular quantitative system that significantly accelerates sentinel node analysis, resulting in reduced operative time and anesthesiologic risk, cost-benefit gain and high accuracy of the result [21, 22, 23, 24]. The first step of the procedure is the homogenization of the collected sentinel nodes in a mRNA-stabilizing solution (Lynorhag, pH 3.5 Sysmex®;), followed by an isothermal (65 C) CK19 amplification using the Lynoamp amplification kit (Sysmex®;) through a reverse transcriptase amplification assay (RT-LAMP) in a gene amplification detector RD-100i (Sysmex®;) [25, 26, 27, 28]. A standard positive control sample and a negative control sample are always used for calibration in every assay and the test results are automatically given in a semi-quantitative way [26, 28, 29, 30]: the result is negative if the CK19 mRNA copy number/l lysate is less than 250/l; micrometastases for copy numbers 250/ l and ¡5000/l; and macrometastases for copy numbers equal or greater than 5000/l.

In the literature, the OSNA method is comparable with both postoperative histological examination and intraoperative frozen section evaluation in terms of overall and disease-free survival, and significantly reduces surgical time from a mean operation length of 69.4 (10.3) minutes when using frozen section to a mean operation length of 41.9 (4.9) minutes when using OSNA [23]. Of course, in order to effectively reduce the overall operation length, it is important to limit the number of excised nodes. As a consequence, both OSNA and frozen section are correlated with fewer excised sentinel nodes than definitive histological examination. Moreover, some authors have also outlined a decrease in the use of CALND after the detection of sentinel node metastases by serial sectioning or immunohistochemistry, probably due to the current trend toward sparing CALND for micrometastases [31].

Furthermore, the OSNA system allows a more efficient detection of micrometastases, thereby reducing the number of false-negative histological examinations resulting from the small size of micrometastases [32]. This may also explain the lower cumulative rate of local recurrences after evaluation with the OSNA method. However, it is not prudent to draw definitive conclusions about local recurrences, due to the overly recent introduction of the OSNA technique and the observation of a peak of local recurrences after SLNB between the third and the sixth year of follow-up [33].

# 4. Non-Sentinel Lymph Node Involvement Prediction

A very controversial topic is the predictability of non-sentinel lymph node status by SLNB negativity or positivity for neoplastic infiltration. In the first case, the contentious subject is the nodal recurrence after negative SLNB. Several different hypothesis have been used to explain this adverse event, such as the "skip metastasis" theory [34], incorrect node excision due to the limited experience of the surgeon [35], or false-negative histological examination resulting from the small size of micrometastases, that may not be included in any microscopical section [32]. With regard to the predictability of axillary, non-sentinel, metastatic nodes in case of SLNB positivity, several nomograms have been designed to predict axillary status and possibly avoid CALND with different degrees of success. [36].

The most famous nomogram for predicting non sentinel node involvement is probably the MSKCC (Memorial Sloan-Kettering Cancer Center), which examines different variables such as pathological size, tumor type, nuclear grade, lymphovascular invasion, multifocality, estrogen receptor status, histopathological method used for sentinel node detection and ratio of the number of positive nodes to the total number of nodes removed [37]. Additional nomograms have been developed at Mayo Clinic [38], MD Anderson Cancer Center [39], and Stanford University [40].

In our population, we observed that 41.57% (69/166) of women who have received CALND had no additional non-sentinel node metastases, which on the contrary were found in 58.43% (97/166) of cases, suggesting the usefulness of CALND in providing additional prognostic information and decreasing axillary recurrences after SLNB positivity [41, 42, 37]. However, when compared with the general breast cancer population, women who have undergone SLNB have a significantly higher prevalence of negative axillary nodes and a lower prevalence of positive nodes of each class of the TNM classification.

Furthermore, the definitive axillary nodal status in women who have received CALND is N1 in 46.99% (78/166), N2 in 7.83% (13/166) and N3 in 3.61% (6/166) of cases. This data suggests the necessity of a more appropriate preoperative ultrasound examination of the axilla, especially in patients with a suspicious axillary clinical finding, or at risk of sentinel node mapping failure, such as elderly or overweight women [43, 33, 44]. In addition to axillary nodes ultrasound [45, 46], the current literature promotes preoperative axillary magnetic resonance imaging [47, 36], while rejects axillary positron emission tomography due to its inadequate reliability [48].

When analyzing the factors which may predict the SLNB positivity, our TNM classification data confirms the linear correlation between the tumor size and the number of metastatic nodes (p¡0.05) [36]. Additionally, women who have undergone SLNB have significantly smaller tumors than the general breast cancer population (p¡0.05), probably reflecting the sensitivity of the current screening, which succeeds in detecting tumors sized mainly between 0.5 and 2 cm [46, 49].

Besides parameters like tumor size and histological type, the tumor nuclear grade also plays an important role in the prediction of axillary nodal status. In particular, axillary lymphatic metastases are significantly more prevalent in tumors with a higher histological grade and negative estrogen-receptor status, being both an expression of less tumor differentiation [50]. Tumor multifocality is not associated with worse axillary nodal status. The literature actually suggests the feasibility of SLNB even in the presence of multiple tumor foci [51].

Age group appears to have a controversial role among indications for SLNB and should not be an absolute exclusion criterion for this procedure. In point of fact, our data gives an evidence that younger age can be a risk factor for lymphatic metastasization [36, 33] and that, despite the size of the tumor, elderly women have a greater prevalence of negative axillary findings. However, our opinion is that young women should also receive SLNB as a primary axillary approach to avoid CALND, when possible [52, 53].

The prediction of non-sentinel node neoplastic involvement is becoming an increasingly important challenge. Several authors have tried to identify eligible patients on whom CALND can be omitted after positive SLNB and, consequently, to prevent unnecessary CALND on future patients at low-risk of axillary recurrence [54, 55]. In this perspective, ACOSOG Z0011 and IBCSG 23-01 trials, which compared patients with positive sentinel node with or without consequent CALND, did not show significant differences between the two groups in terms of both disease-free and overall survival [56, 55].

In addition, the NSABBP B-04 trial showed that metachronous CALND by axillary recurrence after SLNB did not compromise overall survival in comparison with synchronous CALND by non-sentinel node suspected involvement [57]. Studies also concluded that both whole-breast irradiation and systemic adjuvant treatment are comparable to CALND in the case of small-volume lymph node disease [58, 59, 60].

No agreement has indeed been reached on routine use of nomograms in clinical practice, but our experience supports the use of accurate preoperative imaging evaluation of the axilla in order to better select SLNB candidate patients.

## 5. Management of Macrometastases

In a study conducted on women operated on between 1998 and 2005 with a median follow-up of 63 months, no difference was found in loco-regional recurrence or survival between those who underwent SLNB with completion CALND and those who underwent SLNB alone [61]. Similar findings were observed in a review from the Surveillance, Epidemiology, and End Results (SEER) database, where the decrease in CALND for positive sentinel nodes between 1998 and 2004 may have been influenced by the introduction of nomograms to predict non sentinel node involvement [62]. In addition, a review from the Memorial Sloan-Kettering Cancer Center on 287 sentinel node-positive patients who declined CALND showed an axillary relapse rate of 2% in the untreated group compared with a rate of 0.4% in the group that received CALND (p=0.004) [63]. Also, in studies reporting the outcome of patients who declined CALND after positive SLNB there were no recurrences in about 3-year follow-up [64, 65].

Appropriate management of the axilla after a positive sentinel node has been addressed also in a great number of prospective clinical trials. In the ACOSOG Z0011 trial, a prospective Phase III non-inferiority trial that randomized 891 women with clinical T1-T2N0M0 breast cancer with a positive sentinel node to CALND or observation of the axilla, not only non-inferiority was achieved with a high statistical significance (p¡0.008), but also total loco-regional recurrence (3.1% with CALND and 1.6% with SLNB alone), overall survival (91.8% with CALND vs. 92.5% with SLNB alone), and disease-free survival (82.2% with CALND and 83.9% with SLNB alone) were in favor of the SLNB alone group [66, 56].

The findings of the ACOSOG Z0011 trial are still being seen with great disappointment due to a series of biases and controversies. For instance, it reached the planned accrual only by half. In addition, the follow-up is not being considered sufficient. Also, it is thought that there probably was a selection bias in favor of less aggressive cancers with a consequently more favorable outcome. Finally, there was a potential involuntary irradiation of the axillary nodes in the group that did not receive CALND due to whole breast irradiation after conserving surgery, which may have positively influenced the outcome of node-positive patients. In fact, also some landmark historical randomized long-term trials evaluating whether axillary treatment, either in the form of surgery or radiation therapy, affects survival excluded any significant differences in breast cancer-specific or overall survival resulting from axillary nodal treatment [57, 67, 68, 69, 70, 71].

In conclusion, the literature concurs in considering CALND as a treatment of choice in the case of macrometastatic sentinel nodes as it allows an accurate axillary staging, despite its controversial efficacy in loco-regional recurrence reduction.

## 6. Management of Micrometastases and ITCs

The classification of nodal metastases in the case of breast cancer has undergone dramatic changes in recent decades. As a consequence, the presence of neoplastic cells in the sentinel node has then been quantitatively divided into the following entities based on the size of metastatic foci: macrometastases (¿2 mm), micrometastases (0.2-2 mm), and ITCs (¡0.2 mm) [72, 73]. The 7th edition of the AJCC TNM staging system in breast cancer has incorporated changes to reflect the findings on the prognostic significance of micrometastases.

Stage I has been subdivided into Stage IA and Stage IB, where Stage IB includes small tumors (T1) with micrometastases exclusively in the lymph nodes (N1mi).

In the literature, the prevalence of micrometastases and ITCs after SLNB varies between 2% and 23% [33, 74, 75, 76, 77, 78, 79] and between 8.9% and 10.6%, respectively [75, 80, 33], probably due to the fact that frozen section histological examination is recognized to have a higher false-negative rate [81] with a sensitivity of 83.3% for macrometastases, 40% for micrometastases, and only 18.2% for ITCs [82].

For what concerns the clinical significance of ITCs and micrometastases, it has been showed that the size of lymph node metastases is directly related to the probability of non-sentinel lymph node involvement, explaining why patients with sentinel node macrometastases have a worse prognosis than patients with micrometastases or node-negative patients. However, in the literature the probability of non-sentinel lymph node involvement is highly variable: about 0% to 19% in the case of ITCs [83, 80, 84, 85, 86], 0% to 80% in the case of micrometastases [84, 80, 85, 83, 86], and 3% to 80% in the case of macrometastases [80, 84].

If the literature agrees on CALND not being indicated in the case of ITCs [87, 83], its indication in the case of micrometastases is still controversial [74, 88, 58, 59, 87, 89, 83]. In fact, some authors found a 20.9% upstaging risk of micrometastases after CALND, with a prevalence of N1, N2 and N3 at the definitive histological examination of 18.6%, 2.2% and 0.1% respectively [74], but no significant difference was observed about the 5- year overall survival between micrometastatic and node-negative patients [76, 80, 77]. In other studies, CALND for micrometastatic sentinel nodes found further positive non-sentinel nodes in up to 30% of cases [86].

If we have a look at the most numerous and famous trials that evaluated the prognostic role of micrometastases, the ACOSOG Z0010 trial prospectively observed 5184 subjects with stage I-II clinically node-negative invasive breast cancer treated with breast conservation, SLNB, and bilateral iliac crest bone marrow aspirations to determine the prevalence and significance of lymph node and bone marrow metastases identified by immunohistochemistry, and to determine the risk of regional recurrence [90, 91]. The 23.9% of patients had sentinel node metastases identified by routine hematoxylin-eosin, but immunohistochemistry detected an additional 10.5% of metastases, which however did not seem to have a significant impact on the 5-year overall survival. Bone marrow micrometastases were identified by immunocytochemistry in 3% of the cases examined and were significantly associated with worse prognosis.

The IBCSG 23-01 randomized trial that compared CALND with no CALND in 931 patients with clinical T1N0 invasive breast cancer and at least one micrometastasis in the sentinel node, has also found no difference at 5 years in terms of overall and disease-free survival, suggesting that CALND can be safely avoided in patients with early breast cancer and limited nodal involvement [92].

A subset analysis of the NSABP-B32 trial evaluated the prognostic significance of occult metastases in 3887 tissue blocks from histologically negative sentinel nodes that were re-examined with serial sectioning and immunohistochemistry, detecting 15.9% of occult metastases [93]. However, there was no significant difference in terms of overall survival between patients with and without occult metastases (94.6% and 95.8% respectively).

In August 2011, following the reports from ACOSOG Z011 and NSABP-B32 trials, the American Society of Breast Surgeons released a position statement on nodal micrometastases, affirming that sentinel node micrometastases detected only by immunohistochemistry are clinically insignificant and that routine use of immunohistochemical staining of the sentinel node is unnecessary and must be limited to selective use at the discretion of the pathologist. On the other hand, immunohistochemistry is useful to detect metastases from invasive lobular carcinoma which can be difficult to detect with hematoxylin-eosin.

In addition to the size of lymph node metastases, the perinodal extracapsular metastatic invasion is also an important predictive factor of non-sentinel node metastases [94, 95, 96, 37]. In a recent study, a mean of up to 10 non-sentinel nodes resulted metastatic in the case of sentinel node pericapsular invasion [86].

In conclusion, at the current date both ITCs and micrometastases do not represent an indication for CALND, with the consequent reduction of the surgical complications determined by axilla demolition, also considering the fact thet in the literature both metachronous "salvage" CALND and adjuvant treatments seem to be comparable with synchronous CALND in terms of overall survival.

# 7. Special Issues

## 7.1. Ductal Carcinoma in Situ

DCIS should not be able to shed neoplastic cells into the bloodstream and infiltrate the lymphatic net, yet unfortunately there is a variable percentage of DCIS with axillary nodal involvement, showing higher rates in the premammographic era [97, 98, 99, 100, 101, 102]. The most probable explanation for nodal involvement in cases of DCIS is occult microinvasion, defined as the extension of cancer cells sized 1mm beyond the basal membrane into the adjacent tissues [103], although a recent study has hypothesized that tumor cell dissemination may occur also prior to stromal invasion [104].

A histological re-examination of specimens from patients affected by DCIS with nodal metastases has revealed a prevalence of up to 58.3% of occult invasion, and thus significantly higher than the prevalence of occult invasion in specimens from pTisN0 patients [105]. However, microinvasive foci are very difficult to detect, especially in the case of a very large intraductal carcinoma [106, 107].

Taking into consideration in our population 543 pure DCIS, 84 DCIS with microinvasion and 2111 invasive ductal carcinomas operated on between 2002 and 2017, in the case of DCIS without or with microinvasion SLNB was found to be micrometastatic in 1.7% and 6.0% of cases respectively, and macrometastatic in 0.9% and 3.6% of cases respectively. 5-year disease-free survival and overall survival were similar in DCIS with microinvasion and invasive ductal carcinoma, while significantly higher in DCIS. The 5-year local recurrence rate of DCIS without and with microinvasion was respectively 2.5% and 7.9%, and the 5-year distant recurrence rate was respectively 0% and 4%. IDC, tumor grading 2 and lymph node macrometastases were significant predictors of decreased overall survival. In addition, microinvasion, macroscopic nodal metastases and tumor grading 2 were significant predictors of distant metastases. Finally, multifocality/multicentricity, grading 2, ITCs and micrometastases were predictors of microinvasive component in DCIS.

In conclusion, DCIS is significantly more frequent in women who have undergone SLNB (p¡0.05) and appears to be a protective factor against lymphatic metastases. For this reason, the literature suggests that routine SLNB should not be recommended for this histological type [108]. The sole indications for SLNB in the case of DCIS continue to be mastectomy, as the procedure is not reliable after the excision of the whole gland, and the imaging suspicion of microinvasion. Despite their rarity, sentinel node metastases may also occur in the case of DCIS, in the form of micrometastases in most cases. Even in the absence of an evident invasive component, microinvasion should always be suspected in these cases, and its management must be same as for invasive carcinoma.

## 7.2. Sentinel Lymph Node Biopsy during Pregnancy

The contraindications to the use of SLNB have been widely criticized in recent years, and some of them have now been radically abandoned. For example, SLNB is now a routinely performed procedure during pregnancy, a condition in which it has been proved to be safe and effective [109].

Radiotracer injection followed by lymphoscintigraphy is the preferred method for the identification of the sentinel node in pregnant patients because the estimated fetal radiation exposure is calculated to a maximum of 4.3 mGy, which is a quite low value [110]. On the other hand, isosulfan blue dye mapping is not recommended due to concerns about the unknown effects on the fetus as well as the risk of anaphylaxis for the patient.

SLNB sensitivity and specificity in the pregnant women with breast cancer has not been well-established yet. However, it appears to be adequate, in spite of a likely reduction in sentinel node mapping sensitivity without the use of isosulfan blue.

Although breast surgery can be safely performed in all trimesters of pregnancy and no increase in fetal abnormalities due to anesthesia has been observed [111], an increase in the frequency of low- and very-low-birth-weight infants in women undergoing surgery during pregnancy has been shown, but this was attributed to the underlying illness or trauma that required surgery in the first place [112]. Moreover, the preferred timing for surgical intervention recommended by a recent review of surgery in pregnant patients is between 16 and 20 weeks of gestation [113], period after which patients and surgeons may choose to wait until after the $12^{th}$ week of gestation, when the risk of spontaneous abortion is lower [114].

In conclusion, we believe that a prudent and careful clinical evaluation should be conducted preoperatively.

## 7.3. Sentinel Lymph Node Biopsy after Neoadjuvant Treatment

For decades, CALND has represented the traditional axillary treatment after neoadjuvant therapy for staging and regional control. However, as a growing number of patients with operable breast cancer is being offered neoadjuvant systemic treatments, the most appropriate axillary staging procedure and its timing have become an argument of great debate.

Recently, the NSABP-18 trial observed a lower nodal metastases rate after preoperative chemotherapy in comparison with patients who underwent surgery before any chemotherapy had been delivered (40% vs 58%) [115]. In addition, SLNB was suggested as an adequate staging procedure in patients undergoing neoadjuvant chemotherapy, considering that imaging sensitivity is insufficient for detecting subclinical nodal involvement in clinically node-negative patients.

The largest single-institution experience with SLNB in the case of neoadjuvant chemotherapy on patients with clinically node-negative invasive breast cancer studied between 1997 and 2007 3171 patients with SLNB as the first intervention and 575 patients with chemotherapy prior to SLNB [116]. The sentinel node identification rate was 98.5% and not significantly different between the two groups, and was improved by the use of combined mapping techniques. The false-negative rate was not significantly different in the two groups either, 4.1% in the SLNB-first group and 5.9% in the chemotherapy-first group, respectively. Similarly to the NSABP-18 trial, positive sentinel nodes were more prevalent in the SLNB-first group, with a consequent increased incidence of CALND and lymphatic morbidity.

The NSABP-27 multicenter trial conducted on 428 patients with pretreatment clinically node-negative and -positive disease treated with neoadjuvant chemotherapy found a false-negative rate of 11%, which decreased to 8% due to the use of radiocolloid [117]. Another prospective multicenter trial examining the role of SLNB after neoadjuvant chemotherapy in patients with both clinically node-negative and -positive disease showed an identification rate of 90% and a false-negative rate of 11.5%, and found a decreased identification rate and an increased false-negative rate in the case of pretreatment clinically positive nodes [118].

A recent meta-analysis on 21 studies have supported SLNB following neoadjuvant chemotherapy, with identification rates between 72% and 100% and false-negative rates ranging between 0% and 33% [119]. A second meta-analysis on 24 studies have confirmed the previous results and has shown an identification rate of 89.6% and a false-negative rate of 8.4% [120].

The ACOSOG Z1071 phase II trial, which covered women with clinical T0 to T4, N1-2, M0 breast cancer who received neoadjuvant chemotherapy after having node-positive disease documented by fine-needle aspiration cytology or core needle biopsy, concluded that SLNB following chemotherapy was an useful technique for the staging of the axilla after chemotherapy, when same of the surgical standards were used, such as the dual tracer technique and the removal of more than two sentinel nodes [121]. Also in the German SENTINA multicenter trial, which evaluated the timing of SLNB in patients receiving neoadjuvant chemotherapy, the number of removed nodes was a significant predictor of the false-negative rate [122].

Patients with node-positive breast cancer can be converted into node-negative with neoadjuvant chemotherapy, especially through the combined administration of anthracycline- and taxane-based chemotherapy regimens [123, 124], and about 1/4 of patients with HER2-positive disease can be converted to node-negative with the addition of trastuzumab [125]. With the increased complete response rates after neoadjuvant therapy, there has been a growing interest in exploring the role of SLNB following chemotherapy in patients with a confirmed positive node before chemotherapy.

However, the literature still disagrees on the timing of SLNB performance. Some authors support pretreatment axillary surgery, whose accuracy is very similar to that of patients candidates for upfront surgery. Other authors are in favor of posttreatment SLNB, which on the other hand allows a single operation and has the prognostic power to assess response in the axilla after preoperative regimen, lower CALND rates and consequently less morbidity. This second option is very criticized, as not only the effect of chemotherapy on lymphatics is unknown, but the reported false-negative rates are also higher in this setting in comparison with upfront surgery cases.

In conclusion, there is sufficient data to demonstrate that SLNB after neoadjuvant systemic treatment is an appropriate standard of care for clinically node-negative patients before chemotheray, as it improves convenience, reduces costs and CALND rates. In these cases, SLNB should preferably be performed using combined identification techniques and then evaluated with traditional hematoxylin-eosin in order to accurately evaluate the possible nodal response, since the OSNA method precludes any morphological observation. On the other hand, the use of SLNB in patients with clinically node-positive disease who convert to node-negative after neoadjuvant systemic treatment is still controversial. Given the higher false-negative rate of this procedure, it should be used only in selected cases and at most three sentinel nodes should be examined.

### 7.4. Sentinel Lymph Node Biopsy after Previous Axillary Surgery

The current literature shows that SLNB after previous breast conservation and axillary surgery is a safe and effective procedure. Sentinel node identification and false-negative rates for preoperative SLNB are 55% and 9%, respectively [126].

Although it is now possible to offer SLNB to women who have already undergone a previous SLNB [127], more information is necessary before preoperative SLNB is recommended as a routine procedure.

## References

[1] Arnone P., Zurrida S., Viale G., Dellapasqua S., Montagna E., Arnaboldi P., et al. The TNM classification of breast cancer: need for change. *Updates in surgery.* 2010; 62:75–81. doi:10.1007/s13304-010-0014-y.

[2] Veronesi U., Paganelli G., Galimberti V., Viale G., Zurrida S., Bedoni M., et al. Sentinel-node biopsy to avoid axillary dissection in breast cancer with clinically negative lymph-nodes. *Lancet.* 1997;349:1864–1867. doi:10.1016/S0140-6736(97)01004-0.

[3] Veronesi U., Zurrida S., Goldhirsch A., Rotmensz N., Viale G. Breast cancer classification: time for a change. *J Clin Oncol.* 2009;27:2427–2428. doi: 10.1200/JCO.2008.21.2647.

[4] Giuliano A. E., Kirgan D. M., Guenther J. M., Morton D.L. Lymphatic mapping and sentinel lymphadenectomy for breast cancer. *Ann Surg.* 1994;220:391–8; discussion 398–401.

[5] Bass S. S., Cox C. E., Salud C. J., Lyman G. H., McCann C., Dupont E., et al. The effects of postinjection massage on the sensitivity of lymphatic mapping in breast cancer. *J Am Coll Surg.* 2001;192:9–16.

[6] Johnson C. B., Boneti C., Korourian S., Adkins L., Klimberg V. S. Intraoperative injection of subareolar or dermal radioisotope results in predictable identification of sentinel lymph nodes in breast cancer. *Ann Surg.* 2011;254:612–618. doi: 10.1097/SLA.0b013e31823005bf.

[7] Niebling M. G., Pleijhuis R. G., Bastiaannet E., Brouwers A. H., van Dam G. M., Hoekstra H. J. A systematic review and meta-analyses of sentinel lymph node identification in breast cancer and melanoma, a plea for tracer mapping. *European journal of surgical oncology: the journal of the European Society of Surgical Oncology and the British Association of Surgical Oncology.* 2016;42:466–473. doi: 10.1016/j.ejso.2015.12.007.

[8] Reinhart M. B., Huntington C. R., Blair L. J, Heniford B. T, Augenstein V. A. Indocyanine Green: Historical Context, Current Applications, and Future Considerations. *Surgical innovation.* 2016;23:166–175. doi:10.1177/1553350615604053.

[9] Coufal O., Fait V. Use of indocyanine green and the HyperEye system for detecting sentinel lymph nodes in breast cancer within a population of European patients: a pilot study. *World journal of surgical oncology.* 2016;14:299. doi:10.1186/s12957-016-1060-9.

[10] Owens E. A., Lee S., Choi J., Henary M., Choi H. S. NIR fluorescent small molecules for intraoperative imaging. *Wiley interdisciplinary reviews Nanomedicine and nanobiotechnology.* 2015;7:828–838. doi:10.1002/wnan.1337.

[11] Hirano A., Kamimura M., Ogura K., Kim N., Hattori A., Setoguchi Y., et al. A comparison of indocyanine green fluorescence imaging plus blue dye and blue dye alone for sentinel node navigation surgery in breast cancer patients. *Annals of surgical oncology.* 2012;19:4112–4116. doi:10.1245/s10434-012-2478-0.

[12] Tong M., Guo W., Gao W. Use of Fluorescence Imaging in Combination with Patent Blue Dye versus Patent Blue Dye Alone in Sentinel Lymph Node Biopsy in Breast Cancer. *Journal of breast cancer.* 2014;17:250–255. doi:10.4048/jbc.2014.17.3.250.

[13] Guo W., Zhang L., Ji J., Gao W., Liu J., Tong M. Evaluation of the benefit of using blue dye in addition to indocyanine green fluorescence for sentinel lymph node biopsy in patients with breast cancer. *World journal of surgical oncology.* 2014; 12:290. doi:10.1186/1477-7819-12-290.

[14] Pitsinis V., Provenzano E., Kaklamanis L., Wishart G. C., Benson J. R., Indocyanine green fluorescence mapping for sentinel lymph node biopsy in early breast cancer. *Surgical oncology.* 2015;24:375–379. doi:10.1016/j.suronc.2015.10.002.

[15] Toh U., Iwakuma N., Mishima M., Okabe M., Nakagawa S., Akagi Y. Navigation surgery for intraoperative sentinel lymph node detection using Indocyanine green (ICG) fluorescence real-time imaging in breast cancer. *Breast cancer research and treatment.* 2015;153:337–344. doi:10.1007/s10549-015-3542-9.

[16] Ballardini B., Santoro L., Sangalli C., Gentilini O., Renne G., Lissidini G., et al. The indocyanine green method is equivalent to the mTc-labeled radiotracer method for identifying the sentinel node in breast cancer: a concordance and validation study. *European journal of surgical oncology : the journal of the European Society of Surgical Oncology and the British Association of Surgical Oncology.* 2013;39:1332–1336. doi:10.1016/j.ejso.2013.10.004.

[17] Xiong L., Gazyakan E., Yang W., Engel H., Haerbein M., Kneser U., et al. Indocyanine green fluorescence-guided sentinel node biopsy: a meta-analysis on detection rate and diagnostic performance. *European journal of surgical oncology : the journal of the European Society of Surgical Oncology and the British Association of Surgical Oncology.* 2014;40:843–849. doi:10.1016/j.ejso.2014.02.228.

[18] Samorani D., Fogacci T., Panzini I., Frisoni G., Accardi F. G., Ricci M., et al. The use of indocyanine green to detect sentinel nodes in breast cancer: a prospective study. *European journal of surgical oncology: the journal of the European Society of Surgical Oncology and the British Association of Surgical Oncology.* 2015;41:64–70. doi:10.1016/j.ejso.2014.10.047.

[19] Sugie T., Kinoshita T., Masuda N., Sawada T., Yamauchi A., Kuroi K., et al. Evaluation of the Clinical Utility of the ICG Fluorescence Method Compared with the Radioisotope Method for Sentinel Lymph Node Biopsy in Breast Cancer. *Annals of surgical oncology.* 2016;23:44–50. doi:10.1245/s10434-015-4809-4.

[20] Morrow M., Rademaker A. W., Bethke K. P., Talamonti M. S., Dawes L. G., Clauson J., et al. Learning sentinel node biopsy: results of a prospective randomized trial of two techniques. *Surgery.* 1999;126:714–20; discussion 720–2.

[21] DG8. *Introperative tests (RD-100i OSNA system and Metasin test) for detection of sentinel lymph node metastses in breast cancer: guidance.* 7. NICE. 2013.

[22] Chaudhry A., Williams S., Cook J., Jenkins M., Sohail M., Calder C., et al. The real-time intra-operative evaluation of sentinel lymph nodes in breast cancer patients using One Step Nucleic Acid Amplification (OSNA) and implications for clinical decision-making. *European journal of surgical oncology : the journal of the European Society of Surgical Oncology and the British Association of Surgical Oncology.* 2014;40:150–157. doi:10.1016/j.ejso.2013.12.007.

[23] Cattin F., Castriotta L., Zumerle G., Scarpa E., Leo C. A., Semprini G., et al. The breast cancer: a comparison among different diagnostic and therapeutic protocols. *The breast journal.* 2013;19:560–562. doi:10.1111/tbj.12171.

[24] Khaddage A., Berremila S. A., Forest F., Clemenson A., Bouteille C., Seffert P., et al. Implementation of molecular intra-operative assessment of sentinel lymph node in breast cancer. *Anticancer Res.* 2011;31:585–590.

[25] Schem C., Maass N., Bauerschlag D. O., Carstensen M. H., Lening T., Roder C., et al. One-step nucleic acid amplification-a molecular method for the detection of

lymph node metastases in breast cancer patients; results of the German study group. *Virchows Arch.* 2009;454:203–210. doi:10.1007/s00428-008-0703-9.

[26] Pegolo E., Puppin C., Gerometta A., Damante G., Puglisi F., Di Loreto C. One-step nucleic acid amplification (OSNA) for intraoperative evaluation of sentinel lymph node status in breast cancer: a comparative study between CK19 protein expression and CK19 mRNA level in primary tumors and lymph node metastasis. *Virchows Arch.* 2013;463:7–15. doi:10.1007/s00428-013-1440-2.

[27] Tamaki Y., Akiyama F., Iwase T., Kaneko T., Tsuda H., Sato K., et al. Molecular detection of lymph node metastases in breast cancer patients: results of a multicenter trial using the one-step nucleic acid amplification assay. *Clinical cancer research: an official journal of the American Association for Cancer Research.* 2009;15:2879–2884. doi:10.1158/1078-0432.CCR-08-1881.

[28] Tsujimoto M., Nakabayashi K., Yoshidome K., Kaneko T., Iwase T., Akiyama F., et al. One-step nucleic acid amplification for intraoperative detection of lymph node metastasis in breast cancer patients. *Clin Cancer Res.* 2007;13:4807–4816. doi: 10.1158/1078-0432.CCR-06-2512.

[29] Feldman S., Krishnamurthy S., Gillanders W., Gittleman M., Beitsch P. D., Young P. R., et al. A novel automated assay for the rapid identification of metastatic breast carcinoma in sentinel lymph nodes. *Cancer.* 2011;117:2599–2607. doi: 10.1002/cncr.25822.

[30] Snook K. L., Layer G. T., Jackson P. A., de Vries C. S., Shousha S., Sinnett H. D., et al. Multicentre evaluation of intraoperative molecular analysis of sentinel lymph nodes in breast carcinoma. *The British journal of surgery.* 2011;98:527–535. doi: 10.1002/bjs.7347.

[31] Weber W. P., Barry M., Stempel M. M., Junqueira M. J., Eaton A. A., Patil S. M., et al. A 10-year trend analysis of sentinel lymph node frozen section and completion axillary dissection for breast cancer: are these procedures becoming obsolete? *Ann Surg Oncol.* 2012;19:225–232. doi:10.1245/s10434-011-1823-z.

[32] Tanis P. J., van Sandick J. W., Nieweg O. E., Valdes Olmos R. A., Rutgers E. J. T., Hoefnagel C. A., et al. The hidden sentinel node in breast cancer. *Eur J Nucl Med Mol Imaging.* 2002;29:305–311.

[33] Bernardi S., Bertozzi S., Londero A. P., Giacomuzzi F., Angione V., Dri C., et al. Nine years of experience with the sentinel lymph node biopsy in a single Italian center: a retrospective analysis of 1,050 cases. *World J Surg.* 2012;36:714–722. doi:10.1007/s00268-011-1420-0.

[34] McMasters K. M., Tuttle T. M., Carlson D. J., Brown C. M., Noyes R. D., Glaser R. L., et al. Sentinel lymph node biopsy for breast cancer: a suitable alternative to routine axillary dissection in multi-institutional practice when optimal technique is used. *J Clin Oncol.* 2000;18:2560–2566. doi:10.1200/JCO.2000.18.13.2560.

[35] McMasters K. M., Wong S. L., Chao C., Woo C., Tuttle T. M., Noyes R. D., et al. Defining the optimal surgeon experience for breast cancer sentinel lymph node biopsy: a model for implementation of new surgical techniques. *Ann Surg.* 2001; 234:292–9; discussion 299–300.

[36] Bertozzi S., Londero A. P., Giacomuzzi F., Angione V., Carbone A., Petri R., et al. Applicability of two different validated models to predict axillary non-sentinel lymph node status by sentinel node biopsy in a single Italian center. *Breast cancer.* 2015; 22:350–355. doi:10.1007/s12282-013-0485-z.

[37] Van Zee K. J., Manasseh D. M. E., Bevilacqua J. L. B., Boolbol S. K., Fey J. V., Tan L. K., et al. A nomogram for predicting the likelihood of additional nodal metastases in breast cancer patients with a positive sentinel node biopsy. *Ann Surg Oncol.* 2003; 10:1140–1151.

[38] Degnim A. C., Reynolds C., Pantvaidya G., Zakaria S., Hoskin T., Barnes S., et al. Nonsentinel node metastasis in breast cancer patients: assessment of an existing and a new predictive nomogram. *Am J Surg.* 2005;190:543–550. doi: 10.1016/j.amjsurg.2005.06.008.

[39] Mittendorf E. A., Hunt K. K., Boughey J. C., Bassett R., Degnim A. C., Harrell R., et al. Incorporation of sentinel lymph node metastasis size into a nomogram predicting nonsentinel lymph node involvement in breast cancer patients with a positive sentinel lymph node. *Ann Surg.* 2012;255:109–115. doi: 10.1097/SLA.0b013e318238f461.

[40] Kohrt H. E., Olshen R. A., Bermas H. R., Goodson W. H., Wood D. J., Henry S., et al. New models and online calculator for predicting non-sentinel lymph node status in sentinel lymph node positive breast cancer patients. *BMC Cancer.* 2008; 8:66. doi:10.1186/1471-2407-8-66.

[41] Coutant C., Olivier C., Lambaudie E., Fondrinier E., Marchal F., Guillemin F., et al. Comparison of models to predict nonsentinel lymph node status in breast cancer patients with metastatic sentinel lymph nodes: a prospective multicenter study. *Journal of clinical oncology: official journal of the American Society of Clinical Oncology.* 2009;27:2800–2808. doi:10.1200/JCO.2008.19.7418.

[42] Barranger E., Coutant C., Flahault A., Delpech Y., Darai E., Uzan S. An axilla scoring system to predict non-sentinel lymph node status in breast cancer patients with sentinel lymph node involvement. *Breast Cancer Res Treat.* 2005;91:113–119. doi:10.1007/s10549-004-5781-z.

[43] Johnson M. T., Guidroz J. A., Smith B. J., Graham M. M., Scott-Conner C. E. H., Sugg S. L., et al. A single institutional experience of factors affecting successful identification of sentinel lymph node in breast cancer patients. *Surgery.* 2009;146:671–6; discussion 676–7. doi:10.1016/j.surg.2009.06.025.

[44] Hanley J. A., McNeil B. J. A method of comparing the areas under receiver operating characteristic curves derived from the same cases. *Radiology.* 1983;148:839–843. doi:10.1148/radiology.148.3.6878708.

[45] D'Eredita' G., Troilo V. L., Fischetti F., Rubini G., Berardi T. Comparison of two models for predicting non-sentinel lymph node metastases in sentinel lymph node-positive breast cancer patients. *Updates in surgery.* 2011;63:163–170. doi: 10.1007/s13304-011-0079-2.

[46] Driul L., Bernardi S., Bertozzi S., Schiavon M., Londero A. P., Petri R. New surgical trends in breast cancer treatment: conservative interventions and oncoplastic breast surgery. *Minerva Ginecol.* 2013;65:289–296.

[47] Mortellaro V. E., Marshall J., Singer L., Hochwald S. N., Chang M., Copeland E. M., et al. Magnetic resonance imaging for axillary staging in patients with breast cancer. *J Magn Reson Imaging.* 2009;30:309–312. doi:10.1002/jmri.21802.

[48] Pritchard K. I., Julian J. A., Holloway C. M. B., McCready D., Gulenchyn K. Y., George R., et al. Prospective study of 2-[F]fluorodeoxyglucose positron emission tomography in the assessment of regional nodal spread of disease in patients with breast cancer: an Ontario clinical oncology group study. *Journal of clinical oncology: official journal of the American Society of Clinical Oncology.* 2012;30:1274–1279. doi:10.1200/JCO.2011.38.1103.

[49] Cedolini C., Bertozzi S., Londero A. P., Bernardi S., Seriau L., Concina S., et al. Type of breast cancer diagnosis, screening, and survival. *Clin Breast Cancer.* 2014; 14:235–240. doi:10.1016/j.clbc.2014.02.004.

[50] Kim H. J., Son B. H., Park E. W., Lim W. S., Seo J. Y., Jang M. A., et al. Axillary recurrence after negative sentinel lymph node biopsy. *Breast cancer research and treatment.* 2009;114:301–305. doi:10.1007/s10549-008-9994-4.

[51] Bazu C., Coutant C., Antoine M., Moutafoff C., Guillo E., Darae E., et al. [Feasibility of the sentinel node biopsy in breast cancer in case of histological multifocality diagnosis]. *Gynecologie, obstetrique & fertilite.* 2009;37:604–610. doi: 10.1016/j.gyobfe.2009.04.021.

[52] Chen J. J., Huang X. Y., Liu Z. B., Chen T. W., Cheng J. Y., Yang W. T., et al. Sentinel node biopsy and quality of life measures in a Chinese population. *European journal of surgical oncology : the journal of the European Society of Surgical Oncology and the British Association of Surgical Oncology.* 2009;35:921–927. doi: 10.1016/j.ejso.2009.01.009.

[53] Helms G., Kan T., Moser L., Remmel E., Kreienberg R. Shoulder-arm morbidity in patients with sentinel node biopsy and complete axillary dissection–data from a prospective randomised trial. *European journal of surgical oncology: the journal of the European Society of Surgical Oncology and the British Association of Surgical Oncology.* 2009;35:696–701. doi:10.1016/j.ejso.2008.06.013.

[54] Delpech Y., Bricou A., Lousquy R., Hudry D., Jankowski C., Willecocq C., et al. The exportability of the ACOSOG Z0011 criteria for omitting axillary lymph node dissection after positive sentinel lymph node biopsy findings: a multicenter study. *Ann Surg Oncol.* 2013;20:2556–2561. doi:10.1245/s10434-013-2917-6.

[55] Galimberti V., Chifu C., Rodriguez Perez S., Veronesi P., Intra M., Botteri E., et al. Positive axillary sentinel lymph node: is axillary dissection always necessary? *Breast.* 2011;20 Suppl 3:S96–S98. doi:10.1016/S0960-9776(11)70303-4.

[56] Giuliano A. E., McCall L., Beitsch P., Whitworth P. W., Blumencranz P., Leitch A. M., et al. Locoregional recurrence after sentinel lymph node dissection with or without axillary dissection in patients with sentinel lymph node metastases: the American College of Surgeons Oncology Group Z0011 randomized trial. *Ann Surg.* 2010;252:426–32; discussion 432–3. doi:10.1097/SLA.0b013e3181f08f32.

[57] Fisher B., Jeong J. H., Anderson S., Bryant J., Fisher E. R., Wolmark N. Twenty-five-year follow-up of a randomized trial comparing radical mastectomy, total mastectomy, and total mastectomy followed by irradiation. *The New England journal of medicine.* 2002;347:567–575. doi:10.1056/NEJMoa020128.

[58] Pernas S., Gil M., Benatez A., Bajen M. T., Climent F., Pla M. J., et al. Avoiding axillary treatment in sentinel lymph node micrometastases of breast cancer: a prospective analysis of axillary or distant recurrence. *Ann Surg Oncol.* 2010;17:772–777.

[59] Reed J., Rosman M., Verbanac K. M., Mannie A., Cheng Z., Tafra L. Prognostic implications of isolated tumor cells and micrometastases in sentinel nodes of patients with invasive breast cancer: 10-year analysis of patients enrolled in the prospective East Carolina University/Anne Arundel Medical Center Sentinel Node Multicenter Study. *J Am Coll Surg.* 2009;208:333–340. doi:10.1016/j.jamcollsurg.2008.10.036.

[60] Gadd M., Harris J., Taghian A., Hughes K., O'Neill A., S. P., et al. Prospective study of axillary radiation without axillary dissection for breast cancer patients with a positive sentinel node (Abstracts of the 28th Annual San Antonio Breast Cancer Symposium, December 8-11, 2005, San Antonio, Texas, USA). *Breast Cancer Res Treat.* 2005;94 Suppl 1:S1–287.

[61] Bilimoria K. Y., Bentrem D. J., Hansen N. M., Bethke K. P., Rademaker A. W., Ko C. Y., et al. Comparison of sentinel lymph node biopsy alone and completion axillary lymph node dissection for node-positive breast cancer. *Journal of clinical oncology: Official journal of the American Society of Clinical Oncology.* 2009;27:2946–2953. doi:10.1200/JCO.2008.19.5750.

[62] Yi M., Giordano S. H., Meric-Bernstam F., Mittendorf E. A., Kuerer H. M., Hwang R. F., et al. Trends in and outcomes from sentinel lymph node biopsy (SLNB) alone vs. SLNB with axillary lymph node dissection for node-positive breast cancer patients: experience from the SEER database. *Annals of surgical oncology.* 2010;17 Suppl 3:343–351. doi:10.1245/s10434-010-1253-3.

[63] Park J., Fey J. V., Naik A. M., Borgen P. I., Van Zee K. J., Cody H. S. A declining rate of completion axillary dissection in sentinel lymph node-positive breast cancer patients is associated with the use of a multivariate nomogram. *Annals of surgery.* 2007;245:462–468. doi:10.1097/01.sla.0000250439.86020.85.

[64] Hwang R. F., Gonzalez-Angulo A. M., Yi M., Buchholz T. A., Meric-Bernstam F. , Kuerer H. M., et al. Low locoregional failure rates in selected breast cancer patients with tumor-positive sentinel lymph nodes who do not undergo completion axillary dissection. *Cancer.* 2007;110:723–730. doi:10.1002/cncr.22847.

[65] Fant J. S., Grant M. D., Knox S. M., Livingston S. A., Ridl K., Jones R. C., et al. Preliminary outcome analysis in patients with breast cancer and a positive sentinel lymph node who declined axillary dissection. *Annals of surgical oncology.* 2003; 10:126–130.

[66] Giuliano A. E., Hunt K. K., Ballman K. V., Beitsch P. D., Whitworth P. W., Blumencranz P. W., et al. Axillary dissection vs no axillary dissection in women with invasive breast cancer and sentinel node metastasis: a randomized clinical trial. *JAMA.* 2011; 305:569–575. doi:10.1001/jama.2011.90.

[67] Martelli G., Boracchi P., De Palo M., Pilotti S., Oriana S., Zucali R., et al. A randomized trial comparing axillary dissection to no axillary dissection in older patients with T1N0 breast cancer: results after 5 years of follow-up. *Annals of surgery.* 2005; 242:1–6; discussion 7–9.

[68] Louis-Sylvestre C., Clough K., Asselain B., Vilcoq J. R., Salmon R. J., Campana F., et al. Axillary treatment in conservative management of operable breast cancer: dissection or radiotherapy? Results of a randomized study with 15 years of follow-up. *Journal of clinical oncology: official journal of the American Society of Clinical Oncology.* 2004;22:97–101. doi:10.1200/JCO.2004.12.108.

[69] Veronesi U., Orecchia R., Zurrida S., Galimberti V., Luini A., Veronesi P., et al. Avoiding axillary dissection in breast cancer surgery: a randomized trial to assess the role of axillary radiotherapy. *Annals of oncology: official journal of the European Society for Medical Oncology.* 2005;16:383–388. doi:10.1093/annonc/mdi089.

[70] Cancer research campaign (King's/Cambridge) trial for early breast cancer. A detailed update at the tenth year. Cancer Research Campaign Working Party. *Lancet* (London, England). 1980;2:55–60.

[71] Lythgoe J. P., Palmer M. K. Manchester regional breast study–5 and 10 year results. *The British journal of surgery.* 1982;69:693–696.

[72] Ollila D. W., Carey L. A., Sartor C. I. Clinical significance of micrometastatic disease in the era of sentinel node. *Breast disease.* 2001;12:57–67.

[73] Riber-Hansen R., Nyengaard J. R., Hamilton-Dutoit S. J., Steiniche T. Stage migration after minor changes in histologic estimation of tumor burden in sentinel lymph nodes: the protocol trap. *Cancer.* 2009;115:2177–2187. doi:10.1002/cncr.24268.

[74] Wasif N., Maggard M. A., Ko C. Y., Giuliano A. E. Underuse of axillary dissection for the management of sentinel node micrometastases in breast cancer. *Archives of surgery* (Chicago, Ill : 1960). 2010;145:161–166. doi:10.1001/archsurg.2009.269.

[75] Weaver D. L., Le U. P., Dupuis S. L., Weaver K. A. E., Harlow S.P., Ashikaga T., et al. Metastasis detection in sentinel lymph nodes: comparison of a limited widely spaced (NSABP protocol B-32) and a comprehensive narrowly spaced paraffin block sectioning strategy. *The American journal of surgical pathology.* 2009;33:1583–1589. doi:10.1097/PAS.0b013e3181b274e7.

[76] Gobardhan P. D., Elias S. G., Madsen E. V. E, Bongers V., Ruitenberg H. J. M., Perre C. I., et al. Prognostic value of micrometastases in sentinel lymph nodes of patients with breast carcinoma: a cohort study. *Annals of oncology: official journal of the European Society for Medical Oncology.* 2009;20:41–48. doi:10.1093/annonc/mdn535.

[77] Chen S. L., Hoehne F. M., Giuliano A. E. The prognostic significance of micrometastases in breast cancer: a SEER population-based analysis. *Annals of surgical oncology.* 2007;14:3378–3384. doi:10.1245/s10434-007-9513-6.

[78] van der Heiden-van der Loo M., Bezemer P. D., Hennipman A., Siesling S., van Diest P. J., Bongers V., et al. Introduction of sentinel node biopsy and stage migration of breast cancer. *European journal of surgical oncology: the journal of the European Society of Surgical Oncology and the British Association of Surgical Oncology.* 2006; 32:710–714. doi:10.1016/j.ejso.2006.04.001.

[79] van Rijk M. C., Peterse J. L., Nieweg O. E., Oldenburg H. S. A., Rutgers E. J. T., Kroon B. B. R. Additional axillary metastases and stage migration in breast cancer patients with micrometastases or submicrometastases in sentinel lymph nodes. *Cancer.* 2006;107:467–471. doi:10.1002/cncr.22069.

[80] Hansen N. M., Grube B., Ye X., Turner R. R., Brenner R. J., Sim M. S., et al. Impact of micrometastases in the sentinel node of patients with invasive breast cancer. *Journal of clinical oncology: official journal of the American Society of Clinical Oncology.* 2009;27:4679–4684. doi:10.1200/JCO.2008.19.0686.

[81] Tille J. C., Egger J. F., Devillaz M. C., Vlastos G., Pelte M. F. Frozen section in axillary sentinel lymph nodes for diagnosis of breast cancer micrometastasis. *Anticancer research.* 2009;29:4711–4716.

[82] Khalifa K., Pereira B., Thomas V. A., Mokbel K. The accuracy of intraoperative frozen section analysis of the sentinel lymph nodes during breast cancer surgery. *International journal of fertility and women's medicine.* 2004;49:208–211.

[83] Joseph K. A., El-Tamer M., Komenaka I., Troxel A., Ditkoff B. A., Schnabel F. Predictors of nonsentinel node metastasis in patients with breast cancer after sentinel node metastasis. *Archives of surgery* (Chicago, Ill : 1960). 2004;139:648–651. doi: 10.1001/archsurg.139.6.648.

[84] Kim T. , Giuliano A. E., Lyman G. H. Lymphatic mapping and sentinel lymph node biopsy in early-stage breast carcinoma: a metaanalysis. *Cancer.* 2006;106:4–16. doi:10.1002/cncr.21568.

[85] Noguchi M. Avoidance of axillary lymph node dissection in selected patients with node-positive breast cancer. *European journal of surgical oncology : the journal of the European Society of Surgical Oncology and the British Association of Surgical Oncology.* 2008;34:129–134. doi:10.1016/j.ejso.2007.03.026.

[86] Cedolini C., Bertozzi S., Seriau L., Londero A. P., Concina S., Cattin F., et al. Eight-year experience with the intraoperative frozen section examination of sentinel lymph node biopsy for breast cancer in a North-Italian university center. *International journal of clinical and experimental pathology.* 2014;7:364–371.

[87] Lyman G. H., Giuliano A. E., Somerfield M. R., Benson A. B., Bodurka D. C., Burstein H. J., et al. American Society of Clinical Oncology guideline recommendations for sentinel lymph node biopsy in early-stage breast cancer. *Journal of clinical oncology : official journal of the American Society of Clinical Oncology.* 2005; 23:7703–7720. doi:10.1200/JCO.2005.08.001.

[88] Weaver D. L. Pathology evaluation of sentinel lymph nodes in breast cancer: protocol recommendations and rationale. *Modern pathology: an official journal of the United States and Canadian Academy of Pathology,* Inc. 2010;23 Suppl 2:S26–S32. doi: 10.1038/modpathol.2010.36.

[89] Rutledge H., Davis J., Chiu R., Cibull M., Brill Y., McGrath P., et al. Sentinel node micrometastasis in breast carcinoma may not be an indication for complete axillary dissection. *Modern pathology: an official journal of the United States and Canadian Academy of Pathology,* Inc. 2005;18:762–768. doi:10.1038/modpathol.3800394.

[90] Hunt K. K., Ballman K. V., McCall L. M., Boughey J. C., Mittendorf E. A., Cox C. E., et al. Factors associated with local-regional recurrence after a negative sentinel node dissection: results of the ACOSOG Z0010 trial. *Annals of surgery.* 2012; 256:428–436. doi:10.1097/SLA.0b013e3182654494.

[91] Olson J. A., McCall L. M., Beitsch P., Whitworth P. W., Reintgen D. S. , Blumencranz P. W., et al. Impact of immediate versus delayed axillary node dissection on surgical outcomes in breast cancer patients with positive sentinel nodes: results from American College of Surgeons Oncology Group Trials Z0010 and Z0011. *Journal of clinical oncology: official journal of the American Society of Clinical Oncology.* 2008;26:3530–3535. doi:10.1200/JCO.2007.15.5630.

[92] Galimberti V., Cole B. F., Zurrida S., Viale G., Luini A., Veronesi P., et al. Axillary dissection versus no axillary dissection in patients with sentinel-node micrometastases (IBCSG 23-01): a phase 3 randomised controlled trial. *The Lancet Oncology.* 2013;14:297–305. doi:10.1016/S1470-2045(13)70035-4.

[93] Weaver D. L., Ashikaga T., Krag D. N., Skelly J. M., Anderson S. J., Harlow S. P., et al. Effect of occult metastases on survival in node-negative breast cancer. *The New England journal of medicine.* 2011;364:412–421. doi:10.1056/NEJMoa1008108.

[94] Yegiyants S., Romero L. M., Haigh P. I., DiFronzo LA. Completion axillary lymph node dissection not required for regional control in patients with breast cancer who have micrometastases in a sentinel node. *Archives of surgery* (Chicago, Ill : 1960). 2010;145:564–569. doi:10.1001/archsurg.2010.84.

[95] Cserni G., Burzykowski T., Vinh-Hung V., Kocsis L., Boross G., Sinka M., et al. Axillary sentinel node and tumour-related factors associated with non-sentinel node involvement in breast cancer. *Japanese journal of clinical oncology.* 2004;34:519–524.

[96] Degnim A. C., Griffith K. A., Sabel M. S., Hayes D. F., Cimmino V. M., Diehl K. M., et al. Clinicopathologic features of metastasis in nonsentinel lymph nodes of breast carcinoma patients. *Cancer.* 2003;98:2307–2315. doi:10.1002/cncr.11803.

[97] Boler D. E., Cabioglu N., Ince U., Esen G., Uras C. Sentinel Lymph Node Biopsy in Pure DCIS: Is It Necessary? *ISRN surgery.* 2012;2012:394095. doi: 10.5402/2012/394095.

[98] Son B. K., Bong J. G., Park S. H., Jeong Y. J. Ductal carcinoma in situ and sentinel lymph node biopsy. *Journal of breast cancer.* 2011;14:301–307. doi: 10.4048/jbc.2011.14.4.301.

[99] Solin L. J., Kurtz J., Fourquet A., Amalric R., Recht A., Bornstein B. A., et al. Fifteen-year results of breast-conserving surgery and definitive breast irradiation for the treatment of ductal carcinoma in situ of the breast. *Journal of clinical oncology: official journal of the American Society of Clinical Oncology.* 1996;14:754–763. doi: 10.1200/JCO.1996.14.3.754.

[100] Silverstein M. J., Gierson E. D., Colburn W. J., Cope L. M., Furmanski M., Senofsky G. M., et al. Can intraductal breast carcinoma be excised completely by local excision? Clinical and pathologic predictors. *Cancer.* 1994;73:2985–2989.

[101] von Rueden D. G., Wilson R. E. Intraductal carcinoma of the breast. *Surgery, gynecology & obstetrics.* 1984;158:105–111.

[102] Winchester D. P., Menck H. R., Osteen R. T., Kraybill W. Treatment trends for ductal carcinoma in situ of the breast. *Annals of surgical oncology.* 1995;2:207–213.

[103] Singletary S. E., Allred C., Ashley P., Bassett L. W., Berry D., Bland K. I., et al. Revision of the American Joint Committee on Cancer staging system for breast cancer. *Journal of clinical oncology: official journal of the American Society of Clinical Oncology.* 2002;20:3628–3636. doi:10.1200/JCO.2002.02.026.

[104] Banys M., Gruber I., Krawczyk N., Becker S., Kurth R., Wallwiener D., et al. Hematogenous and lymphatic tumor cell dissemination may be detected in patients

diagnosed with ductal carcinoma in situ of the breast. *Breast cancer research and treatment.* 2012;131:801–808. doi:10.1007/s10549-011-1478-2.

[105] Osako T., Iwase T., Kimura K., Horii R., Akiyama F. Detection of occult invasion in ductal carcinoma in situ of the breast with sentinel node metastasis. *Cancer science.* 2013;104:453–457. doi:10.1111/cas.12095.

[106] Schulz S., Sinn P., Golatta M., Rauch G., Junkermann H., Schuetz F., et al. Prediction of underestimated invasiveness in patients with ductal carcinoma in situ of the breast on percutaneous biopsy as rationale for recommending concurrent sentinel lymph node biopsy. *Breast* (Edinburgh, Scotland). 2013;22:537–542. doi: 10.1016/j.breast.2012.11.002.

[107] Fisher E. R. Pathobiological considerations relating to the treatment of intraductal carcinoma (ductal carcinoma in situ) of the breast. *CA: a cancer journal for clinicians.* 1997;47:52–64.

[108] Takacs T., Paszt A., Szentpali K., Ormandi K., Lazar M., Palka I., et al. Importance of sentinel lymph node biopsy in surgical therapy of in situ breast cancer. *Pathology oncology research*: POR. 2009;15:329–333. doi:10.1007/s12253-008-9123-z.

[109] Matrai Z., Banhidy F., Taglas M., Kovacs E., Savolt A., Udvarhelyi N., et al. [Sentinel lymph node biopsy in pregnancy-associated breast cancer]. *Orvosi hetilap.* 2013;154:1991–1997. doi:10.1556/OH.2013.29771.

[110] Spanheimer P. M., Graham M. M., Sugg S. L., Scott-Conner C. E. H., Weigel R. J. Measurement of uterine radiation exposure from lymphoscintigraphy indicates safety of sentinel lymph node biopsy during pregnancy. *Annals of surgical oncology.* 2009;16:1143–1147. doi:10.1245/s10434-009-0390-z.

[111] Duncan P. G., Pope W. D., Cohen M. M., Greer N. Fetal risk of anesthesia and surgery during pregnancy. *Anesthesiology*. 1986;64:790–794.

[112] Mazze R. I., Kallan B. Reproductive outcome after anesthesia and operation during pregnancy: a registry study of 5405 cases. *American journal of obstetrics and gynecology.* 1989;161:1178–1185.

[113] Kizer N. T., Powell M. A. Surgery in the pregnant patient. *Clinical obstetrics and gynecology.* 2011;54:633–641. doi:10.1097/GRF.0b013e318236eb0d.

[114] Loibl S., von Minckwitz G., Gwyn K., Ellis P., Blohmer J. U., Schlegelberger B., et al. Breast carcinoma during pregnancy. International recommendations from an expert meeting. *Cancer.* 2006;106:237–246. doi:10.1002/cncr.21610.

[115] Fisher B., Brown A., Mamounas E., Wieand S., Robidoux A., Margolese R. G., et al. Effect of preoperative chemotherapy on local-regional disease in women with operable breast cancer: findings from National Surgical Adjuvant Breast and Bowel Project B-18. *Journal of clinical oncology: official journal of the American Society of Clinical Oncology*. 1997;15:2483–2493. doi:10.1200/JCO.1997.15.7.2483.

[116] Hunt K. K., Yi M., Mittendorf E. A., Guerrero C., Babiera G. V., Bedrosian I., et al. Sentinel lymph node surgery after neoadjuvant chemotherapy is accurate and reduces the need for axillary dissection in breast cancer patients. *Annals of surgery.* 2009; 250:558–566. doi:10.1097/SLA.0b013e3181b8fd5e.

[117] Mamounas E. P., Brown A., Anderson S., Smith R., Julian T., Miller B., et al. Sentinel node biopsy after neoadjuvant chemotherapy in breast cancer: results from National Surgical Adjuvant Breast and Bowel Project Protocol B-27. *Journal of clinical oncology: official journal of the American Society of Clinical Oncology.* 2005; 23:2694–2702. doi:10.1200/JCO.2005.05.188.

[118] Classe J. M., Bordes V., Campion L., Mignotte H., Dravet F., Leveque J., et al. Sentinel lymph node biopsy after neoadjuvant chemotherapy for advanced breast cancer: results of Ganglion Sentinelle et Chimiotherapie Neoadjuvante, a French prospective multicentric study. *Journal of clinical oncology: official journal of the American Society of Clinical Oncology*. 2009;27:726–732. doi:10.1200/JCO.2008.18.3228.

[119] Xing Y., Foy M, Cox D. D., Kuerer H. M., Hunt K. K., Cormier J. N. Meta-analysis of sentinel lymph node biopsy after preoperative chemotherapy in patients with breast cancer. *The British journal of surgery.* 2006;93:539–546. doi: 10.1002/bjs.5209.

[120] Kelly A. M., Dwamena B., Cronin P., Carlos R. C. Breast cancer sentinel node identification and classification after neoadjuvant chemotherapy-systematic review and meta analysis. *Academic radiology*. 2009;16:551–563. doi: 10.1016/j.acra.2009.01.026.

[121] Boughey J., Suman V., Mittendorf E., Ahrendt G., Wilke L., Taback B., et al. Abstract S2-1: The role of sentinel lymph node surgery in patients presenting with node positive breast cancer (T0-T4, N1-2) who receive neoadjuvant chemotherapy – results from the ACOSOG Z1071 trial:. *Cancer Research.* 2012;72:S2–1–S2–1. doi:10.1158/0008-5472.sabcs12-s2-1.

[122] Kuehn T., Bauerfeind I., Fehm T., Fleige B., Helms G., Lebeau A., et al. Abstract S2-2: Sentinel Lymph Node Biopsy Before or After Neoadjuvant Chemotherapy - Final Results from the Prospective German, multiinstitutional SENTINA-Trial -. *Cancer Research.* 2012;72:S2–2–S2–2. doi:10.1158/0008-5472.sabcs12-s2-2.

[123] Kuerer H. M., Sahin A. A., Hunt K. K., Newman L. A., Breslin T. M., Ames F. C., et al. Incidence and impact of documented eradication of breast cancer axillary lymph node metastases before surgery in patients treated with neoadjuvant chemotherapy. *Annals of surgery*. 1999;230:72–78.

[124] Bear H. D., Anderson S., Brown A., Smith R., Mamounas E. P., Fisher B., et al. The effect on tumor response of adding sequential preoperative docetaxel to preoperative doxorubicin and cyclophosphamide: preliminary results from National Surgical Adjuvant Breast and Bowel Project Protocol B-27. *Journal of clinical oncology: official journal of the American Society of Clinical Oncology.* 2003;21:4165–4174. doi:10.1200/JCO.2003.12.005.

[125] Dominici L. S., Negron Gonzalez V. M., Buzdar A. U., Lucci A., Mittendorf E. A., Le-Petross H. T., et al. Cytologically proven axillary lymph node metastases are eradicated in patients receiving preoperative chemotherapy with concurrent trastuzumab for HER2-positive breast cancer. *Cancer.* 2010;116:2884–2889. doi: 10.1002/cncr.25152.

[126] Port E. R., Garcia-Etienne C. A., Park J., Fey J., Borgen P. I., Cody H. S. Reoperative sentinel lymph node biopsy: a new frontier in the management of ipsilateral breast tumor recurrence. *Annals of surgical oncology*. 2007;14:2209–2214. doi: 10.1245/s10434-006-9237-z.

[127] Ikeda T. Re-sentinel node biopsy after previous breast and axillary surgery. *Surgery today.* 2014;44:2015–2021. doi:10.1007/s00595-013-0783-2.

In: The Sentinel Lymph Node
Editors: A. Londero, S. Bertozzi and C. Cedolini
ISBN: 978-1-53614-557-1


*Chapter 5*

# Breast Cancer Nodal Staging

***Luigi Viola*[1,*], *Ambrogio P. Londero*[2], *Serena Bertozzi*[3] and *Gianluca Gatta*[1]**
[1]Radiology Department,
University of Campania "Luigi Vanvitelli", Naples, Italy,
[2]Clinic of Obstetrics and Gynecology, University Hospital of Udine, Italy
[3]Breast Unit, University Hospital of Udine, Italy

**Abstract**

In patients with breast cancer, an accurate assessment of the status of regional lymph node is crucial to provide valuable information in order to choose the best treatment for the patient. Lymph node status is established to be one of the most critical prognostic indicators, being the axillary nodal involvement a sign of aggressive biologic behavior, and consequently, an indicator of poor prognosis. Clinical staging of nodes is based on clinical or imaging findings and aims at identifying suspicious nodes in the axilla or extra-axillary regions. In contrast, pathological staging is based on the number of axillary nodes involved determined during surgery. Over the last few decades, nodal staging has experienced drastic changes. Sentinel lymph node biopsy is now the standard of care for the detection of metastatic disease in clinically node-negative breast cancer patients. Supported by the results of numerous randomized clinical trials conducted worldwide, is actually the current reference standard and has clinically replaced the more radical and harmful complete axillary lymph node dissection. In parallel, radiological staging of the axilla has become increasingly useful and the imaging techniques have consistently improved. In clinical staging, preoperative axillary ultrasound and ultrasound-guided biopsy are increasingly being used to identify metastases within axillary lymph nodes. Despite progress in estimating prognosis and predicting response to adjuvant systemic therapy, axillary nodal status remains a critical component in initial surgical planning and determining therapeutic strategies for breast cancer patients.

**Keywords:** lymph node status, breast cancer, mammography, ultrasound, computed tomography, magnetic resonance imaging

*Corresponding Author E-mail: luigiviola19@libero.it.

# 1. Introduction

Almost 100 years ago, routine removal of axillary nodes, known as complete axillary lymph node dissection (CALND), became part of the standard surgical treatment for breast cancer after the publication of the autopsy studies conducted by the German pathologist Rudolf Virchow's (1821-1902). Virchow hypothesized that breast cancer had a centrifugal expansion by first invading the axillary nodes and then spreading to other sites after exceeding the loading capacity of the axillary nodal stations. A few years later, William Stewart Halsted (1852-1922) described the importance of axillary contents removal to reduce local recurrence rates in women with breast cancer [1, 2].

In 1970 the Mayo Clinic provided firm evidence of the prognostic significance of axillary nodal metastases. Axillary nodal involvement was identified as the primary determinant of survival, with 5-year survival rates of 86% in node-negative patients compared to 50% in node-positive patients [3].

CALND is a radical procedure whereby all axillary nodes are excised, allowing each node to be individually assessed for metastases by the pathologist. Although this procedure is effective in assessing axillary disease burden, it may be associated with significant long-term morbidity, including ipsilateral arm lymphedema and paresthesia, as well as short-term postoperative complications, such as wound infection and seroma [4].

In the 1940s, studies by Gilchrist, Zeidman and Buss showed that metastatic cells spread through the regional lymphatics in an orderly and reproducible manner, paving the way for the evolution of sentinel lymph node biopsy (SLNB).Thus, routine staging by CALND has been progressively replaced by SLNB, which is a minimally invasive operation and aims at excising only the axillary sentinel node [5, 6, 7].

The sentinel node is defined as the first node that drains lymph from the breast and is the first node where breast cancer metastases ought to be detectable. The SLNB procedure mimics the physiological spread of cancer cells from the neoplastic lesion to the lymph nodes, by migration within the lymphatic net of a tracer injected adjacent to the lesion.

Before being validated and applied in breast cancer, SLNB has been shown to be feasible in penile cancer and melanoma. The existence of one or more breast sentinel nodes has been demonstrated by Kett and colleagues and Krag and colleagues using two different injection techniques. The feasibility of identifying the sentinel node in breast cancer and the ability to accurately predict the status of the entire axillary basin through its biopsy was demonstrated by Giuliano and colleagues in 1994 [8, 9, 10, 11]. SLNB now represents the standard staging procedure among patients with clinically node-negative (cN0) breast cancer, being an appropriate, safe and effective approach for this group of patients.

Over the past two decades, several randomized studies comparing different techniques for lymphatic mapping (blue dye or radiocolloid or their combination) have been conducted. The purpose was to determine whether SLNB should be part of the standard of care for specific subsets of breast cancer patients. In these trials, the investigators randomized patients to SLNB vs CALND or to SLNB followed by CALND vs SLNB alone. Some of the most important trials are the National Surgical Adjuvant Breast and Bowel Project B-32 (NSABP B-32) trial, the Sentinella-Gruppo Interdisciplinare Veneto di Oncologia Mammaria (Sentinella-GIVOM) trial, the Axillary Lymphatic Mapping Against Nodal Axillary Clearance (ALMANAC) trial, the Instituto Nazionale per la Ricerca sul Cancro trial, the Royal

Australian College of Surgeons Sentinel Node vs Axillary Clearance (RACS SNAC) trial, the NCT00970983 trial (The Milan Study) and the Cambridge/East Anglia Study Group trial [12, 13, 14, 15, 16, 17, 18, 19, 20].

The results of these and other studies show that SLNB is comparable with CALND in terms of disease-free survival, overall survival, axillary recurrence and morbidity rates. In terms of quality of life, SLNB has significantly lower rates of arm lymphedema, numbness, shoulder movement deficits and wound seroma than CALND. In addition, these studies produced sentinel node identification rates of approximately 74% to 94% and false negative rates of up to 13%. In most of these studies, the sentinel node detection rate was above 95% and the false negative rate below 10% [5, 21, 22, 15, 14, 23, 24, 25, 26, 20]. However, although SLNB is a minimally invasive procedure, it is still associated with some morbidity, including a lymphedema risk of 5% at 5 years [1, 4].

SLNB alone has been incorporated into clinical practice also for selected patients with low-volume axillary metastases, based on the results of the ACOSOG Z0011 trial [27, 28]. This phase III non-inferiority trial, initiated in 1999 by the American College of Surgeons Oncology Group (ACOSOG) as a prospective randomized multicenter trial, evaluated whether completion CALND would improve overall survival in patients with T1-T2 estrogen receptor-positive invasive breast cancer, clinically negative axilla and 1 to 2 sentinel nodes containing either micrometastases or macrometastases, undergoing breast-conserving surgery. Although the enrolment target was 1,900 patients, this trial was closed early, after reaching about a fifth of the 500 deaths required to support the study, due to slow accrual and a very low event rate. All patients received post-lumpectomy whole-breast irradiation, but high breast tangents were used frequently and regional nodal radiotherapy was used in 19% of patients [26]. The results of the trial suggest that there are no statistically significant differences in terms of mortality, disease-free survival and recurrence rate in patients with 1 or 2 positive lymph nodes undergoing either SLNB or CALND followed by breast conserving surgery and whole-breast irradiation.

Prior to the Z0011 trial, radiologists attempted to identify axillary metastases preoperatively, allowing patients with early breast cancer to proceed directly to complete axillary dissection [29, 30]. In any case, adequate preoperative imaging evaluation of axillary nodes should always be performed in order to select clinically node-negative patients, candidates for SLNB.

## 2. Anatomy of the Axilla

The axilla is a pyramidal space located between the upper aspect of the thoracic wall and the medial aspect of the arm. The contents of the axilla consist of the axillary artery and the axillary vein, together with their branches; intercostal nerves and nerves coming from the brachial plexus; and lymph nodes, fibrous tissue, adipose tissue and vestigial breast glandular tissue. At mammography, the standard axilla has a density similar to that of the adipose tissue and sometimes exhibits small reactive lymph nodes and accessory breast tissue. However, mammography is not considered reliable for the evaluation of axillary nodes, as certain parts of the axillary area may not be visualized by routine mammograms.

During ultrasound examination, it is of great importance to examine all the contents of the axilla, as well as of the axillary tail, which is posterior to the space where the pectoralis major muscle crosses the cranial edge of the breast gland and is a common location for the sentinel node.

The axillary lymph nodes, which are inferolateral to the pectoralis minor muscle, are divided into levels I, II, and III. The level is determined by the lymph node location in relation to the pectoralis minor muscle. Level I includes the lymph nodes located below the inferolateral border of the pectoralis minor muscle; level II, the lymph nodes that are located posteriorly to and between the lateral and medial borders of the pectoralis minor muscle; level III, the lymph nodes located medially to the superior border of the pectoralis minor muscle (including the infra-clavicular nodes). Axillary lymphatic drainage follows a precise anatomical order, from level I to III, and ultimately into the thorax [31, 32, 33, 34, 35, 36].

## 3. The TNM Classification for Nodal Staging of Breast Cancer

The TNM classification for nodal staging of breast cancer is divided into clinical and pathological staging. Clinical nodal staging (cN) is used for patients with suspected cancer on the basis of an imaging study or a clinical examination other than lymphoscintigraphy, a cytologic examination using ultrasound-guided fine needle aspiration cytology (FNAC), or an ultasound-guided core needle biopsy (CNB). The designation cN1 refers to ipsilateral lymph node metastases at level I-II axillary nodes. The cN2 category is divided into subcategories cN2a (ipsilateral level I-II axillary lymph nodes clinically matted to one another or to other structures) and cN2b (clinically detected ipsilateral internal mammary lymph nodes without clinically evident axillary lymph node metastases). The cN3 category, which includes level III metastases (infraclavicular) and supraclavicular nodal stations, is divided into subcategories cN3a, cN3b, and cN3c. cN3a includes ipsilateral infraclavicular lymph node metastases with or without level I-II axillary involvement; cN3b includes ipsilateral internal mammary lymph node metastases with level I-II axillary nodal involvement; and cN3c ipsilateral supraclavicular lymph node metastases with or without level I-II axillary involvement.

On the other hand, pathological nodal staging (pN) is based on the number of positive lymph nodes by post-operative histological examination. The pathological stages are pN1, pN2, and pN3, where pN1 is 1 to 3 positive nodes, pN2 is 4 to 9 metastatic lymph nodes and are pN3 is 10 or more metastatic lymph nodes. However, many recent studies have shown that the prognosis of breast cancer is influenced not only by the anatomic extent of the tumor, but also by biological characteristics. Thus, biological characteristics such as estrogen and progesterone receptors, human epidermal receptor-2 and multigene expression profiles should in the future be incorporated into the traditional TNM staging system [31, 32, 37, 38, 39].

## 4. Rationale of Preoperative Axillary Nodes Evaluation

In Europe and the UK, all newly diagnosed patients will have an axillary ultrasound to stage the axilla, even when the clinical examination of the axilla is regular. Equivocal, suspicious or abnormal axillary lymph nodes are biopsied. Biopsy can be performed by both conventional CNB or FNAC. If the biopsy is benign, the patient is managed with

SLNB and, only in the presence of metastases in the sentinel node, with CALND.

On the other hand, in the Unites States, guidelines recommend that an axillary ultrasound should only be performed in patients with clinically palpable axillary lymph nodes, although clinical palpation has a false-negative rate of 30-50%. Two recent meta-analyses suggest that routine preoperative axillary ultrasound combined with CNB or FNAC correctly identifies nodal metastases in 50-55% of breast cancer patients. It has been shown that one in four patients with negative axillary ultrasound, with or without biopsy, have metastatic lymph nodes on subsequent SLNB. In view of this, SLNB is currently considered the gold standard intraoperative procedure for axillary staging in clinically node-negative patients.

SLNB consists in a set of actions designed to locate, identify, excise and assess one or more sentinel nodes for metastases. Most SLNB procedures use a radiotracer as a means of locating and identifying the sentinel node, but vital dyes or fluorescent dyes can also be used, alone or in combination. If the sentinel node does not contain metastases, it implies that the rest of the axilla is also considered disease-free and there is no benefit in submitting the patient to subsequent CALND.

Technically, prior to the surgical procedure, radiotracer (technetium-99) or vital dye (i.e. isosulfan blue, methylene blue, or patent blue) is subdermally injected into the periareolar region or close to the neoplastic lesion, whereupon it enters the lymphatics and drains to the sentinel node. The surgeon identifies the position of the sentinel node by using a handheld gamma camera to detect radioactivity prior to making the incision or by visually inspecting the blue stained nodes. In any case, it is not yet clear whether the objective of SLNB procedure is to assess at least one sentinel node or all sentinel nodes.

The detection rate is a reasonably accurate estimate of the number of patients in whom at least one sentinel node is identified. SLNB has a high detection rate of 95% in patients with breast cancer or melanoma, especially when using the combination of blue dye and radioisotope. However, the dual tracer technique may not be widely available worldwide due to its high costs and the logistical difficulty of obtaining medical radioisotopes. Many centers use blue dye as the sole tracer, even though it is inferior to the dual technique and has experienced some problems such as a risk of anaphylaxis of 0.9%. SLNB is also a surgical procedure, and although it has less morbidity than CALND it is associated with debilitating complications at 12 months, such as sensory loss (11%) and arm lymphedema (5%) [40, 41, 42, 43, 44, 45, 46, 47, 48, 49, 15].

Preoperative identification of high-volume metastatic axillary nodes would allow the patient to proceed directly with CALND, obviating a two-stage surgical procedure. Alternatively, if axillary metastases can be excluded it would spare the patient from axillary surgery and the potential complications and associated morbidity. Therefore, accurate diagnosis and quantification of the axillary disease in an outpatient setting could lead to individualized appropriate treatment plans, where only the affected nodes are excised or monitored, or where non-surgical treatment regimens are undertaken through accurate outpatient staging and review.

## 5. Technical Aspects of Intraoperative Sentinel Node Identification

It is possible to replace radiotracers and blue dyes with other tracers, which would probably also require the development and use of other imaging and detection technologies. In view of the logistical challenges associated with the use of radioisotopes, their limited availability and the risk of anaphylactic reactions from blue dye, alternative techniques for sentinel node identification are being studied. The two most promising techniques are based on indocyanine green fluorescence and superparamagnetic iron oxide nanoparticles. Indocyanine green dye is injected intraoperatively, and a simultaneous transcutaneous fluorescent lymphography can be performed for lymphatic mapping. The potential benefits of superparamagnetic iron oxide nanoparticles include their long half-life, which allows their shipment to remote locations worldwide [12, 29, 50, 51, 52, 53, 54, 55]. However, a systematic review concluded that these new procedures cannot put into question the current clinical standard of care.

The most used tracer in the world remains the technetium-99-labeled colloid. In the United States, the most used radiotracer is usually sulfur colloid (50-1000 nm), mostly a filtered sulfur colloid (30-50 nm); in Europe, a human serum albumin nanocolloid (3-23 nm); in Australia, antimony trisulfide (7-23 nm); and in Japan, calcium phytate (150-1500 nm or 150-200 nm). Other tracers include rhenium sulfide (8-68 nm), tin colloid (33-255 nm) and stannous or stannic hydroxide (30-200 nm) [45]. All of the aforementioned radiotracers are significantly smaller than cancer cells, 15-20 times smaller in size, and all migrate simply via lymphatic flow. They all serve as means of locating the sentinel node and have all been successfully used for the SLNB in the management of thousands of breast cancer or melanoma patients.

In addition, the Food and Drug Administration (FDA)-approved an alternative radiotracer to radiolabeled colloid in the United States, technetium-99-tilmanocept. This radiotracer is explicitly approved by the FDA for SLNB in patients with melanoma, breast cancer or squamous cell carcinoma of the oral cavity. Compared to radiolabeled colloid, technetium-99-tilmanocept features a different receptor-based uptake mechanism. In particular, it targets the CD206 receptor on the surface of macrophages and dendritic cells [12, 56, 57, 53, 58, 59, 60, 61, 62, 63].

## 6. Technical Aspects of Intraoperative Axillary Nodes Evaluation

Pathologists have used new technologies such as immunohistochemistry, serial sectioning, and molecular techniques, including polymerase chain reaction, to detect disease in lymph nodes that would otherwise have gone undetected during routine histopathological examination. This led to the detection of metastases in up to one third of patients who would otherwise have been classified as pN0 at routine histological examination [5, 64].

The American Joint Committee on Cancer, for its 7$^{th}$ edition, based on the assessment of smaller nodal metastases evaluated by hematoxylin-eosin or immunohistochemistry, classified metastases as follows: pN0 is defined by the presence of malignant cells aggregates in regional lymph nodes 0.2 mm (ITCs); pN1mi is defined by the presence of micrometastases (¿0.2 mm and/or more than 200 cells, but none ¿2.0 mm) in regional lymph nodes.

The relevance of these small deposits (ITCs and micrometastases) has been debated extensively. In their presence, the initial guidelines used to recommend completion CALND. However, studies have shown that, thanks to the modern adjuvant therapy regimens, additional surgical treatment of the axilla does not confer any advantage to the overall or disease-free survival of these patients.

Two large studies, the American College of Surgeons Oncology Group (ACOSOG) Z0010 trial and NSABP-32 trial, focused on the prognostic impact of ITCs and micrometastases. In the ACOSOG Z0010 trial, a prospective observational study, occult metastases were detected by immunohistochemical examination in the sentinel nodes of an additional 10.5% of patients who were reported negative on routine hematoxylin-eosin staining. Furthermore, this did not imply a worsening of survival for patients with cT1/T2 N0M0 disease. Meanwhile, NSABP B-32 is the largest trial conducted to evaluate the efficacy of SLNB in early breast cancer. In this trial, occult metastases were detected by immunohistochemistry in a further 15-16% of patients, who had negative sentinel nodes on routine histological staining. However, the presence of occult metastases in the sentinel nodes was not a negative prognostic factor for the overall survival, in line with the findings of the ACOSOG Z0010 study. The findings of these two trials confirm that completion CALND is not required for patients with occult sentinel lymph node metastases (¡2.0 mm) [5, 27, 13, 28].

It is well-established that axillary surgery can cause significant shoulder and arm morbidity. Participants in the ALMANAC trial (SNLB vs CALND), reported high rates of reduction in shoulder flexion and abduction at one month after surgery, but most returned almost to baseline at one year. Arm pain and numbness are more frequently persistent, with almost one third of patients reporting some degree of these symptoms at one year. These symptoms are severe in only a minority of cases. Lymphedema following CALND remains one of the most feared complications. The reported rates vary between 11% and 20% based on data from recent studies such as Z0011, NSABP B32, and ALMANAC [27, 15].

# 7. Diagnostic Imaging Techniques for Preoperative Axillary Lymph Node Evaluation

## 7.1. Mammography

Mammography is the standard screening imaging technique for breast disease. However, as previously mentioned, mammography is not considered reliable for axillary node evaluation, as certain parts of the axillary area may not be visualized by routine mammograms.

Mammography is limited in its ability to distinguish between malignant and benign lymph nodes, especially when they are small or the lymph node involvement is at an early stage, in which case non-specific imaging findings may be found. In addition, there are no consistent criteria for classifying a lymph node as abnormal. In general, mammographic findings suspicious for nodal involvement include enlarged nodes with ill-defined margins and homogeneously dense lymph nodes without a fatty hilum.

The sensitivity and specificity of this technique have been reported to be 31% and 97%, respectively, when using a size larger than 33 mm in the long axis as a criterion for a suspicious node showing homogeneous density with no fatty hilum on mammography. Certainly, the sensitivity and specificity of mammography for the detection of positive lymph nodes in breast cancer patients have been reported at 21% and 99.5%, respectively, with an accuracy of 79.5% [32, 35, 65, 66, 67].

## 7.2. Ultrasound

In addition to clinical palpation of the axilla, the evaluation of regional nodes with axillary ultrasound, using a high-frequency linear-array transducer (7.57 - 17 MHz), has recently been proven to be a useful imaging technique to evaluate both axillae during the assessment of patients with symptoms and signs suspicious for breast cancer. Axillary ultrasound is integrated into the clinical practice guidelines in all dedicated breast units as an instrument of significant clinical utility.

The patient should be in a supine-oblique position with his arm abducted and rotated externally. It is essential to examine the full extent of the axillary contents. A normal lymph node generally has a reniform shape, an uniformly hypoechoic cortex with a maximal thickness of less than 3 mm, smooth margins and an intact central fatty hilum. On the other hand, suspicious findings of axillary nodes include a cortical thickness in excess of 3 mm, an eccentric thickening, irregular margins and an encroachment or displacement of the fatty hilum [32, 68, 69].

Patients with abnormal or suspicious nodes at axillary ultrasound, i.e. nodes showing loss of their fatty hilum, considerable enlargement, cortical thickening or a combination of these factors, are typically subjected to an ultrasound-guided FNAC or CNB. Following an ultrasound-guided biopsy-proven regional spread of the primary breast cancer, the axilla is considered clinically positive and the patient is routinely subjected to CALND, without the need for SLNB as a staging procedure.

It has been indicated that axillary ultrasound and subsequent biopsy represent a feasible, efficient and economically viable staging strategy in preoperative axillary staging. In an updated meta-analysis, preoperative ultrasound and biopsy in early breast cancer had a sensitivity of 50%, a positive predictive value of 100% and a false negative rate of 25%. However, SLNB remains the standard of care if ultrasound does not detect axillary nodal involvement [70, 71, 72, 73, 47, 74, 75].

A systematic literature review reported that ultrasound sensitivity has a wide range for the representation of non-palpable metastatic lymph nodes of 49-87% when based on size and 26-76% when based on morphologic criteria. The specificity was of 55-97% when based on size, and 88-98% when based on morphologic features.

The SOUND trial (Sentinel node vs. Observation after axillary UltrasouND), started in 2012 at the European Institute of Oncology, will assess whether ultrasound staging of the axilla can replace SLNB. This prospective, multicenter, randomized controlled study is enrolling patients with breast cancers smaller than 2 cm (cT1N0) and suitable for breast conserving surgery and SLNB, who are subjected to preoperative axillary ultrasound to exclude suspicion of nodal involvement. Patients with a single indeterminate lymph node are given an ultrasound-guided FNAC. Patients with negative cytology of the single indeterminate lymph node or negative axillary ultrasound are randomized into conventional management (SLNB CALND) or no axillary surgical staging. In the conventional arm,

CALND is performed only in the presence of macrometastases, but not of isolated tumor cells or micrometastases. The primary endpoint is the distant disease-free survival, which will act as a proxy for the overall survival, allowing results to be obtained in a shorter period of time than the overall survival. Secondary endpoints will be the cumulative incidence of distant and axillary recurrences, disease-free survival and overall survival [1, 76].

High-resolution ultrasound is useful for the evaluation of palpable lymph nodes at all levels and non-palpable axillary nodes at low levels. However, results may vary depending by the operator. In addition to axillary lymph nodes detection, magnetic resonance imaging (MRI) can help detect internal mammary and supraclavicular adenopathy. The abnormal cortex of a suspicious lymph node should be biopsied for the maximum possible outcome to determine if any metastases are present. The most suspicious lymph node should be biopsied, as the nodal stage affects overall staging, surgical management, eligibility for various chemotherapy trials and radiation therapy planning [31, 77].

Preoperative axillary ultrasound is widely used to stage breast cancer patients, providing an evaluation of node morphology and allowing targeted biopsy of abnormal nodes. This is important for deciding which patients should proceed directly to CALND and which should first be subjected to SLNB. However, grey-scale ultrasound alone is not flawless and may overestimate or underestimate axillary disease.

Other ultrasound techniques using contrast agents such as microbubbles can help improve diagnostic reliability in the visual evaluation of axillary nodes. Sever and colleagues have shown that contrast-enhanced ultrasound using intradermal injection of phospholipid-stabilized microbubbles containing sulphur hexafluoride gas with a mean diameter of 2.5 m into the breast can be very useful. Ultrasound techniques using microbubbles has demonstrated great ability to locate and biopsy the ultrasound-guided sentinel lymph node and increase the likelihood that such techniques may in the future avoid the need for surgical SLNB in selected patients [50, 78, 79].

Contrast-enhanced ultrasound is well-established in abdominal imaging, but as far as the axilla is concerned it is a relatively new technique that was first introduced in humans by Omoto and colleagues to identify ultrasound-guided sentinel lymph nodes, using 25% albumin solution as a contrast agent. In short, the current procedure is performed with the standard sterile technique of injecting approximately 2 ml of 1% lidocaine into the upper outer quadrant of the breast, adjacent to the nipple. Subsequently, 1 ml of the ultrasound contrast agent is injected intradermally using a 1-ml tuberculin syringe to raise a small bleb in the skin. Then, the breast is gently massaged to help absorb microbubbles into the lymphatic system. Subsequently, using contrast pulse sequencing, breast ultrasound is performed from the periareolar region in search of the microbubbles in the lymphatic channel. Once the microbubbles are seen in the lymphatics, their flow to the axilla is monitored in real time. The first axillary lymph node to fill with the ultrasound contrast agent is presumed to be the sentinel lymph node. Finally, a biopsy of this lymph node is performed and a clip is inserted in the lymph node.

This technology has advanced with the development of second-generation ultrasound contrast agents such as Sonazoid (GE Healthcare, Oslo, Norway), SonoVue (Bracco, Milano, Italy) and Definity (marketed in North America as Luminity by Lantheus Medical Imaging, North Billerica, MA, USA). These newer products stabilize the microbubbles by using an inert gas instead of air, which increases the transit time. This allows for real-time high-resolution imaging of both the arterial and parenchymal enhancement phases within the lymph nodes [40, 80, 81].

### 7.3. Computed Tomography

Computed tomography (CT) is not generally used in the evaluation of axillary nodal status in breast cancer patients. However, it is useful for assessing the extent of the disease as well as distant metastases in patients with advanced breast cancer. Computed tomography can be used to examine the breasts and axillae simultaneously, and is also useful for identifying internal mammary and supraclavicular lymphadenopathy [32, 31].

### 7.4. Magnetic Resonance Imaging

MRI is used primarily for the preoperative assessment of newly diagnosed breast cancer patients and to assess the response to chemotherapy. Preoperative contrast-enhanced breast MRI is useful for detecting cancer foci or metastatic lymph nodes that are not detectable using other preoperative imaging techniques such as mammography or ultrasound. Findings indicating metastases include lymph node cortical thickening, cortical irregularity, loss of fatty hilum and round shape and are similar to ultrasonographic findings [32, 82].

## Conclusion

Ultrasound preoperative assessment of the axilla and potential ultrasound-guided biopsy provide additional information to aid the patient, the surgeon and rest of the multidisciplinary team in the decision-making process and should be used to guide the team towards the best possible management of each individual patient.

Many imaging techniques can be used to preoperatively evaluate axillary nodal status. A detailed knowledge of the diagnostic characteristics and the advantages of combining some of these modalities can be useful for the proper staging of the axillary nodal status and for avoiding unnecessary CALND [32].

Where axillary ultrasound does not suggest a high-volume metastatic disease, but a microbubble-guided lymph node core biopsy contains metastases smaller than 2 mm, for example, the multidisciplinary team may still recommend SLNB (perhaps with a wire-hook or radio-guided localization of the biopsied node) to the informed patient.

In addition, we must not overlook the fact that our imaging capabilities continue to evolve. Perhaps we have not yet reached the limits of what radio-diagnostics can offer. The microbubble technique offers exciting potential to be able to target the sentinel node preoperatively and, with further refinements and experience, we may be able to avoid sentinel lymph node excision and subsequent CALND in selected patients.

Finally, axillary management strategies have evolved rapidly, and it is important that radiologists are familiar with current developments [50].

## References

[1] Ozmen T., Huff Vinyard A., Avisar E. Management of the Positive Axilla in 2017. *Cureus. 2017*;9:e1216. doi:10.7759/cureus.1216.

[2] Virchow R., Chance F. Cellular Pathology: As Based Upon Physiological and Pathological Histology. *Twenty Lectures Delivered in the Pathological Institute of Berlin During the Months of February, March and April, 1858.* R. M. De Witt. 1860.

[3] Hunt K. K., Ballman K. V., McCall L. M., Boughey J. C., Mittendorf E. A., Cox C. E., et al. Factors associated with local-regional recurrence after a negative sentinel node dissection: results of the ACOSOG Z0010 trial. *Ann Surg. 2012*;256:428–436. doi:10.1097/SLA.0b013e3182654494.

[4] McLaughlin S. A., Wright M. J., Morris K. T., Giron G. L., Sampson M. R., Brockway J. P., et al. Prevalence of lymphedema in women with breast cancer 5 years after sentinel lymph node biopsy or axillary dissection: objective measurements. *J Clin Oncol. 2008*;26:5213–5219. doi:10.1200/JCO.2008.16.3725.

[5] Zahoor S., Haji A., Battoo A., Qurieshi M., Mir W., Shah M. Sentinel Lymph Node Biopsy in Breast Cancer: A Clinical Review and Update. *J Breast Cancer. 2017*; 20:217–227. doi:10.4048/jbc.2017.20.3.217.

[6] Gilchrist R. K. Fundamental factors governing lymphatic spread of carcinoma. *Ann Surg. 1940*;111:630–639.

[7] Zeidman I., Buss J. M. Experimental studies on the spread of cancer in the lymphatic system. I. Effectiveness of the lymph node as a barrier to the passage of embolic tumor cells. *Cancer Res. 1954*;14:403–405.

[8] D'Angelo-Donovan D. D., Dickson-Witmer D., Petrelli N. J. Sentinel lymph node biopsy in breast cancer: a history and current clinical recommendations. *Surg Oncol. 2012*;21:196–200. doi:10.1016/j.suronc.2011.12.005.

[9] Kett K., Varga G., Lukacs L. Direct lymphography of the breast. *Lymphology. 1970*; 3:2–12.

[10] Krag D. N., Weaver D. L., Alex J. C., Fairbank J. T. Surgical resection and radiolocalization of the sentinel lymph node in breast cancer using a gamma probe. *Surg Oncol. 1993*;2:335–9; discussion 340.

[11] Giuliano A. E., Kirgan D. M., Guenther J. M., Morton D. L. Lymphatic mapping and sentinel lymphadenectomy for breast cancer. *Ann Surg. 1994*;220:391–8; discussion 398–401.

[12] Moncayo V. M., Alazraki A. L., Alazraki N. P., Aarsvold J. N. Sentinel Lymph Node Biopsy Procedures. *Semin Nucl Med. 2017*;47:595–617. doi: 10.1053/j.semnuclmed.2017.06.004.

[13] Krag D. N., Anderson S. J., Julian T. B., Brown A. M., Harlow S. P., Costantino J. P., et al. Sentinel-lymph-node resection compared with conventional axillary-lymph-node dissection in clinically node-negative patients with breast cancer: overall survival findings from the NSABP B-32 randomised phase 3 trial. *Lancet Oncol. 2010*;11:927–933. doi:10.1016/S1470-2045(10)70207-2.

[14] Zavagno G. , De Salvo G. L., Scalco G., Bozza F., Barutta L., Del Bianco P., et al. A Randomized clinical trial on sentinel lymph node biopsy versus axillary lymph node dissection in breast cancer: results of the Sentinella/GIVOM trial. *Ann Surg. 2008*; 247:207–213. doi:10.1097/SLA.0b013e31812e6a73.

[15] Mansel R. E., Fallowfield L., Kissin M., Goyal A., Newcombe R. G., Dixon J. M., et al. Randomized multicenter trial of sentinel node biopsy versus standard axillary treatment in operable breast cancer: the ALMANAC Trial. *J Natl Cancer Inst. 2006*; 98:599–609. doi:10.1093/jnci/djj158.

[16] Canavese G., Bruzzi P., Catturich A., Tomei D., Carli F., Garrone E., et al. Sentinel Lymph Node Biopsy Versus Axillary Dissection in Node-Negative Early-Stage Breast Cancer: 15-Year Follow-Up Update of a Randomized Clinical Trial. *Ann Surg Oncol. 2016*;23:2494–2500. doi:10.1245/s10434-016-5177-4.

[17] Gill P. G. Sentinel lymph node biopsy versus axillary clearance in operable breast cancer: The RACS SNAC trial, a multicenter randomized trial of the Royal Australian College of Surgeons (RACS) Section of Breast Surgery, in collaboration with the National Health and Medical Research Council Clinical Trials Center. *Ann Surg Oncol. 2004*;11:216S–221S.

[18] Ung O. A. Australasian experience and trials in sentinel lymph node biopsy: the RACS SNAC trial. *Asian J Surg. 2004*;27:284–290. doi:10.1016/S1015-9584(09)60052-X.

[19] Veronesi U., Viale G., Paganelli G., Zurrida S., Luini A., Galimberti V., et al. Sentinel lymph node biopsy in breast cancer: ten-year results of a randomized controlled study. *Ann Surg. 2010*;251:595–600. doi:10.1097/SLA.0b013e3181c0e92a.

[20] Purushotham A. D., Upponi S., Klevesath M. B., Bobrow L., Millar K., Myles J. P., et al. Morbidity after sentinel lymph node biopsy in primary breast cancer: results from a randomized controlled trial. *J Clin Oncol. 2005*;23:4312–4321. doi: 10.1200/JCO.2005.03.228.

[21] Mamounas E. T. P. Optimal Management of the Axilla: A Look at the Evidence. *Adv Surg. 2016*;50:29–40. doi:10.1016/j.yasu.2016.03.003.

[22] Veronesi U., Paganelli G., Viale G., Luini A., Zurrida S., Galimberti V., et al. A randomized comparison of sentinel-node biopsy with routine axillary dissection in breast cancer. *N Engl J Med. 2003*;349:546–553. doi:10.1056/NEJMoa012782.

[23] Gill G., of the Royal Australasian College of Surgeons (RACS) STG, Centre NCT. Sentinel-lymph-node-based management or routine axillary clearance? One-year outcomes of sentinel node biopsy versus axillary clearance (SNAC): a randomized controlled surgical trial. *Ann Surg Oncol. 2009*;16:266–275. doi:10.1245/s10434-008-0229-z.

[24] Krag D. N., Anderson S. J., Julian T. B., Brown A. M., Harlow S. P., Ashikaga T., et al. Technical outcomes of sentinel-lymph-node resection and conventional axillary-lymph-node dissection in patients with clinically node-negative breast cancer: results from the NSABP B-32 randomised phase III trial. *Lancet Oncol. 2007*;8:881–888. doi:10.1016/S1470-2045(07)70278-4.

[25] Canavese G., Catturich A., Vecchio C., Tomei D., Gipponi M., Villa G., et al. Sentinel node biopsy compared with complete axillary dissection for staging early breast cancer with clinically negative lymph nodes: results of randomized trial. *Ann Oncol. 2009*;20:1001–1007. doi:10.1093/annonc/mdn746.

[26] Del Bianco P., Zavagno G., Burelli P., Scalco G., Barutta L., Carraro P., et al. Morbidity comparison of sentinel lymph node biopsy versus conventional axillary lymph node dissection for breast cancer patients: results of the sentinella-GIVOM Italian randomised clinical trial. *Eur J Surg Oncol. 2008*;34:508–513. doi: 10.1016/j.ejso.2007.05.017.

[27] McCartan D., Gemignani M. L. Current Management of the Axilla. *Clin Obstet Gynecol. 2016*;59:743–755. doi:10.1097/GRF.0000000000000232.

[28] Giuliano A. E., Hunt K. K., Ballman K. V., Beitsch P. D., Whitworth P. W., Blumencranz P. W., et al. Axillary dissection vs no axillary dissection in women with invasive breast cancer and sentinel node metastasis: a randomized clinical trial. *JAMA. 2011*; 305:569–575. doi:10.1001/jama.2011.90.

[29] Mamounas E. P., Kuehn T., Rutgers E. J. T., von Minckwitz G. Current approach of the axilla in patients with early-stage breast cancer. *Lancet. 2017*;doi:10.1016/S0140-6736(17)31451-4.

[30] Jagsi R., Chadha M., Moni J., Ballman K., Laurie F., Buchholz T. A., et al. Radiation field design in the ACOSOG Z0011 (Alliance) Trial. *J Clin Oncol. 2014*;32:3600–3606. doi:10.1200/JCO.2014.56.5838.

[31] Lee S. C., Jain P. A., Jethwa S. C., Tripathy D., Yamashita M. W. Radiologist's role in breast cancer staging: providing key information for clinicians. *Radiographics. 2014*; 34:330–342. doi:10.1148/rg.342135071.

[32] Choi H. Y., Park M., Seo M., Song E., Shin S. Y., Sohn Y. M. Preoperative Axillary Lymph Node Evaluation in Breast Cancer: Current Issues and Literature Review. *Ultrasound Q. 2017*;33:6–14. doi:10.1097/RUQ.0000000000000277.

[33] Macéa J. R., Fregnani J. H. T. G. Anatomy of the Thoracic Wall, Axilla and Breast. *Int J Morphol. 2006*;24. doi:10.4067/s0717-95022006000500030.

[34] Dialani V., James D. F., Slanetz P. J. A practical approach to imaging the axilla. *Insights Imaging. 2015*;6:217–229. doi:10.1007/s13244-014-0367-8.

[35] Shetty M. K., Carpenter W. S. Sonographic evaluation of isolated abnormal axillary lymph nodes identified on mammograms. *J Ultrasound Med. 2004*;23:63–71.

[36] Rahbar H., Partridge S. C., Javid S. H., Lehman C. D. Imaging axillary lymph nodes in patients with newly diagnosed breast cancer. *Curr Probl Diagn Radiol. 2012*;41:149–158. doi:10.1067/j.cpradiol.2011.08.002.

[37] Ecanow J. S., Abe H., Newstead G. M., Ecanow D. B., Jeske J. M. Axillary staging of breast cancer: what the radiologist should know. *Radiographics. 2013*;33:1589–1612. doi:10.1148/rg.336125060.

[38] Orucevic A., Chen J., McLoughlin J. M., Heidel R. E., Panella T., Bell J. Is the TNM staging system for breast cancer still relevant in the era of biomarkers and emerging personalized medicine for breast cancer - an institution's 10-year experience. *Breast J. 2015*;21:147–154. doi:10.1111/tbj.12367.

[39] Edge S. B., Compton C. C. The American Joint Committee on Cancer: the 7th edition of the AJCC cancer staging manual and the future of TNM. *Ann Surg Oncol. 2010*; 17:1471–1474. doi:10.1245/s10434-010-0985-4.

[40] Sharma N., Cox K. Axillary Nodal Staging with Contrast-Enhanced Ultrasound. *Curr Breast Cancer Rep. 2017*;9:259–263. doi:10.1007/s12609-017-0258-3.

[41] NICE (National Institute for Health and Care Excellence). *Early and locally advanced breast cancer: diagnosis and treatment (CG80).* Available from: https://www.nice.org.uk/guidance/cg80/, publishen on February 2009, last updated March 2017, accessed on 18/05/2018.

[42] Senkus E., Kyriakides S., Penault-Llorca F., Poortmans P., Thompson A., Zackrisson S., et al. Primary breast cancer: ESMO Clinical Practice Guidelines for diagnosis, treatment and follow-up. *Ann Oncol. 2013*;24 Suppl 6:vi7–v23. doi: 10.1093/annonc/mdt284.

[43] Gradishar W. J., Anderson B. O., Balassanian R., Blair S. L., Burstein H. J., Cyr A., et al. NCCN Guidelines Insights: Breast Cancer, Version 1.2017. *J Natl Compr Canc Netw. 2017*;15:433–451.

[44] Rajesh Y. S., Ellenbogen S., Banerjee B. Preoperative axillary ultrasound scan: its accuracy in assessing the axillary nodal status in carcinoma breast. *Breast. 2002*; 11:49–52. doi:10.1054/brst.2001.0352.

[45] Specht M. C., Fey J. V., Borgen P. I., Cody H. S. Is the clinically positive axilla in breast cancer really a contraindication to sentinel lymph node biopsy? *J Am Coll Surg. 2005*;200:10–14. doi:10.1016/j.jamcollsurg.2004.09.010.

[46] Diepstraten S. C. E., Sever A. R., Buckens C. F. M., Veldhuis W. B., van Dalen T., van den Bosch M. A. A. J., et al. Value of preoperative ultrasound-guided axillary lymph node biopsy for preventing completion axillary lymph node dissection in breast cancer: a systematic review and meta-analysis. *Ann Surg Oncol. 2014*;21:51–59. doi: 10.1245/s10434-013-3229-6.

[47] Houssami N., Ciatto S., Turner R. M., Cody H. S., Macaskill P. Preoperative ultrasound-guided needle biopsy of axillary nodes in invasive breast cancer: meta-analysis of its accuracy and utility in staging the axilla. *Ann Surg. 2011*;254:243–251. doi:10.1097/SLA.0b013e31821f1564.

[48] Pesek S., Ashikaga T., Krag L. E., Krag D. The false-negative rate of sentinel node biopsy in patients with breast cancer: a meta-analysis. *World J Surg. 2012*;36:2239–2251. doi:10.1007/s00268-012-1623-z.

[49] Barthelmes L., Goyal A., Newcombe R. G., McNeill F., Mansel R. E., START N., et al. Adverse reactions to patent blue V dye - The NEW START and ALMANAC experience. *Eur J Surg Oncol. 2010*;36:399–403. doi:10.1016/j.ejso.2009.10.007.

[50] Lowes S., Leaver A., Cox K., Satchithananda K., Cosgrove D., Lim A. Evolving imaging techniques for staging axillary lymph nodes in breast cancer. *Clin Radiol. 2018*;73:396–409. doi:10.1016/j.crad.2018.01.003.

[51] Mokbel K., Mostafa A. The role of subareolar blue dye in identifying the sentinel node in patients with invasive breast cancer. *Curr Med Res Opin. 2001*;17:93–95.

[52] Rescigno J., Zampell J. C, Axelrod D. Patterns of axillary surgical care for breast cancer in the era of sentinel lymph node biopsy. *Ann Surg Oncol. 2009*;16:687–696. doi:10.1245/s10434-008-0195-5.

[53] Ahmed M., Purushotham A. D., Douek M. Novel techniques for sentinel lymph node biopsy in breast cancer: a systematic review. *Lancet Oncol. 2014*;15:e351–e362. doi: 10.1016/S1470-2045(13)70590-4.

[54] Ballardini B., Santoro L., Sangalli C., Gentilini O., Renne G., Lissidini G., et al. The indocyanine green method is equivalent to the mTc-labeled radiotracer method for identifying the sentinel node in breast cancer: a concordance and validation study. *Eur J Surg Oncol. 2013*;39:1332–1336. doi:10.1016/j.ejso.2013.10.004.

[55] Wishart G. C., Loh S. W., Jones L., Benson J. R. A feasibility study (ICG-10) of indocyanine green (ICG) fluorescence mapping for sentinel lymph node detection in early breast cancer. *Eur J Surg Oncol. 2012*;38:651–656. doi:10.1016/j.ejso.2012.05.007.

[56] Jimenez I. R., Roca M., Vega E., Garcia M. L., Benitez A., Bajan M., et al. Particle sizes of colloids to be used in sentinel lymph node radiolocalization. *Nucl Med Commun. 2008*;29:166–172. doi:10.1097/MNM.0b013e3282f258d9.

[57] Cardinal Health 414, LLC. *Lymphoseek prescribing information.* Available from: https://www.lymphoseek.com/content/dam/lymphoseek/web/documents/product-literature/lymphoseek-package-insert.pdf, accessed on 18/05/2018.

[58] Giammarile F., Alazraki N., Aarsvold J. N., Audisio R. A., Glass E., Grant S. F., et al. The EANM and SNMMI practice guideline for lymphoscintigraphy and sentinel node localization in breast cancer. *Eur J Nucl Med Mol Imaging. 2013*;40:1932–1947. doi:10.1007/s00259-013-2544-2.

[59] Wallace A. M., Hoh C. K., Limmer K. K., Darrah D. D., Schulteis G., Vera D. R. Sentinel lymph node accumulation of Lymphoseek and Tc-99m-sulfur colloid using a "2-day" protocol. *Nucl Med Biol. 2009*;36:687–692. doi: 10.1016/j.nucmedbio.2009.04.007.

[60] Baker J. L., Pu M., Tokin C. A., Hoh C. K., Vera D. R., Messer K., et al. Comparison of [(99m)Tc]tilmanocept and filtered [(99m)Tc]sulfur colloid for identification of SLNs in breast cancer patients. *Ann Surg Oncol. 2015*;22:40–45. doi:10.1245/s10434-014-3892-2.

[61] Unkart J. T., Baker J. L., Hosseini A., Hoh C. K., Wallace M. S., Vera D. R., et al. Comparison of Post-injection Site Pain Between Technetium Sulfur Colloid and Technetium Tilmanocept in Breast Cancer Patients Undergoing Sentinel Lymph Node Biopsy. *Ann Surg Oncol. 2015*;22 Suppl 3:S559–S565. doi:10.1245/s10434-015-4802-y.

[62] Wallace A. M., Han L. K., Povoski S. P., Deck K., Schneebaum S., Hall N. C., et al. Comparative evaluation of [(99m)tc]tilmanocept for sentinel lymph node mapping in breast cancer patients: results of two phase 3 trials. *Ann Surg Oncol. 2013*;20:2590–2599. doi:10.1245/s10434-013-2887-8.

[63] Shahrzad M., Moncayo V., Malko J., Halkar R. Rate of sentinel lymph node visualization in fatty breasts: Tc-99m Tilmanocept versus Tc-99m filtered sulfur colloid (abstract N 1481). *J Nucl Med. 2016*;57:1481.

[64] Chagpar A. B. Clinical significance of minimal sentinel node involvement and management options. *Surg Oncol Clin N Am. 2010*;19:493–505. doi: 10.1016/j.soc.2010.03.002.

[65] Kalisher L., Chu A. M, Peyster R. G. Clinicopathological correlations of xeroradiography in determining involvement of metastic axillary nodes in female breast cancer. *Radiology. 1976*;121:333–335. doi:10.1148/121.2.333.

[66] Walsh R., Kornguth P. J., Soo M. S., Bentley R., DeLong D. M. Axillary lymph nodes: mammographic, pathologic, and clinical correlation. *AJR Am J Roentgenol. 1997*;168:33–38. doi:10.2214/ajr.168.1.8976915.

[67] Valente S. A., Levine G. M., Silverstein M. J., Rayhanabad J. A., Weng-Grumley J. G., Ji L., et al. Accuracy of predicting axillary lymph node positivity by physical examination, mammography, ultrasonography, and magnetic resonance imaging. *Ann Surg Oncol. 2012*;19:1825–1830. doi:10.1245/s10434-011-2200-7.

[68] Alvarez S., Aiorbe E., Alcorta P., Lopez F., Alonso I., Cortes J. Role of sonography in the diagnosis of axillary lymph node metastases in breast cancer: a systematic review. *AJR Am J Roentgenol. 2006*;186:1342–1348. doi:10.2214/AJR.05.0936.

[69] Net J. M., Mirpuri T. M., Plaza M. J., Escobar C. A., Whittington E. E., Collado-Mesa F., et al. Resident and fellow education feature: US evaluation of axillary lymph nodes. *Radiographics. 2014*;34:1817–1818. doi:10.1148/rg.347140081.

[70] Charalampoudis P., Markopoulos C., Kovacs T. Controversies and recommendations regarding sentinel lymph node biopsy in primary breast cancer: A comprehensive review of current data. *Eur J Surg Oncol. 2018*;44:5–14. doi: 10.1016/j.ejso.2017.10.215.

[71] Houssami N., Turner R. M. Staging the axilla in women with breast cancer: the utility of preoperative ultrasound-guided needle biopsy. *Cancer Biol Med. 2014*;11:69–77. doi:10.7497/j.issn.2095-3941.2014.02.001.

[72] Houssami N., Diepstraten S. C. E., Cody H. S., Turner R. M., Sever A. R. Clinical utility of ultrasound-needle biopsy for preoperative staging of the axilla in invasive breast cancer. *Anticancer Res. 2014*;34:1087–1097.

[73] Schipper R. J., van Roozendaal L. M., de Vries B., Pijnappel R. M., Beets-Tan R. G. H, Lobbes M. B. I., et al. Axillary ultrasound for preoperative nodal staging in breast cancer patients: is it of added value? *Breast. 2013*;22:1108–1113. doi: 10.1016/j.breast.2013.09.002.

[74] Tucker N. S., Cyr A. E., Ademuyiwa F. O., Tabchy A., George K., Sharma P. K., et al. Axillary Ultrasound Accurately Excludes Clinically Significant Lymph Node Disease in Patients With Early Stage Breast Cancer. *Ann Surg. 2016*;264:1098–1102. doi:10.1097/SLA.0000000000001549.

[75] Nwaogu I. Y., Yan Y., Appleton C. M., Cyr A. E., Margenthaler J. A. Predictors of false negative axillary ultrasound in breast cancer. *J Surg Res. 2015*;198:351–354. doi:10.1016/j.jss.2015.03.057.

[76] Gentilini O., Veronesi U. Abandoning sentinel lymph node biopsy in early breast cancer? A new trial in progress at the European Institute of Oncology of Milan (SOUND: Sentinel node vs Observation after axillary UltraSouND). *Breast. 2012*;21:678–681. doi:10.1016/j.breast.2012.06.013.

[77] Damera A., Evans A. J., Cornford E. J., Wilson A. R. M., Burrell H. C., James J. J., et al. Diagnosis of axillary nodal metastases by ultrasound-guided core biopsy in primary operable breast cancer. *Br J Cancer. 2003*;89:1310–1313. doi: 10.1038/sj.bjc.6601290.

[78] Sever A., Jones S., Cox K., Weeks J., Mills P., Jones P. Preoperative localization of sentinel lymph nodes using intradermal microbubbles and contrast-enhanced ultrasonography in patients with breast cancer. *Br J Surg. 2009*;96:1295–1299. doi: 10.1002/bjs.6725.

[79] Sever A. R., Mills P., Jones S. E., Cox K., Weeks J., Fish D., et al. Preoperative sentinel node identification with ultrasound using microbubbles in patients with breast cancer. *AJR Am J Roentgenol. 2011*;196:251–256. doi:10.2214/AJR.10.4865.

[80] Chung Y. E., Kim K. W. Contrast-enhanced ultrasonography: advance and current status in abdominal imaging. *Ultrasonography. 2015*;34:3–18. doi:10.14366/usg.14034.

[81] Omoto K., Hozumi Y., Omoto Y., Taniguchi N., Itoh K., Fujii Y., et al. Sentinel node detection in breast cancer using contrast-enhanced sonography with 25 *J Clin Ultrasound. 2006*;34:317–326. doi:10.1002/jcu.20241.

[82] He N., Xie C., Wei W., Pan C., Wang W., Lv N., et al. A new, preoperative, MRI-based scoring system for diagnosing malignant axillary lymph nodes in women evaluated for breast cancer. *Eur J Radiol. 2012*;81:2602–2612. doi:10.1016/j.ejrad.2012.03.019.

In: The Sentinel Lymph Node
Editors: A. Londero, S. Bertozzi and C. Cedolini
ISBN: 978-1-53614-557-1


*Chapter 6*

# SENTINEL LYMPH NODE BIOPSY IN MELANOMA

***Roberta Di Vora*[1], *Carla Cedolini*[1], *Cinzia Bulligan*[2], *Fabrizio De Biasio*[3], *Pier Camillo Parodi*[3] and *Serena Bertozzi*[1,*]**
[1]Breast Unit, DAME, University of Udine,
University Hospital of Udine,
[2]Clinic of Dermatology, DAME, University of Udine,
University Hospital of Udine,
[3]Clinic of Plastic Surgery, DAME, University of Udine,
University Hospital of Udine

**Abstract**

The sentinel lymph node biopsy for melanoma is a standard procedure for clinically and imaging node-negative patients. In particular, this procedure is indicated for melanomas thicker than 1mm in any case, and for those thinner than 1mm in the presence of unfavorable prognostic factors. The most commonly used detection technique is the radiocolloid injection, but also indocyanine green seems to be a promising tool. The evaluation of the sentinel node is usually carried out by traditional postoperative histological examination, as the sentinel lymph node biopsy is usually performed under local anesthesia. Macrometastases are an absolute indication for complete regional lymph node dissection, whereas the management of micrometastases is still being disputed. However, it has to be discussed on a case-by-case basis, evaluating all the prognostic factors, and treated prudentially with radical dissection in dubious cases. The region to be completely dissected depends on the location of the sentinel node; it may be the axilla in the case of a positive axillary sentinel node, the inguinal-ilio-obturatory region in the case of a positive inguinal node or the neck region in the case of head and neck melanomas.

**Keywords:** melanoma, sentinel lymph node biopsy, management, macrometastases, micrometastases

---

*Corresponding Author E-mail: dr.bertozzi@gmail.com.

# 1. Introduction

Approximately 85% of melanomas diagnosed worldwide affect the populations of North America, Europe and Oceania [1]. In Italy, melanoma is the second most frequent tumor among men aged less than 50 and the third among women aged less than 50, and is one of the most frequent cancers in young age. Fortunately, despite a progressive increase in melanoma incidence, its mortality appears to be stable, causing around 1% of cancer deaths in both genders [2].

About 2% of melanomas is associated with a genetic mutation. In particular, around 10% of patients with malignant melanoma have an evident familial history, with at least one first-degree relative affected by the same neoplastic disease. Approximately 20% of these familial cases are mutation carriers in a susceptibility gene. The most important genes involved in melanoma onset are CDKN2A, which encodes for two proteins that have a negative control on the cell cycle, and CDK4, which also implies a dysregulation of the cell cycle [3, 4]. Currently, genetic testing is recommended in patients with multiple melanomas, as well as in those with familial history, defined as the presence of at least two first-degree relatives affected by melanoma [5, 6].

Along with the personal or familial history of melanoma, the most significant risk factors for melanoma are the prolonged intermittent exposure to sun or UV radiations and the very light skin phenotype, which strongly influences also the geographical distribution of this neoplastic disease. The prolonged sun exposure in youth results at higher risk than the sun exposure in adulthood [7, 8, 9].

Dermatoscopy, combined with objective examination, represents the main diagnostic tool for melanoma diagnosis [10]. Every lesion ¿6mm with asymmetry, irregular borders or color, or any kind of evolution in time must be histologically analyzed [11, 12]. The prognostic factors that the pathologist must always describe are the following:

- histological subtype (superficial diffusion, nodular, lentigo maligna, acral lentiginous, desmoplastic, nevoid, spitzoid): it is not currently considered an independent prognostic factor [13, 14];
- growth phase: vertical growth is unfavorable if compared with radial growth as it is the phase in which melanoma acquires metastatic capacity [15, 16];
- Breslow thickness: thickness in millimeters is the most significant prognostic factor, and is measured from the granulous layer or, in the case of ulcerated melanoma, from the ulceration base to the maximal infiltration point [16, 17];
- Clark level: describes the skin layers involvement, and is an adjuncted value to Breslow thickness, but is not included in the $8^{th}$ edition of AJCC guidelines [18, 19];
- mitotic index: is the count of mitosis/mmq in the hot spot with major mitotic activity;
- ulceration: it is a predictive factor of metastatic capacity of melanoma to the bone and viscera [20];
- tumor infiltrating lymphocytes (absent, brisk, non brisk): they are predictive factors of lymph node involvement [21];

- regression: it should be measured in terms of percentage of extention, and may involve an underestimation of tumor size and incorrect tumor downstaging [16, 15, 22];
- microsatellites: their prognosis does not seem to differ from the prognosis of melanomas with macrosatellites [23];
- lymphovascular invasion: it is correlated with an increased risk of local relapse or development of in transit metastases [24];
- TNM stage: it is described in the 8$^{th}$ edition of AJCC [25];
- lateral and deep margin status after surgical excision: it is of fundamental importance for assessing the correctness of surgical extension;
- BRAF V600 mutation: specific mutation present in 50% of melanomas [26] that implies a dysfunction in a gene that encodes for a kinase involved in the signal transmission pathway of RAS/RAF/MEK/ERK mitogenic kinases, responsible for cellular proliferation, invasion and survival [27];
- NRAS mutation: mutation present in about 15-20% of melanomas and, as for the BRAF mutation, which must be searched in patients with III or IV stage inoperable melanomas [26];
- cKIT mutation: mutation present in only 1-3% of melanomas but, as for BRAF and NRAS mutations, which must be searched in patients with III or IV stage inoperable melanomas [26].

These factors are also crucial in the therapeutic decision-making process, as they are necessary in the choice of surgical and non-surgical indications.

In the following sections, we will discuss the role of the sentinel node in the treatment of melanoma, its indications, the technical aspects of its detection and analysis, and, finally, the predictive and prognostic value of lymph node metastases.

## 2. Rationale of Sentinel Lymph Node Biopsy in Melanoma

The lymph node status represents a milestone in the field of oncological staging, as tumors tend to spread through both the lymphatic system and bloodstream. The surgical excision of locoregional lymph nodes is fundamental also in the case of malignant melanoma, to exclude its possible lymphatic diffusion.

Postulating that migrating tumor cells from the primary tumor would first metastasize to a single node, or a selected few nodes, before continuing on the rest of the nodal basin and beyond, when examining the sentinel node it is possible to spare the residual nodes, if negative for metastatic involvement. Subsequently, as in the case of other cancers, in order to reduce the overtreatment that occurred in the past by performing elective regional node dissections on clinically node-negative patients, the sentinel lymph node biopsy (SLNB) has become the technique of choice for evaluating lymph node status in the case of melanoma in patients who have been diagnosed with negative nodes during the preoperative clinical and imaging examination.

While the diagnostic skin biopsy allows only an initial prognostic framing, the description of the aforementioned prognostic factors together with the wide local excision and the evaluation of the sentinel lymph node are fundamental to achieving surgical radicality and adequate staging of the disease [28].

The size of the wide local excision is substantially guided by the tumor infiltration and thickness, with the aim of finding possible microsatellites. In particular, in situ melanoma deserves a margin of 5 mm, whereas invasive melanoma with a thickness 2 mm or ¿2 mm requires a margin of 1 cm or 2 cm respectively [29]. An exception to this kind of procedure can only be made in the case of important aesthetic compromise.

The risk of lymph node involvement is directly proportional to the tumor thickness and the amount of mitosis [30, 31, 32, 33, 34]. In particular, nodal involvement is extremely uncommon for melanomas thinner than 0,75 mm, while it may be present in about 25% of cases for melanomas between 1.5 and 4 mm thick and in even 60% of cases for melanomas thicker than 4mm [33, 34].

Thereafter, melanomas thicker than 1 mm are always an indication for SLNB, whereas melanomas thinner than 0.75 mm are not an indication for SLNB, applied exclusively to selected cases where other unfavorable prognostic factors are present, such as the presence of mitosis or lymphocyte infiltration. There is also evidence that extensive regression (¿75% of the lesion), ulceration, under-40 age group and Clark level IV increase the risk of sentinel node micrometastases, and thus constitute indications for SLNB regardless of tumor thickness [28, 35, 36, 37]. Melanomas between 0.75 mm and 1 mm thick are also an indication for SLNB, except in cases where the procedure has more risks than benefits, such as very deep or difficult lymph node localizations (i.e. deep cervical, intra-abdominal, intra-thoracic nodes). In these cases the performance of the procedure has to be discussed with the patient while acquiring their informed consent [38].

Furthermore, some studies have observed that patients with melanoma between 1.2 and 3.5 mm thick who underwent SLNB have a longer disease-free survival than patients who did not undergo SLNB. In particular, patients who promptly received a complete regional lymph node dissection for positive sentinel node appear to have a longer disease-free survival than those who received a complete nodal dissection after nodal recurrence [28]. The same holds true of patients with melanomas thicker than 4 mm. In more detail, SLNB in melanomas between 1.2 and 3.5 mm thick and in melanomas thicker than 4 mm is shown to prevent nodal recurrence in 7% and 12%, respectively, of patients.

Finally, to better tailor the lymph node surgical approach, every patient must preoperatively undergo an accurate objective examination and imaging evaluation of the regional nodes, in order to exclude their clinical macroscopic involvement, also with the use of cytology or biopsy in suspicious nodes. However, despite the accuracy of ultrasound, especially if combined with physical examination, this technique is limited by the small size of metastastic deposits within the lymph nodes [39].

In summary, current evidence supports the use of SLNB as only about 15-20% of patients harbor regional node metastases that may portend a significantly worse prognosis [20]. The procedure is strongly supported in the case of melanomas thicker than 1 mm, while is suggested in the case of melanomas thinner than 1 mm if associated with the presence of other unfavorable prognostic factors [28, 38].

# 3. Technical Aspects

SLNB is considered a minimally invasive procedure to accurately stage the disease, and was first introduced for melanoma in 1989.

In contrast to other tumors, this type of procedure for melanoma has caused a series of controversies. On one hand, it is not always easy to unequivocally detect the lymph node drainage. For example, in the case upper and lower limb melanoma the sentinel node is usually found in the axilla and groin respectively, but no prediction can be made in the case of head or trunk melanoma.

On the other hand, the significance of small amount of metastatic cells within the sentinel lymph node is still a matter of debate.

In the next sections, we will discuss the technical aspects of the SLNB in melanoma and the clinical implications of the eventual presence of sentinel node metastases.

## 3.1. Sentinel Lymph Node Detection Techniques

After the initial use of vital dye to detect the sentinel node, today the most preferred detection method is the preoperative dynamic lymphoscintigraphy after radiotracer injection, as the radiocolloid use has been shown to be significantly superior than the use of vital dye in the sentinel node identification, reaching about 87% to 100% of successful detection rates [40, 41, 42, 43].

Despite the high detection rate by radiocolloid injection, the predictive factors of the non-visualization of the sentinel node at the preoperative lymposcintigraphy are age, head or neck tumor location and previous surgery on any adjacent site [44]. In the case of failed or controversial sentinel node identification, a single photon emission computed tomography (SPECT) can be performed to better define which sentinel node or nodes deserve surgical excision [45].

Recently, new radiotracers have been tested, such as tilmanocept, as well as new additional technologies, including indocyanine green and superparamagnetic iron oxide tracer [46, 47, 48]. In particular, indocyanine green has been of great help in finding occult sentinel nodes in about 24% of patients, potentially able to have an impact on the reduction of the false-negative rate. [49].

A recent meta-analysis provided data that favors the use of radiocolloid by experienced surgeons on account of the multiple disadvantages of vital dye, and considers indocyanine green as a promising technique for the near future [50].

SLNB is feasible also during pregnancy without increasing adverse events, but it is desirable to wait until the 12th week of gestation to conjointly reduce the anesthesiological risk [51], and not to use vital dye because of its possible teratogenic effects and its 1% risk of anaphylaxis [52].

## 3.2. Sentinel Lymph Node Evaluation Techniques

Since SLNB is usually performed at the same time of the wide local excision, the operation is carried out under local anesthesia only or supported by a mild sedation. The excised nodes are then sent to definitive histological examination and usually analyzed by classical histological examination. In detail, the formalin-fixed and paraffin-embedded specimen is hematoxylin-eosin-stained and cut into 0.15-mm-spaced sections, which are then morphologically evaluated.

In the case of melanoma, OSNA method is not applied, no due to the lack of a valid mRNA marker, but because there is no need for a rapid lymph node analysis. In fact, patients are usually operated under local anesthesia and the specimen examination can be performed comfortably after surgery, without changing any intraoperative choice.

In the lymph node histological examination it is recommended to remark the following characteristics:

- maximal size of metastatatic foci
- site of metastatatic foci (capsular, subcapsular, parenchimal, mixed)
- eventual extracapsular extension
- nevic cells presence
- invasion depth by Starz, measured from the inner layer of the lymph node capsula to the deepest infiltration point in the lymph node parenchima [53]

### 3.3. Complications of the Sentinel Lymph Node Biopsy

The purpose of SLNB is to reduce lymphadenectomy morbidity by maintaining an adequate prognostic value. In particular, if complete regional dissections are associated with a rate of complications of 65%, including wound dehiscence, cellulitis, hematoma, seroma, lymphedema, and nerve injuring [54, 55, 56], the overall complication rate of SLNB alone is about 5%, usually due to seroma, hematoma, lymphocele or infection [57].

The rate of complications also varies from site to site. In fact, if axillary lymph node dissection has a complication rate of 4.6%, inguinal dissection can reach a complication rate of about 31.5%, while neck dissection up to about 40%.

Very rarely SLNB may be a cause of lymphedema in patients with previous lymphatic defects due to deep wounds or additional radio- and chemotherapy.

## 4. Prediction of the Non-Sentinel Lymph Node Status

Although SLNB represents a valuable staging and prognostic tool, there is a small percentage of patients with negative sentinel node that later develop a nodal recurrence in the dissected nodal basin, likely due to a missed microscopic nodal disease. This percentage is called false-negative rate and in the literature ranges between 0% and 34% with a weighted summary estimate value of 12.5% [42].

In the literature, additional non-sentinel nodal involvement is around 15-20% in case of positive sentinel node, and nodal recurrence varies between 4% and 15% [58, 59]. Several histological features of metastatic melanoma in the sentinel node have been shown to predict non-sentinel node involvement, such as the increasing size or depth of tumor deposits and the intranodal non-subcapsular location [60, 61, 62, 63]. Over time, several different classification systems have been developed to predict non sentinel nodal disease, but none of them is universally accepted [64, 65, 66, 67].

Thereafter, primary complete dissection is recommended for regional disease control in the case of positive sentinel node. However, although immediate complete nodal dissection for positive sentinel node improves the survival rate and significantly reduces the complication rate of patients compared with rescue radical dissection after recurrence, there is no direct evidence that complete dissections definitely impart a survival benefit [68, 28, 69].

Moreover, recent studies have focused on biomolecular markers that may predict lymph nodes metastases, by increasing tissutal angiogenetic and lymphoangiogenetic capability, modifying the local immune environment and increasing intra-tumoral interstitial fluid pressure causing widened inter-endothelial openings [70, 71, 72]. Finally, studies on melanoma gene expression profile have identified a wide variety of genetic, epigenetic and proteomic markers that could help predict nodal involvement disease in the future, such as higher expression levels of NCOA3, SPP1 or RGS proteins [73, 74, 75].

# 5. Management of the Macrometastases

Lymph node macrometastases are an indication for complete regional lymph node dissection, which results in a significant improvement of local disease control and correlation with longer disease-free survival [76, 77]. In addition, in the case of nodal macrometastases it is strongly recommended to evaluate the presence of BRAF, NRAS and c-KIT gene mutations [78].

The dissection site and extension are related to the anatomical region of melanoma. Next, we will describe the complete dissection procedure based on the localization of the sentinel node [79, 80].

## 5.1. Complete Axillary Lymph Node Dissection

Positive axillary sentinel node is an indication for complete axillary dissection. The axilla is a quadrangular space limited superiorly by the axillary vein, medially by the chest wall, laterally by the axillary skin, anteriorly by the pectoralis major and minor muscles, and posteriorly by the latissimus dorsi, the teres major, and the subcapularis muscles. Although the nodes are in a continuum, they can be anatomically divided into three levels based on the relation of the tissue to the pectoralis minor muscle (Figure 1). An adequate axillary dissection must include all three levels and should remove all the nodes and fat from this space, with a minimum of 12 lymph nodes [79].

Although SLNB can be carried out under local anesthesia, complete axillary dissection is preferably performed under general anesthesia. Additional local anesthetics may be injected around the axillary incision site and can be instilled directly into the remaining axillary structures. Patients are placed in a supine position, with the arm abducted at 90 degrees from the chest wall on an armboard. The surgical site is usually shaved with electric clippers.

Subsequently, axillary dissection is performed through an incision of about 5-6 cm in the axillary cavity. Often, the surgeon's preference is for a skin crease incision just below the axillary hairline extending from the posterior edge of the pectoral fold to the posterior axillary line. Dissection is carried out past the edge of the pectoralis major muscle. The retraction of the pectoralis major medially exposes the pectoralis minor muscle and the clavipectoral fascia, which is then incised to allow entry into the axilla. Consequently, axillary fat is also incised and the contained nodes are removed en bloc.

Dissection is carried out superiorly along the edge of the pectoralis minor muscle to reach the inferior edge of the axillary vein. Once the axillary vein has been identified, it is followed medially to reach the axillary apex, where the axillary vein crosses the lateral border of the first rib. The axillary content is then separated from the lateral thoracic wall, exposing the long thoracic nerve, which supplies the serratus anterior muscle, and should be spared when possible to prevent scapular winging.

While carrying out the dissection, the branches of the intercostobrachial nerve will also be identified, as they cross the axilla after emerging from the intercostal spaces. The larger trunks should be preserved if possible, as well as the thoracodorsal nerve and vessels, which are usually visualized and identified after the ligation and division of the smaller tributaries of the axillary vein and which reach the subscapular and the latissimus dorsi muscles posteriorly.

The axillary fat and nodal tissue between the long thoracic nerve and the subscapular vascular bundle are carefully dissected. Often, this procedure is performed as a single en bloc specimen, although it sometimes can occur separately if there is an extensive nodal involvement. The dissection is then carried out towards the apex to include the level III nodes that are medial to the pectoralis minor muscle, and this maneuver may be facilitated by the flexion at the shoulder of the free draped arm. The axillary fat and nodes are then separated from the axillary tail of the breast to allow direct excision of the specimen. Finally, after a careful hemostasis control and the positioning of a drainage within the excision bed, the wound is closed by layers.

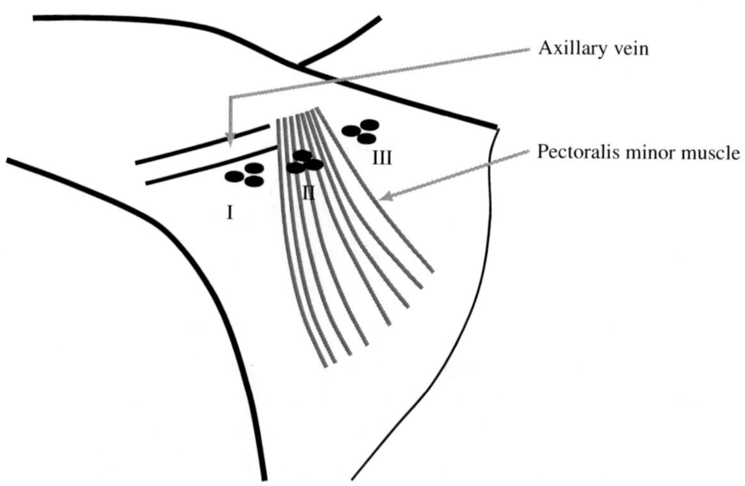


Figure 1. Axilla lymph nodes (drawing by SB and APL).

## 5.2. Complete Neck Lymph Node Dissection

In the case of positive latero-cervical sentinel nodes, radical neck dissection is indicated and it must include at least 4 levels and 14 lymph nodes. This procedure was first described in 1906 and until recently was considered the standard procedure for the management of both occult and clinically positive neck disease [81]. In the past few decades, there has been a shift towards the use of more conservative surgical procedures, as the conservation of non-lymphatic structures yields equivalent oncologic outcomes by improving the functional results, and also as the specific nodal groups at risk for metastatic disease are reliably predictable on the basis of size, location, and other features of the primary tumor [82, 83, 84, 85, 86].

The lymphatic drainage of the mucosal surfaces and other head and neck tissues is directed to the lymph nodes located within the fibroadipose tissue between the superficial layer of the deep fascia and the visceral and prevertebral layers underneath it. In this space, lymph nodes tend to be aggregated around certain neural and vascular structures, such as the internal jugular vein, the spinal accessory nerve, and the transverse cervical artery [87], and are currently grouped, according to the Memorial Sloan Kettering Cancer Center classification, into 5 levels corresponding to: submandibular and submental nodes (level I); upper, middle, and lower jugular nodes (levels II, III, IV); posterior triangle nodes (level V) (Figure 2). Level VI has been then introduced to describe mid-anterior lymph nodes of the neck.

Radical neck lymph node dissection is an en bloc clearance of all the fibrous-fatty tissue from one side of the neck, including all the lymph nodes from levels I to V and the lymph nodes that surround the tail of the parotid gland, the spinal accessory nerve, the internal jugular vein and the sternocleidomastoid muscle. Modified radical neck dissection involves the removal of the same nodal groups, while preserving some non-lymphatic structures, such as the spinal accessory nerve, the internal jugular vein, and the sternocleidomastoid muscle [88]. On the other hand, extended neck dissection, usually used in the case of advanced neck disease, in order to obtain negative margins, includes certain lymphatic or non-lymphatic structures not routinely considered in the aforementioned dissections, such as retropharyngeal lymph nodes, the hypoglossal nerve, portions of the prevertebral musculature, or the carotid artery.

However, taking into consideration the specific location of the primary tumor, the lymph node groups most likely to be involved with metastatic disease can be excised and consequently the lymph node groups which carry negligible risk of involvement can be preserved. Although a great variety of surgical procedures have been described, the American Academy of Otolaryngology-Head and Neck Surgery (AAO-HNS) and the Committee for Head and Neck Surgery and Oncology have developed an universally accepted classification system for neck dissections that was lastly modified in 2008 [89, 90, 91, 92, 93]: supraomohyoid neck dissection (levels I, II, III), lateral neck dissection (levels II, III, IV), anterior compartment neck dissection (VI), and posterolateral neck dissection (levels II, III, IV, V).

Selective posterolateral neck dissection (II-V, postauricular, suboccipital) was initially described in 1962 for cutaneous malignancies of the scalp, postauricular or suboccipital regions. This operation is performed with the patient in the lateral decubitus position and consists of an en bloc removal of the lymph nodes of the suboccipital, postauricular, upper, middle, and lower jugular nodes, along with the posterior triangle nodes situated superior to the accessory nerve [94]. In cancers arising in the preauricular and anterior scalp or in the temporal region the elective neck dissection of choice is selective neck dissection (II,

III, Va, parotid, facial, external jugular nodes).

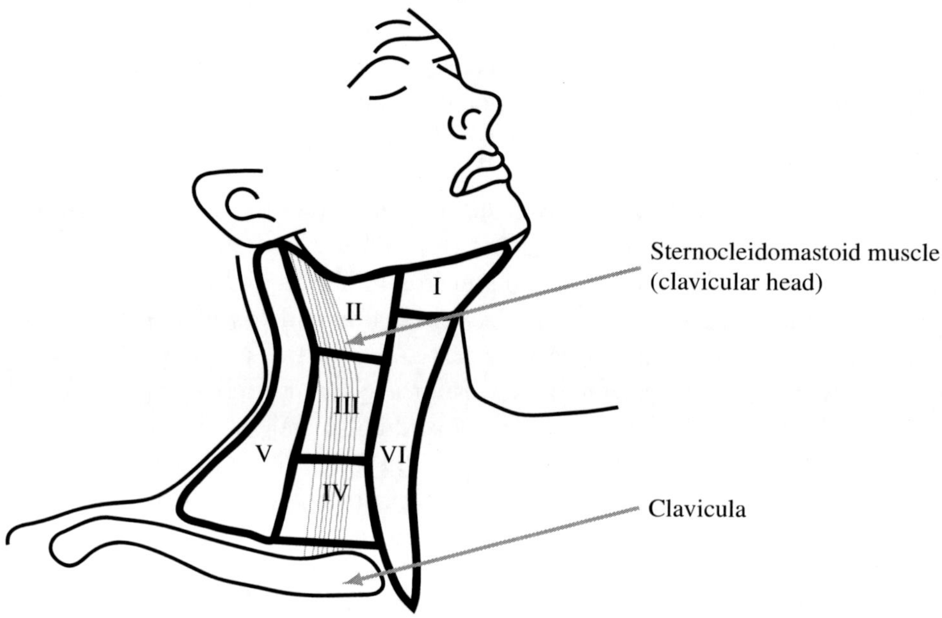


Figure 2. Cervical lymph nodes (drawing by SB and APL).

## 5.3. Complete Inguino-Iliaco-Obturatory Lymph Node Dissection

The presence of a positive inguinal sentinel node implies the need for an ipsilateral complete inguinal-ilio-obturatory dissection, which must include at least 13 nodes, in spite of the fact that this kind of procedure is still characterized by clinical uncertainty in addition to high morbidity [95] (Figure 3).

The superficial inguinal nodes, which are located superficially to the fascia lata within the boundaries of the femoral triangle, receive afferent superficial lymphatics from the lower extremity, the scrotum, the penis, the vulva, the clitoris, the anus, and the infra-umbilical region of the anterior abdominal wall. The femoral triangle is delimited by the inguinal ligament superiorly, the adductor longus medially, and the sartorius laterally. Its roof and floor are constituted by the fascia lata and by the iliopsoas and pectineus, respectively.

The six to eight deep inguinal nodes are located deeply to the fascia lata and medially to the femoral vein, and include the Cloquet's node, which is situated at the apex of the femoral canal. They receive afferents from the superficial inguinal nodes and from the deep lymphatic trunks associated with the femoral vessels draining the popliteal nodes, and drain the lymph into the external iliac nodes.

The ilio-obturatory lymph nodes are located inside the abdomen along the course of the iliac vein up to the obturatory foramen. The boundaries of ilio-obturatory dissection are the genito-femoralis nerve and the ileo-psoas muscle laterally, the internal iliac artery and the caudal-lateral umbilical legament medially, the bifurcation of the common iliac artery cranially, the deep iliac circumflex vein caudally.

For the inguinal-ilio-obturatory dissection, the patient is positioned supine. The incision must depart from about 5 cm under the crossing point of the femoral vein and the inguinal ligament and, passing through it, reach a point on the first third of the line between the upper anterior iliac spina and the umbilicus. Recent studies have shown that multiple small incisions rather than a large inguinal-abdominal incision reduce the postoperative complications resulting from excessive tissue removal [96].

The superficial and deep inguinal nodes are removed through a lower incision under the inguinal ligament, while the ilio-obturatory nodes are removed through an upper incision after having shifted the peritoneum medially. In the case of the possible opening of the peritoneum, it must be immediately sutured to avoid delays in subsequent postoperative feeding. After an accurate control of hemostasis, two drainages are usually placed. The iliac drainage may pass through the inguinal ligament and exit close to the inguinal one.

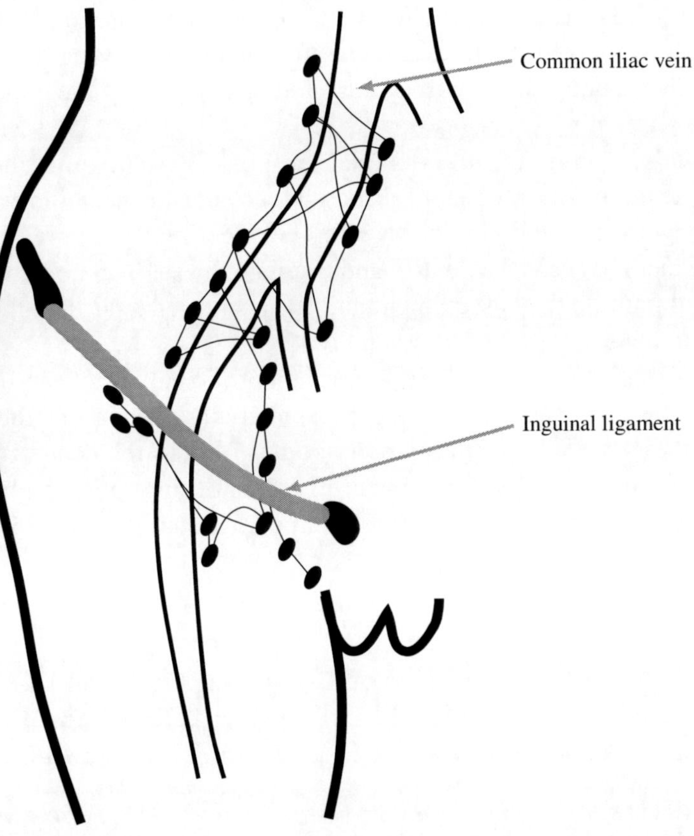


Figure 3. Inguinal-ilio-obturatory dissection (drawing by SB and APL).

## 6. Management of the Micrometastases

Unlike other cancers, in the case of melanoma, small amounts of metastatic cells are a very unfavorable prognostic factor. In fact, if a negative sentinel node predicts the negative status of the remaining nodes in at least 96% of cases [97, 98, 99, 28], the presence of micrometastases predicts an involvement of the other nodes in around 20% of cases [100, 101]. Also, cancer cell dissemination to the sentinel node may be considered a quantitative risk factor for melanoma-related mortality, especially if combined with other unfavorable prognostic factors, such as thickness and ulceration [102].

Some authors have shown that deposits of less than 0,1 mm are correlated with outcomes similar to those of negative sentinel nodes [103, 104, 105, 106, 77]. In any case, more recently, other authors have shown that even very small deposits (¡0,1 mm) of metastatic melanoma in the sentinel node cannot be safely regarded as negative due to their association with adverse clinical outcomes [65, 107].

In addition, there are many other factors that may affect the prognosis of patients with melanoma [102], as well as other technical limitations that may have an impact on the detection and measurement of small deposits, with a consequent risk of underestimation [104, 108, 109, 110]. For example, the most appropriate staining and sectioning protocol is not clear from the available literature, and classifying and measuring these parameters can be extremely difficult, depending on the nature and distribution of the tumor deposits in the sentinel node [104].

Therefore, with the presence of a minimal level of metastatic tumor burden in the sentinel node, despite the negligible risk of disease recurrence or melanoma-related mortality, subsequent management could be facilitated by considering the natural history of disease progression, the methods used to identify and evaluate the sentinel node, the inter-observer reproducibility of pathological assessment and the issues related to the therapies administered as well as to the subsequent follow-up [104].

Furthermore, studies about the micro-morphometric analysis of the intra-nodal distribution of metastatic cells have found that the Starz's classification of the invasion depth, measured from the inner layer of the lymph node capsula to the deepest infiltration point in the lymph node parenchima, was very helpful in identifying patients who would actually benefit from a complete regional dissection for a positive sentinel node [53, 111].

# References

[1] Ferlay J., Shin H. R., Bray F., Forman D., Mathers C., Parkin D. M. GLOBOCAN 2008, cancer incidence and mortality worldwide: IARC CancerBase No. 10 [Internet]. Lyon, France: *International Agency for Research on Cancer. 2010*;2.

[2] AIOM-AIRTUM. I *numeri del cancro in Italia 2016. [Cancer numbers in Italy 2016.]* Il Pensiero Scientifico Editore. 2016.

[3] Goldstein A. M., Chan M., Harland M., Hayward N. K., Demenais F., Bishop D. T., et al. Features associated with germline CDKN2A mutations: a GenoMEL study of melanoma-prone families from three continents. *J Med Genet. 2007*;44:99–106. doi:10.1136/jmg.2006.043802.

[4] Kefford R., Bishop J. N., Tucker M., Bressac-de Paillerets B., Bianchi-Scarri G., Bergman W., et al. Genetic testing for melanoma. *Lancet Oncol. 2002*;3:653–654.

[5] American Society of Clinical Oncology. American Society of Clinical Oncology policy statement update: genetic testing for cancer susceptibility. *J Clin Oncol. 2003*; 21:2397–2406. doi:10.1200/JCO.2003.03.189.

[6] Bruno W., Ghiorzo P., Battistuzzi L., Ascierto P. A., Barile M., Gargiulo S., et al. Clinical genetic testing for familial melanoma in Italy: a cooperative study. *J Am Acad Dermatol. 2009*;61:775–782. doi:10.1016/j.jaad.2009.03.039.

[7] Ivry G. B., Ogle C. A., Shim E. K. Role of sun exposure in melanoma. *Dermatol Surg. 2006*;32:481–492. doi:10.1111/j.1524-4725.2006.32101.x.

[8] Gandini S., Sera F., Cattaruzza M. S., Pasquini P., Picconi O., Boyle P., et al. Meta-analysis of risk factors for cutaneous melanoma: II. Sun exposure. *Eur J Cancer. 2005*;41:45–60. doi:10.1016/j.ejca.2004.10.016.

[9] Whiteman D. C., Whiteman C. A., Green A. C. Childhood sun exposure as a risk factor for melanoma: a systematic review of epidemiologic studies. *Cancer Causes Control. 2001*;12:69–82.

[10] Vestergaard M. E., Macaskill P., Holt P. E., Menzies S. W. Dermoscopy compared with naked eye examination for the diagnosis of primary melanoma: a meta-analysis of studies performed in a clinical setting. *Br J Dermatol. 2008*;159:669–676. doi: 10.1111/j.1365-2133.2008.08713.x.

[11] Healsmith M. F., Bourke J. F., Osborne J. E., Graham-Brown R. A. An evaluation of the revised seven-point checklist for the early diagnosis of cutaneous malignant melanoma. *Br J Dermatol. 1994*;130:48–50.

[12] Abbasi N. R, Shaw H. M., Rigel D. S., Friedman R. J., McCarthy W. H., Osman I., et al. Early diagnosis of cutaneous melanoma: revisiting the ABCD criteria. *JAMA. 2004*;292:2771–2776. doi:10.1001/jama.292.22.2771.

[13] Scolyer R. A., Long G. V., Thompson J. F. Evolving concepts in melanoma classification and their relevance to multidisciplinary melanoma patient care. *Molecular oncology. 2011*;5:124–136. doi:10.1016/j.molonc.2011.03.002.

[14] Callender G. G., Egger M. E., Burton A. L., Scoggins C. R., Ross M. I., Stromberg A. J., et al. Prognostic implications of anatomic location of primary cutaneous melanoma of 1 mm or thicker. *Am J Surg. 2011*;202:659–64; discussion 664–5. doi:10.1016/j.amjsurg.2011.06.048.

[15] Clark W. H., Elder D. E., Guerry D., Braitman L. E., Trock B. J., Schultz D., et al. Model predicting survival in stage I melanoma based on tumor progression. *J Natl Cancer Inst. 1989*;81:1893–1904.

[16] Guerry D., Synnestvedt M., Elder D. E., Schultz D., Lessons from tumor progression: the invasive radial growth phase of melanoma is common, incapable of metastasis, and indolent. *J Invest Dermatol. 1993*;100:342S–345S.

[17] Breslow A. Thickness, cross-sectional areas and depth of invasion in the prognosis of cutaneous melanoma. *Ann Surg. 1970*;172:902–908.

[18] Gimotty P. A., Elder D. E., Fraker D. L., Botbyl J., Sellers K., Elenitsas R., et al. Identification of high-risk patients among those diagnosed with thin cutaneous melanomas. *J Clin Oncol. 2007*;25:1129–1134. doi:10.1200/JCO.2006.08.1463.

[19] Battner P., Garbe C., Bertz J., Burg G., d'Hoedt B., Drepper H., et al. Primary cutaneous melanoma. Optimized cutoff points of tumor thickness and importance of Clark's level for prognostic classification. *Cancer. 1995*;75:2499–2506.

[20] Balch C. M., Gershenwald J. E., Soong S. J., Thompson J. F., Atkins M. B., Byrd D. R., et al. Final version of 2009 AJCC melanoma staging and classification. *J Clin Oncol. 2009*;27:6199–6206. doi:10.1200/JCO.2009.23.4799.

[21] Azimi F. , Scolyer R. A., Rumcheva P., Moncrieff M., Murali R., McCarthy S. W., et al. Tumor-infiltrating lymphocyte grade is an independent predictor of sentinel lymph node status and survival in patients with cutaneous melanoma. *J Clin Oncol. 2012*;30:2678–2683. doi:10.1200/JCO.2011.37.8539.

[22] Ribero S., Osella-Abate S., Sanlorenzo M., Savoia P., Astrua C., Cavaliere G., et al. Favourable prognostic role of regression of primary melanoma in AJCC stage I-II patients. *Br J Dermatol. 2013*;169:1240–1245. doi:10.1111/bjd.12586.

[23] Bartlett E. K., Gupta M., Datta J., Gimotty P. A., Guerry D., Xu X., et al. Prognosis of patients with melanoma and microsatellitosis undergoing sentinel lymph node biopsy. *Ann Surg Oncol. 2014*;21:1016–1023. doi:10.1245/s10434-013-3388-5.

[24] Stucky C. C. H., Gray R. J., Dueck A. C., Wasif N., Laman S. D., Sekulic A., et al. Risk factors associated with local and in-transit recurrence of cutaneous melanoma. *Am J Surg. 2010*;200:770–4; discussion 774–5. doi:10.1016/j.amjsurg.2010.07.025.

[25] Amin M. B., Edge S. B., Greene F. L., Byrd D. R., Brookland R. K., Washington M. K., et al., editors. *AJCC Cancer Staging Manual.* Springer International Publishing. 2017. doi:10.1007/978-3-319-40618-3.

[26] Long G. V., Menzies A. M., Nagrial A. M., Haydu L. E., Hamilton A. L., Mann G. J., et al. Prognostic and clinicopathologic associations of oncogenic BRAF in metastatic melanoma. *J Clin Oncol. 2011*;29:1239–1246. doi:10.1200/JCO.2010.32.4327.

[27] Network CGA. Genomic Classification of Cutaneous Melanoma. *Cell. 2015*; 161:1681–1696. doi:10.1016/j.cell.2015.05.044.

[28] Morton D. L., Thompson J. F., Cochran A. J., Mozzillo N., Nieweg O. E., Roses D. F., et al. Final trial report of sentinel-node biopsy versus nodal observation in melanoma. *N Engl J Med. 2014*;370:599–609. doi:10.1056/NEJMoa1310460.

[29] Sladden M. J., Balch C., Barzilai D. A., Berg D., Freiman A., Handiside T., et al. Surgical excision margins for primary cutaneous melanoma. *Cochrane Database Syst Rev. 2009*;CD004835. doi:10.1002/14651858.CD004835.pub2.

[30] Cordeiro E., Gervais M. K., Shah P. S., Look Hong N. J., Wright F. C., Sentinel Lymph Node Biopsy in Thin Cutaneous Melanoma: A Systematic Review and Meta-Analysis. *Ann Surg Oncol. 2016*;23:4178–4188. doi:10.1245/s10434-016-5137-z.

[31] Stankard C., Cruse C. W., Cox C., Wells K. E., King J., Reintgen D. S., The concept of lymph node dissections in patients with malignant melanoma. *Ann Plast Surg. 1992*;28:33–38.

[32] Balch C. M. The John Wayne Clinical Research Lecture. Surgical management of melanoma: results of prospective randomized trials. *Ann Surg Oncol. 1998*;5:301–309.

[33] Veronesi U., Adamus J., Bandiera D. C., Brennhovd I. O., Caceres E., Cascinelli N., et al. Stage I melanoma of the limbs. Immediate versus delayed node dissection. *Tumori. 1980*;66:373–396.

[34] McCarthy W. H., Shaw H. M., Cascinelli N., Santinami M., Belli F. Elective lymph node dissection for melanoma: two perspectives. *World J Surg. 1992*;16:203–213.

[35] Maurichi A., Miceli R., Camerini T., Mariani L., Patuzzo R., Ruggeri R., et al. Prediction of survival in patients with thin melanoma: results from a multi-institution study. *J Clin Oncol. 2014*;32:2479–2485. doi:10.1200/JCO.2013.54.2340.

[36] Mitteldorf C., Bertsch H. P., Jung K., Thomas K. M., Schaun M. P., Tronnier M., et al. Sentinel node biopsy improves prognostic stratification in patients with thin (pT1) melanomas and an additional risk factor. *Ann Surg Oncol. 2014*;21:2252–2258. doi:10.1245/s10434-014-3641-6.

[37] Ribero S., Gualano M. R., Osella-Abate S., Scaioli G., Bert F., Sanlorenzo M., et al. Association of Histologic Regression in Primary Melanoma With Sentinel Lymph Node Status: A Systematic Review and Meta-analysis. *JAMA dermatology. 2015*; 151:1301–1307. doi:10.1001/jamadermatol.2015.2235.

[38] Mozzillo N., Pennacchioli E., Gandini S., Caraci C., Crispo A., Botti G., et al. Sentinel node biopsy in thin and thick melanoma. *Ann Surg Oncol. 2013*;20:2780–2786. doi:10.1245/s10434-012-2826-0.

[39] Pilko G., Zgajnar J., Music M., Hocevar M. Lower tumour burden and better overall survival in melanoma patients with regional lymph node metastases and negative preoperative ultrasound. *Radiology and oncology. 2012*;46:60–68. doi:10.2478/v10019-011-0028-1.

[40] Morton D. L., Thompson J. F., Essner R., Elashoff R., Stern S. L., Nieweg O. E., et al. Validation of the accuracy of intraoperative lymphatic mapping and sentinel lymphadenectomy for early-stage melanoma: a multicenter trial. Multicenter Selective Lymphadenectomy Trial Group. *Ann Surg. 1999*;230:453–63; discussion 463–5.

[41] Liu L. C., Parrett B. M., Jenkins T., Lee W., Morita E., Treseler P., et al. Selective sentinel lymph node dissection for melanoma: importance of harvesting nodes with

lower radioactive counts without the need for blue dye. *Ann Surg Oncol. 2011*; 18:2919–2924. doi:10.1245/s10434-011-1689-0.

[42] Valsecchi M. E., Silbermins D., de Rosa N., Wong S. L., Lyman G. H., Lymphatic mapping and sentinel lymph node biopsy in patients with melanoma: a meta-analysis. *J Clin Oncol. 2011*;29:1479–1487. doi:10.1200/JCO.2010.33.1884.

[43] Uhara H., Yamazaki N., Takata M., Inoue Y., Sakakibara A., Nakamura Y., et al. Applicability of radiocolloids, blue dyes and fluorescent indocyanine green to sentinel node biopsy in melanoma. *J Dermatol. 2012*;39:336–338. doi:10.1111/j.1346-8138.2011.01340.x.

[44] Schuitevoerder D., Grinlington L., Stevens J., Nance R., Fortino J., Vetto J. T. Nonvisualized sentinel lymph nodes on lymphoscintigraphy in melanoma: predictive factors and surgical outcomes. *Nucl Med Commun. 2017*;38:383–387. doi: 10.1097/MNM.0000000000000658.

[45] Stoffels I., Dissemond J., Pappel T., Schadendorf D., Klode J. Intraoperative Fluorescence Imaging for Sentinel Lymph Node Detection: Prospective Clinical Trial to Compare the Usefulness of Indocyanine Green vs Technetium Tc 99m for Identification of Sentinel Lymph Nodes. *JAMA surgery. 2015*;150:617–623. doi: 10.1001/jamasurg.2014.3502.

[46] Sondak V. K., King D. W., Zager J. S., Schneebaum S., Kim J., Leong S. P. L., et al. Combined analysis of phase III trials evaluating [mTc]tilmanocept and vital blue dye for identification of sentinel lymph nodes in clinically node-negative cutaneous melanoma. *Ann Surg Oncol. 2013*;20:680–688. doi:10.1245/s10434-012-2612-z.

[47] Pouw J. J., Grootendorst M. R., Bezooijen R., Klazen C. A. H., De Bruin W. I., Klaase J. M., et al. Pre-operative sentinel lymph node localization in breast cancer with superparamagnetic iron oxide MRI: the SentiMAG Multicentre Trial imaging subprotocol. *Br J Radiol. 2015*;88:20150634. doi:10.1259/bjr.20150634.

[48] Polom K., Murawa D., Nowaczyk P., Rho Y. S., Murawa P. Breast cancer sentinel lymph node mapping using near infrared guided indocyanine green and indocyanine green–human serum albumin in comparison with gamma emitting radioactive colloid tracer. *Eur J Surg Oncol. 2012*;38:137–142. doi:10.1016/j.ejso.2011.11.004.

[49] Fujisawa Y., Nakamura Y., Kawachi Y., Otsuka F. Indocyanine green fluorescence-navigated sentinel node biopsy showed higher sensitivity than the radioisotope or blue dye method, which may help to reduce false-negative cases in skin cancer. *J Surg Oncol. 2012*;106:41–45. doi:10.1002/jso.23045.

[50] Niebling M. G., Pleijhuis R. G., Bastiaannet E., Brouwers A. H., van Dam G. M., Hoekstra H. J. A systematic review and meta-analyses of sentinel lymph node identification in breast cancer and melanoma, a plea for tracer mapping. *Eur J Surg Oncol. 2016*;42:466–473. doi:10.1016/j.ejso.2015.12.007.

[51] Andtbacka R. H. I, Donaldson M. R., Bowles T. L., Bowen G. M., Grossmann K., Khong H., et al. Sentinel lymph node biopsy for melanoma in pregnant women. *Ann Surg Oncol. 2013*;20:689–696. doi:10.1245/s10434-012-2633-7.

[52] Cragan J. D. Teratogen update: methylene blue. *Teratology. 1999*;60:42–48. doi: 10.1002/(SICI)1096-9926(199907)60:1¡42::AID-TERA12¿3.0.CO;2-Z.

[53] Starz H., Siedlecki K., Balda B. R. Sentinel lymphonodectomy and s-classification: a successful strategy for better prediction and improvement of outcome of melanoma. *Ann Surg Oncol. 2004*;11:162S–168S.

[54] Brouns E., Donceel P., Stas M. Quality of life and disability after ilio-inguinal lymphadenectomy. *Acta Chir Belg. 2008*;108:685–690.

[55] de Vries M., Hoekstra H. J., Hoekstra-Weebers J. E. H. M. Quality of life after axillary or groin sentinel lymph node biopsy, with or without completion lymph node dissection, in patients with cutaneous melanoma. *Ann Surg Oncol. 2009*;16:2840–2847. doi:10.1245/s10434-009-0602-6.

[56] Kretschmer L., Thoms K. M., Peeters S., Haenssle H., Bertsch H. P., Emmert S. Postoperative morbidity of lymph node excision for cutaneous melanoma-sentinel lymphonodectomy versus complete regional lymph node dissection. *Melanoma Res. 2008*;18:16–21. doi:10.1097/CMR.0b013e3282f2017d.

[57] Wrightson W. R., Wong S. L., Edwards M. J., Chao C., Reintgen D. S., Ross M. I., et al. Complications associated with sentinel lymph node biopsy for melanoma. *Ann Surg Oncol. 2003*;10:676–680.

[58] Wong S. L., Morton D. L., Thompson J. F., Gershenwald J. E., Leong S. P. L., Reintgen D. S., et al. Melanoma patients with positive sentinel nodes who did not undergo completion lymphadenectomy: a multi-institutional study. *Ann Surg Oncol. 2006*; 13:809–816. doi:10.1245/ASO.2006.03.058.

[59] Morton D. L., Cochran A. J., Thompson J. F., Elashoff R., Essner R., Glass E. C., et al. Sentinel node biopsy for early-stage melanoma: accuracy and morbidity in MSLT-I, an international multicenter trial. *Ann Surg. 2005*;242:302–11; discussion 311–3.

[60] Reeves M. E., Delgado R., Busam K. J., Brady M. S., Coit D. G. Prediction of nonsentinel lymph node status in melanoma. *Ann Surg Oncol. 2003*;10:27–31.

[61] Francischetto T., Spector N., Neto Rezende J. F., de Azevedo Antunes M., de Oliveira Romano S., Small I. A., et al. Influence of sentinel lymph node tumor burden on survival in melanoma. *Ann Surg Oncol. 2010*;17:1152–1158. doi: 10.1245/s10434-009-0884-8.

[62] Younan R., Bougrine A., Watters K., Mahboubi A., Bouchereau-Eyegue M., Loutfi A., et al. Validation study of the s classification for melanoma patients with positive sentinel nodes: the Montreal experience. *Ann Surg Oncol. 2010*;17:1414–1421. doi: 10.1245/s10434-009-0876-8.

[63] Wright E. H., Stanley P. R. W., Roy A. Evaluation of sentinel lymph nodes positive for melanoma for features predictive of non-sentinel nodal disease and patient prognosis: a 49 patient series. *J Plast Reconstr Aesthet Surg. 2010*;63:e500–e502. doi:10.1016/j.bjps.2009.07.043.

[64] Murali R., Desilva C., Thompson J. F., Scolyer R. A., Non-Sentinel Node Risk Score (N-SNORE): a scoring system for accurately stratifying risk of non-sentinel node positivity in patients with cutaneous melanoma with positive sentinel lymph nodes. *J Clin Oncol. 2010*;28:4441–4449. doi:10.1200/JCO.2010.30.9567.

[65] Murali R., Scolyer R. A., Thompson J. F., Can we better identify thin cutaneous melanomas that are likely to metastasize and cause death? *Ann Surg Oncol. 2012*; 19:3310–3312. doi:10.1245/s10434-012-2470-8.

[66] Wiener M., Acland K. M., Shaw H. M., Soong S. J., Lin H. Y., Chen D. T., et al. Sentinel node positive melanoma patients: prediction and prognostic significance of nonsentinel node metastases and development of a survival tree model. *Ann Surg Oncol. 2010*;17:1995–2005. doi:10.1245/s10434-010-1049-5.

[67] van der Ploeg A. P. T., van Akkooi A. C. J., Rutkowski P., Nowecki Z. I., Michej W., Mitra A., et al. Prognosis in patients with sentinel node-positive melanoma is accurately defined by the combined Rotterdam tumor load and Dewar topography criteria. *J Clin Oncol. 2011*;29:2206–2214. doi:10.1200/JCO.2010.31.6760.

[68] Han D., Thomas D. C., Zager J. S., Pockaj B., White R. L., Leong S. P. Clinical utilities and biological characteristics of melanoma sentinel lymph nodes. *World J Clin Oncol. 2016*;7:174–188. doi:10.5306/wjco.v7.i2.174.

[69] Faries M. B., Thompson J. F., Cochran A., Elashoff R., Glass E. C., Mozzillo N., et al. The impact on morbidity and length of stay of early versus delayed complete lymphadenectomy in melanoma: results of the Multicenter Selective Lymphadenectomy Trial (I). *Ann Surg Oncol. 2010*;17:3324–3329. doi:10.1245/s10434-010-1203-0.

[70] Christianson D. R., Dobroff A. S., Proneth B., Zurita A. J., Salameh A., Dondossola E., et al. Ligand-directed targeting of lymphatic vessels uncovers mechanistic insights in melanoma metastasis. *Proc Natl Acad Sci U S A. 2015*;112:2521–2526. doi:10.1073/pnas.1424994112.

[71] Nathanson S. D., Shah R., Rosso K. Sentinel lymph node metastases in cancer: causes, detection and their role in disease progression. *Semin Cell Dev Biol. 2015*; 38:106–116. doi:10.1016/j.semcdb.2014.10.002.

[72] Nathanson S. D., Insights into the mechanisms of lymph node metastasis. *Cancer. 2003*;98:413–423. doi:10.1002/cncr.11464.

[73] Leong S. P. L., Witte M. Biomarkers of cancer metastasis through the lymphovascular system: future perspectives. *Clin Exp Metastasis. 2012*;29:861–864. doi: 10.1007/s10585-012-9522-0.

[74] Leong S. P. L., Biomarkers of cancer metastasis through the lymphovascular system. Editorial. *Clin Exp Metastasis. 2012*;29:639–640. doi:10.1007/s10585-012-9509-x.

[75] Torabian S., Kashani-Sabet M. Biomarkers for melanoma. *Curr Opin Oncol. 2005*; 17:167–171.

[76] Faries M. B., Thompson J. F., Cochran A. J., Andtbacka R. H., Mozzillo N., Zager J. S., et al. Completion Dissection or Observation for Sentinel-Node Metastasis in Melanoma. *N Engl J Med. 2017*;376:2211–2222. doi:10.1056/NEJMoa1613210.

[77] Leiter U., Stadler R., Mauch C., Hohenberger W., Brockmeyer N., Berking C., et al. Complete lymph node dissection versus no dissection in patients with sentinel lymph node biopsy positive melanoma (DeCOG-SLT): a multicentre, randomised, phase 3 trial. *Lancet Oncol. 2016*;17:757–767. doi:10.1016/S1470-2045(16)00141-8.

[78] Moreau S., Saiag P., Aegerter P., Bosset D., Longvert C., Halias-Rodzewicz Z., et al. Prognostic value of BRAF(V) mutations in melanoma patients after resection of metastatic lymph nodes. *Ann Surg Oncol. 2012*;19:4314–4321. doi:10.1245/s10434-012-2457-5.

[79] Rossi C. R., Mozzillo N., Maurichi A., Pasquali S., Macripi G., Borgognoni L., et al. Number of excised lymph nodes as a quality assurance measure for lymphadenectomy in melanoma. *JAMA surgery. 2014*;149:700–706. doi: 10.1001/jamasurg.2013.5676.

[80] Rossi C. R., Mozzillo N., Maurichi A., Pasquali S., Quaglino P., Borgognoni L., et al. The number of excised lymph nodes is associated with survival of melanoma patients with lymph node metastasis. *Ann Oncol. 2014*;25:240–246. doi: 10.1093/annonc/mdt510.

[81] Hemmat S., Wang S. J., Ryan W. R. How, when, and from whom neck dissection operative technique is learned: An international survey on neck dissection education among head and neck oncologic surgeons. *Am J Otolaryngol. 2016*;37:431–435. doi:10.1016/j.amjoto.2016.04.002.

[82] Bocca E., Pignataro O., Oldini C., Cappa C. Functional neck dissection: an evaluation and review of 843 cases. *Laryngoscope. 1984*;94:942–945.

[83] Gavilan C., Gavilan J. Five-year results of functional neck dissection for cancer of the larynx. *Arch Otolaryngol Head Neck Surg. 1989*;115:1193–1196.

[84] Shah J. P. Patterns of cervical lymph node metastasis from squamous carcinomas of the upper aerodigestive tract. *Am J Surg. 1990*;160:405–409.

[85] Lindberg R. Distribution of cervical lymph node metastases from squamous cell carcinoma of the upper respiratory and digestive tracts. *Cancer. 1972*;29:1446–1449.

[86] Fisch U. P, Sigel M. E. Cervical lymphatic system as visualized by lymphography. *Ann Otol Rhinol Laryngol. 1964*;73:870–882.

[87] Akutsu Y., Matsubara H. Lymph node dissection for esophageal cancer. *Gen Thorac Cardiovasc Surg. 2013*;61:397–401. doi:10.1007/s11748-013-0237-1.

[88] Dua A., Desai S. S. Utility of internal jugular vein reconstruction in modified radical neck dissection. *Vascular. 2014*;22:81–84. doi:10.1177/1708538113476024.

[89] Ferlito A., Rinaldo A., Robbins K. T., Silver C. E. Neck dissection: past, present and future? *J Laryngol Otol. 2006*;120:87–92. doi:10.1017/S0022215105004512.

[90] Robbins K. T. Classification of neck dissection: current concepts and future considerations. *Otolaryngol Clin North Am. 1998*;31:639–655.

[91] Robbins K. T., Clayman G., Levine P. A., Medina J., Sessions R., Shaha A., et al. Neck dissection classification update: revisions proposed by the American Head and Neck Society and the American Academy of Otolaryngology-Head and Neck Surgery. *Arch Otolaryngol Head Neck Surg. 2002*;128:751–758.

[92] Robbins K. T., Medina J. E., Wolf G. T., Levine P. A., Sessions R. B., Pruet C. W. Standardizing neck dissection terminology. Official report of the Academy's Committee for Head and Neck Surgery and Oncology. *Arch Otolaryngol Head Neck Surg. 1991*;117:601–605.

[93] Robbins K. T., Shaha A. R., Medina J. E., Califano J. A., Wolf G. T., Ferlito A., et al. Consensus statement on the classification and terminology of neck dissection. *Arch Otolaryngol Head Neck Surg. 2008*;134:536–538. doi:10.1001/archotol.134.5.536.

[94] Diaz E. M., Austin J. R., Burke L. I., Goepfert H. The posterolateral neck dissection. Technique and results. *Arch Otolaryngol Head Neck Surg. 1996*;122:477–480.

[95] Dzwierzynski W. W. Complete lymph node dissection for regional nodal metastasis. *Clin Plast Surg. 2010*;37:113–125. doi:10.1016/j.cps.2009.07.002.

[96] Delman K. A., Kooby D. A., Ogan K., Hsiao W., Master V. Feasibility of a novel approach to inguinal lymphadenectomy: minimally invasive groin dissection for melanoma. *Ann Surg Oncol. 2010*;17:731–737. doi:10.1245/s10434-009-0816-7.

[97] Gershenwald J. E., Colome M. I., Lee J. E., Mansfield P. F., Tseng C., Lee J. J., et al. Patterns of recurrence following a negative sentinel lymph node biopsy in 243 patients with stage I or II melanoma. *J Clin Oncol. 1998*;16:2253–2260. doi: 10.1200/JCO.1998.16.6.2253.

[98] Gershenwald J. E., Thompson W., Mansfield P. F., Lee J. E., Colome M. I., Tseng C. H., et al. Multi-institutional melanoma lymphatic mapping experience: the prognostic value of sentinel lymph node status in 612 stage I or II melanoma patients. *J Clin Oncol. 1999*;17:976–983. doi:10.1200/JCO.1999.17.3.976.

[99] McMasters K. M., Reintgen D. S., Ross M. I., Gershenwald J. E., Edwards M. J., Sober A., et al. Sentinel lymph node biopsy for melanoma: controversy despite widespread agreement. *J Clin Oncol. 2001*;19:2851–2855. doi: 10.1200/JCO.2001.19.11.2851.

[100] Leong S. P. L., Mihm M. C., Murphy G. F., Hoon D. S. B., Kashani-Sabet M., Agarwala S. S., et al. Progression of cutaneous melanoma: implications for treatment. *Clin Exp Metastasis. 2012*;29:775–796. doi:10.1007/s10585-012-9521-1.

[101] Leung A. M., Morton D. L., Ozao-Choy J., Hari D. M., Shin-Sim M., Difronzo A. L., et al. Staging of regional lymph nodes in melanoma: a case for including nonsentinel lymph node positivity in the American Joint Committee on Cancer staging system. *JAMA surgery. 2013*;148:879–884. doi:10.1001/jamasurg.2013.3044.

[102] Ulmer A., Dietz K., Hodak I., Polzer B., Scheitler S., Yildiz M., et al. Quantitative measurement of melanoma spread in sentinel lymph nodes and survival. *PLoS Med. 2014*;11:e1001604. doi:10.1371/journal.pmed.1001604.

[103] Murali R., Thompson J. F., Scolyer R. A., Sentinel lymph node biopsy for melanoma: aspects of pathologic assessment. *Future Oncol. 2008*;4:535–551. doi: 10.2217/14796694.4.4.535.

[104] Scolyer R. A., Murali R., Satzger I., Thompson J. F., The detection and significance of melanoma micrometastases in sentinel nodes. *Surg Oncol. 2008*;17:165–174. doi: 10.1016/j.suronc.2008.06.005.

[105] van Akkooi A. C. J., de Wilt J. H. W., Verhoef C., Schmitz P. I. M., van Geel A. N., Eggermont A. M. M., et al. Clinical relevance of melanoma micrometastases (¡0.1 mm) in sentinel nodes: are these nodes to be considered negative? *Ann Oncol. 2006*; 17:1578–1585. doi:10.1093/annonc/mdl176.

[106] Satzger I., Valker B., Meier A., Kapp A., Gutzmer R. Criteria in sentinel lymph nodes of melanoma patients that predict involvement of nonsentinel lymph nodes. *Ann Surg Oncol. 2008*;15:1723–1732. doi:10.1245/s10434-008-9888-z.

[107] Scheri R. P., Essner R., Turner R. R., Ye X., Morton D. L., Isolated tumor cells in the sentinel node affect long-term prognosis of patients with melanoma. *Ann Surg Oncol. 2007*;14:2861–2866. doi:10.1245/s10434-007-9472-y.

[108] Abrahamsen H. N., Hamilton-Dutoit S. J., Larsen J., Steiniche T. Sentinel lymph nodes in malignant melanoma: extended histopathologic evaluation improves diagnostic precision. *Cancer. 2004*;100:1683–1691. doi:10.1002/cncr.20179.

[109] Riber-Hansen R., Sjoegren P., Hamilton-Dutoit S. J., Steiniche T. Extensive pathological analysis of selected melanoma sentinel lymph nodes: high metastasis detection rates at reduced workload. *Ann Surg Oncol. 2008*;15:1492–1501. doi: 10.1245/s10434-008-9847-8.

[110] Spanknebel K., Coit D. G., Bieligk S. C., Gonen M., Rosai J., Klimstra D. S. Characterization of micrometastatic disease in melanoma sentinel lymph nodes by enhanced pathology: recommendations for standardizing pathologic analysis. *Am J Surg Pathol. 2005*;29:305–317.

[111] Migliano E., Bellei B., Govoni F. A., Paolino G., Catricali C., Bucher S., et al. SLN melanoma micrometastasis predictivity of nodal status: a long term retrospective study. *J Exp Clin Cancer Res. 2013*;32:47. doi:10.1186/1756-9966-32-47.

In: The Sentinel Lymph Node
Editors: A. Londero, S. Bertozzi and C. Cedolini
ISBN: 978-1-53614-557-1


*Chapter 7*

# Complications of the Sentinel Lymph Node Biopsy for Breast Cancer and Melanoma

***Carla Cedolini[1], Serena Bertozzi[1,*], Luca Seriau[1], Luigino Noce[2] and Ambrogio P. Londero[3]***
[1]Breast Unit, University Hospital of Udine, Italy
[2]Clinic of Surgery, University Hospital of Udine, Italy
[3]Clinic of Obstetrics and Gynecology, University Hospital of Udine, Italy

**Abstract**

The increased sensibility of both clinicians and patients to the postoperative quality of life after oncological surgery has drawn attention to a number of postoperative complications, which in the past have probably been misdiagnosed or underestimated. The extent of locoregional surgery, the number of excised lymph nodes, the age and comorbidities of patients are the most important risk factors for the occurrence of postoperative complications. In addition to common early hemorrhagic or infective complications, some late complications may occur after the excision of one or more locoregional lymph nodes, such as scar defects, lymphatic drainage failure, axillary web syndrome, chronic pain, sensory or motor deficits. Unfortunately, the majority of late sequelae are usually chronic, difficult to prevent due to the necessity of an adequate surgical approach to the disease, and almost never completely solvable through standard treatments. Their management usually consists in symptom control through drug administration, physioterapist treatments and, only in very selected cases and with dubious results, surgical re-intervention. Finally, patients should always be aware of the possible complications to be encountered and be fully informed about the available therapeutic options.

**Keywords:** surgical complications, sentinel lymph node biopsy, axillary web syndrome, lymphedema

*Corresponding Author E-mail: dr.bertozzi@gmail.com.

# 1. Introduction

Sentinel lymph node biopsy (SLNB) is a minimally invasive surgical technique, which is burdened with a minimum complication rate, much lower than the complication rate of complete lymph node dissection. On the other hand, there does not seem to be any difference between therapeutic and completion dissections [1].

In the literature, the complication incidence of SLNB varies between 1.8% and 30% [2, 3, 4, 5, 6, 7], raising suspicion of a likely underestimation. In fact, some authors report only complications that require a second intervention, and generally there is no homogeneity in the definition of the various complications.

A Cochrane Collaboration systematic review showed an overall complication incidence after SLNB for melanoma of 11.3% [8]. A subsequent large international, multicenter trial determined a seroma incidence of 7.1%, a hematoma incidence of 1.4%, a infection incidence of 1% and a nerve injury incidence of 0.2% within the first month of intervention, and a lymphedema incidence of 7.9% at 6 months [9]. A more recent meta-analysis calculated an overall complication incidence of 11.3%, including a seroma incidence of 5.1%, a infection incidence of 2.9%, a lymphedema incidence of 1.3%, a hematoma incidence of 0.5% and a nerve injury incidence of 0.3% [10]. No statistical difference was found between the pooled estimated complication rates across continents.

As with any surgical procedure, there may be early and late complications. The most common early complications include seroma, bleeding and infection, which usually occur within a few days of surgery and resolve spontaneously. Other complications, such as lymphocele or web syndrome, may appear about 10 to 15 days after surgery and most cases they also resolve spontaneously.

There may also be some other complications with a later onset, but usually a chronic course that can be controlled, such as lymphedema or paresthesia, yet usually do not have a definitive resolution.

The most frequent lymph node surgery complications will be discussed in the following sections, addressing their incidence, risk factors and treatment. We will focus on the complications of neck and axillary lymph node excision, as the complications of inguinal and pelvic lymph node excision will be discussed in another chapter.

# 2. Early Complications

Early complications resemble those of any surgical intervention, are not uncommon but at the same time very mild, being usually treated conservatively.

Bleeding consists of the collection of blood in the excision bed of the lymph nodes. In the case of SLNB, it is very limited due to the small size of the excised tissue, while it may be greater in the case of complete lymphadenectomy. In the latter case, a drainage tube is usually inserted into the excision cavity so that the bleeding is drained rather than collected, and it is also easy to measure the extent of bleeding. Bleeding usually stops and reabsorbs spontaneously, and only in very few cases is a re-intervention required, with the aim of reducing the compression of vascular and nervous structures, improving the healing process and avoiding later scar defects (Figure 1).

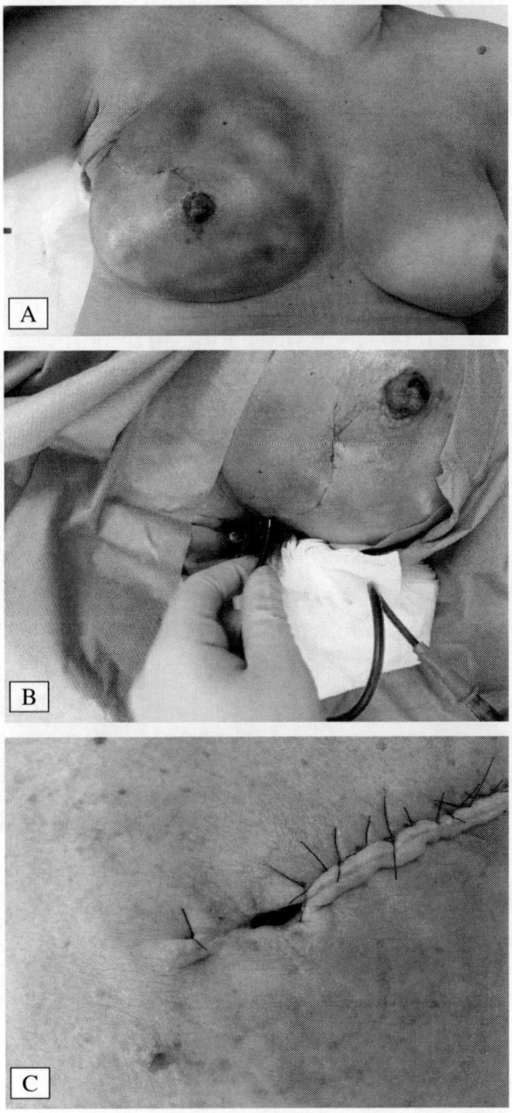


Figure 1. Panel A) Breast Hematoma after axilla and breast surgery. Panel B) Percutaneous hematoma drainage. Panel C) Scar dehiscence.

Serum and lymph may also collect in the excision bed along with the blood, forming seroma and lymphocele, respectively. Also the collection of these fluids rarely requires an evacuative puncture or surgical removal, because they usually reabsorb spontaneously. Evacuation of the collection is only indicated in the presence of symptoms such as pain, local discomfort, or functional limitations.

Another early complication of lymph node excision is infection. Manifestations of infection are pain, reddening and swelling, and more rarely fever. To reduce further complications early treatment is essential and is actually very accessible given the availability of numerous antibiotics. The bacteria most frequently involved in surgical wound infection after lymph node excision are gram positive cocci, which usually inhabits the skin, but other bacteria can also cause infections through a hematogenous spread. The medical therapy may avail of an antibiogram performed on the purulent collection, when present. In fact, in the case of antibiotic therapy inefficiency, after an initial empirical treatment with penicillins, the antibiogram can determine the choice of a more effective drug.

## 3. Lymphatic Complications

The main complications of lymph node dissection include postoperative discomfort, locoregional edema and functional impotence. The excision of a single node usually does not imply any of these complications, but due to the anatomic variability and individual pain perception, some patients undergoing SLNB may have a large number of subjective or objective symptoms.

Typical symptoms of lymphatic drainage failure are lymphocele, a collection of lymph in the axillary cavity, and lymphedema, a swelling of the upper limb due to the intra-tissutal collection of lymph. However, due to the increased sensibility of patients and clinicians to the postoperative quality of life, other complications have emerged, probably previously underestimated, such as axillary web syndrome. This condition is characterized by a painful limitation of the motility of the upper limb caused by the development of tenacious fibrotic chords within the axilla.

Lymphedema and axillary web syndrome presentation, risk factors and management will be described in the next sections.

### 3.1. Lymphedema

Lymphedema is the most dreaded long-term complication of axillary surgery (Figure 2). It is a chronic process that cannot be reliably prevented and has a significant negative impact on women's quality of life [11, 12]. It can contribute to musculoskeletal pain, reduced shoulder motility and limitations of daily activity performance. In addition, an outdated and neglected lymphedema may cause elephantiasis or angiosarcoma in the so-called Stewart-Treves syndrome.

Although the medical community has devoted little time and attention to lymphedema research and despite the resources needed for an effective treatment, a trend in reducing the surgical impact on the breast through breast conserving surgery and the widespread adoption of SLNB as the standard of care for axillary staging, have fortunately contributed to significantly reducing the incidence of lymphedema. However, this incidence is still variable, between 7% and 37% in patients undergoing complete axillary lymph node dissection and between 0% to 7% after SLNB [13, 14, 15, 16, 17]. This great variability reflects differences in measurement techniques and the lack of a standardized definition of lymphedema, which imply a great homogeneity among articles with regard to lymphedema prevalence.

Although lymphedema usually occurs within 3 years of treatment [18, 19], approximately 1% of annual risk persists for many years to come. In particular, it may develop even after many years of surgery in the case of any acute event, which is usually negligible for patients who have not undergone any axillary surgery. For instance, it may occur after

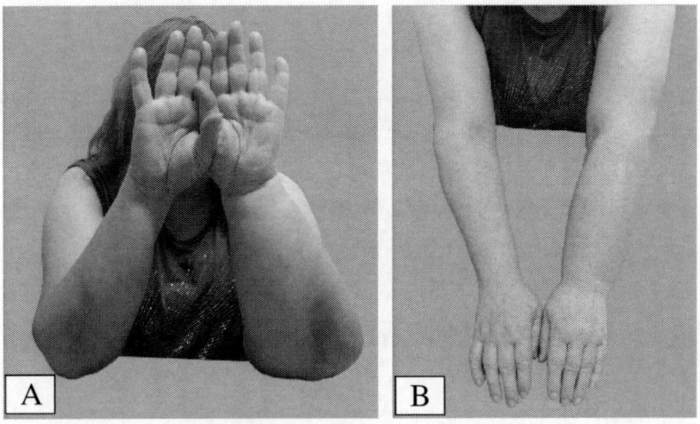


Figure 2. Lymphedema of the left arm in two different views (panel A and B).

a venous blood sampling in the operated arm or after an accidental trauma to the ipsilateral arm. Moreover, it may also occur after one or two decades without any reported event, as a result of progressive lymphatic failure with age.

Risk factors for lymphedema include age over 65, obesity, infection or injury in the ipsilateral upper extremity, a large number of removed nodes or a large extension of axillary surgery, reflecting the amount of lymphatic destruction, additional chemotherapy and radiotherapy at the lymph node stations [20, 1, 21, 22, 23]. In particular, chemotherapy leads to 4- to 5-fold increase in hazard ratio for lymphedema compared with no treatment, especially in the case of ipsilateral arm chemotherapy infusions, while nodal irradiation has a documented synergistic effect with surgery, which results in a 3.5- to 10-fold higher risk of lymphedema compared with surgery alone, increasing, for example, the incidence of lymphedema up to 65% after radical mastectomy [24].

The underlying mechanism that promotes lymphedema development during or immediately after adjuvant treatments is a progressive lesion of the lympho-vascular structures of the limb. For example, the infusion of antiblastic drugs is recognized to damage the venous net at the injection site due to both direct cytotoxic action and indirect weakening of proliferating tissues. One possible solution to prevent this kind of occurrence is to insert an infuse-a-port into a large vein, such as the internal jugular or the subclavian vein, which are less sensitive to this type of damage.

As far as radiotherapy is concerned, lymphatic damage is correlated with the burn effect on the target tissues, which consequently establishes a sort of reparative mechanism that thickens and stiffens the tissues and also reduces the elasticity of the blood and lymphatic vessels. There is of course a higher risk of lymphedema associated with axillary lymph nodes irradiation than with residual breast irradiation in conservative surgery. This observation may also explain the evident increased risk of lymphedema in patients with a greater extent of nodal involvement, for whom radiotherapy is consequently more indicated.

The evaluation of lymphedema is carried out with the patient sitting with their arms first outstretched, then flexed and finally resting on the hips to detect any circumferential difference, particularly at the olecranon process, at the styloid process of the ulnar head, and on the extensor tendons of the hand, as well as the presence of pitting or non-pitting edema or any imprints of tight-fitting shirt sleeves, watches, or jewelry.

Patient-perceived lymphedema is uncommon after SLNB alone, but its prevalence increases with the increasing number of sentinel nodes excised [25]. Although lymphedema is usually determined by measuring the limb circumference, even in the absence of visible limb swelling, patients may perceive a limb enlargement causing great discomfort during common daily activities. In fact, some authors suggest that factors other than limb enlargement, such as sensory nerve injury resulting from multiple nodes retrieval and the laterality of surgery, may play a significant role in patients' perception of lymphedema after SLNB.

Early detection and intervention can reduce or resolve lymphedema progression [18, 26], as otherwise 48% of patients with mild lymphedema tend to progress toward a more severe lymphedema by 5 years of follow-up [27]. While studies agree on the importance of early identification and intervention, there is less agreement on the type of intervention to be pursued. The treatment of lymphedema focuses on the chronic nature of the disease and aims to prevent lymphedema progression and recurrent infection and to facilitate the return to normal function.

Complex decongestant therapy remains the standard of care for long-term treatment of lymphedema and for limiting tissue fibrosis and pain, and includes compression garments, short stretch bandages and manual lymphatic drainage. Medical therapy can also be undertaken, which usually consists of the administration of oral diuretic drugs to drain the accumulation of peripheral fluids.

Regardless of the volume of axillary surgery, women are always instructed to move their arm from the immediate postoperative period. They are given specific exercises to do in order to prevent the potential lymphatic failure. In addition, they are given advice on general behaviors that may improve lymphatic drainage, such as holding the limb raised by applying a cushion under the arm during the hours of rest, and avoiding any arm strain or activities that can worsen the lymphatic stasis.

Only in very selected cases of severe lymphedema that does not respond to any decongestant therapy, microvascular surgery techniques may be applied in order to connect the microscopic lymphatic vessels to the axillary venous system and to restore the locoregional lymphatic drainage as a result. However, this type of surgery requires a lot of advanced skills, is performed only in highly specialized centers, and still encounters controversial success.

### 3.2. Axillary Web Syndrome

Less known but increasingly frequent is the axillary web syndrome, which consists of the presence of visible webs of axillary skin overlying palpable anelastic cords of tissue that are made stiff and painful by shoulder abduction and as a result hinder the physiologic movements of the upper limb (Figure 3). They developed just below the skin, frequently in the axillary cavity, but are also found in the cubital fossa, and less frequently at the base of the thumb or in the pectoral region [28].

The incidence of web syndrome after complete axillary lymph node dissection is about 6%. Among patient operated for breast cancer generally varies between 4% and 85%, but there is no clear data about its incidence after SLNB [28, 29]. In fact, this syndrome is probably underestimated, due to difficult recognition of symptoms, lack of patient knowledge, and timing of onset and release of symptoms. In particular, this complication usually

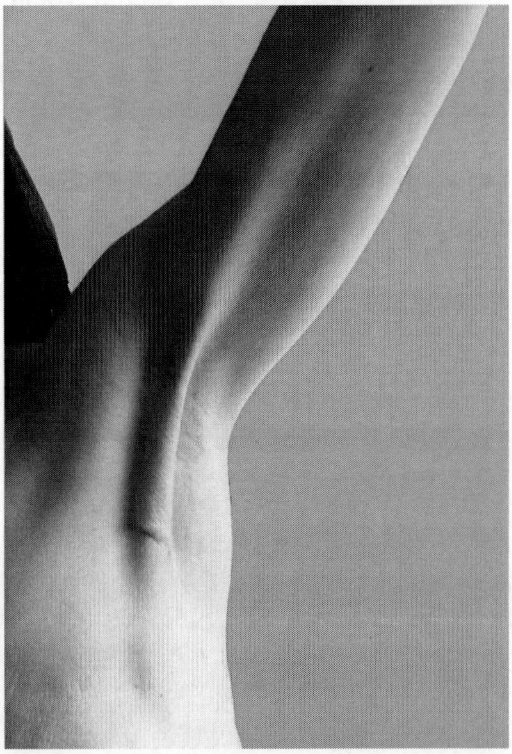

Figure 3. Web syndrome, which consists of the presence of visible webs of axillary skin overlying palpable anelastic cords of tissue.

develops about 7-10 days after surgery and as a consequence after discharge from hospital, because this type of patients hardly remain hospitalized for more than a few days. Moreover, symptoms often disappear spontaneously within 2-10 weeks after their onset.

Some authors have reported an overall incidence of axillary web syndrome after breast surgery of 28.1% [30]. In association with this type of complication, they have also reported an incidence of pain in the ipsilateral upper limb of 5.4% and an incidence of shoulder joint restriction of 11.4%. The authors of the study have concluded that axillary web syndrome was significantly associated with the surgical extent, and therefore more frequent in the case of complete axillary lymph node dissection, and numbness of the arm more frequent after intercostobrachial nerve injury. In any case, this condition is very disabling for patients, because it affects their common domestic activities due to pain and movements limitation.

Very few studies have reported a detailed histopathological description of the axillary web syndrome, showing a dilatation of lymphatic vessels and their occlusion by fibrin clots, along with venous thrombosis [28]. These features resemble an axillary variant of the Mondor's disease, which is a superficial thrombophlebitis of thoracoepigastric vein after surgery or trauma [31, 32]. In particular, some authors have found dilated lymphatic vessels surrounded by fibrosis, suggesting that the axillary web syndrome is the result of scars of the connective tissue that encloses the blood vessels. Other authors have found a thrombophlebitic inflammatory process that suggest both lymphatic and venous involvement [28, 29, 33, 34, 35]. In any case, the initially hypothesized role of the intercostobrachial nerve entrapment seems to be excluded.

In addition, there seems to be no association between axillary web syndrome and the rate of positive axillary dissections [28]. In fact, it may occur even after a very limited and targeted removal of lymph nodes in the case of SLNB, because even a limited lymph node excision can disrupt an important lymphatic drainage of the medial arm, supporting the hypothesis of an angio-lymphatic etiology.

There is controversial data also regarding the risk factors of axillary web syndrome, due to its low incidence rate and even lower identification rate. However, repeated axillary surgery, axillary radiotherapy and chemotherapy have been observed to increase the incidence of axillary web syndrome, probably because of lesions to the locoregional lymphatic system, resulting in lympho-venous stasis and hyper-coagulability. In addition, the use of modern dissection devices has also been reported to play a role in the development of axillary web syndrome. In fact, these new instruments combine heat with ultrasound or radiofrequency to achieve a faster and more efficient coagulation and cutting, and may somehow affect the residual lymphatic structures. In any case, there is no evidence to support this theory, also because randomized studies to detect risk factors for axillary web syndrome have not yet been conducted.

In most cases, axillary web syndrome disappears spontaneously within a few weeks of its onset. If not, the main option for treatment is the scar tissue massage. Patients are usually well-informed on when and how to massage their scars after hospital discharge. In particular, it is recommended to start approximately two weeks after surgery or after the scabs from the surgical wound have fallen. Physiotherapy examination is offered to patients who have undergone complete axillary lymph node dissection, and also to patients who have undergone SLNB in the case of lymphatic complications occurring at any time after surgery.

In addition to simple massage, other complementary treatments have been described, such as manual cord disruption, analgesic and anti-inflammatory administration, and surgical excision of the cord with or without immediate autologous fat grafting [36, 37, 38]. In the event of a very disabling movement limitation, surgical excision of an abundant part of the cord is also recommended to reduce pain and immobility, followed by a physiotherapist massage. However, there are no randomized trials on the treatment of axillary web syndrome, and for this reason there is certainly little homogeneity in the treatment options offered in the various centers.

## 4. Nerve Complications

Surgical excision of the sentinel node may also imply nerve injuries, with both sensory and motor consequences. For example, in the case of axillary lymph node excision, there may be different types of nerve lesions. The lesion of the long thoracic nerve usually causes an arm range of motion and internal rotation deficit, but these actions are usually compensated by the properly innervated agonist muscles, such as the pectoralis major muscle. The lesion of the intercostobrachial nerve causes a sense of compression under the armpit, altered sensitivity and functional limitation. These changes can sometimes also be perceived in the medial region of the arm and forearm. As for the lesion of the thoracodorsalis nerve, it implies a shoulder range of motion and internal rotation deficit.

Sensory dysfunction affects 0.1% to 32% of patients who have undergone SLNB for melanoma, and up to 82% of those who have undergone complete lymph node dissection. It has been shown to correlate with the extent of surgery, as a larger excision increases the probability of including nerve structures [39]

Another factor correlated with nerve complications is definitely the lymph node excision site. In fact, there are anatomical regions at high risk of nerve injury, such as the neck. In particular, the surgeon should always be aware of a high potential risk of spinal accessory nerve injury in the case of lymph node excision in the posterior cervical triangle [40]. Another delicate region is the parotid region, where a nerve stimulator should be used during selective SLNB to minimize facial and spinal accessory nerve injury [41, 42].

A frequent sensory complication is persistent postoperative pain, which affects about 1-14% of patients who have undergone SLNB for melanoma, and up to 34% of patients who have undergone complete lymph node dissection [43]. This type of neuropathic pain, which frequently persists for months after surgery, has been suggested to result from nerve injury [44]. Different patterns of sensory profiles have been observed in individual patients, suggesting individual heterogeneous sensory processing. However, further studies are needed to better explain its onset and optimize its management.

The current medical treatment of chronic pain or discomfort related to nervous injury is based on a combination of different antalgic drugs. The main analgesic anti-inflammatory drugs include cortisone derivatives and non-steroidal anti-inflammatory drugs derived from acetyl-salicylic acid. The advantage of these drugs is their anti-inflammatory power that helps reduce the effects of an excessive healing process, which can cause redundant fibrosis and consequent nerve entrapment. Another option is the use of paracetamol, which has only analgesic properties but not anti-inflammatory ones, or morphine derivatives. The latter has certainly a more powerful antalgic activity and can be administered in many different ways, such as lollipops or comfortable intra-dermal patches. However, morphine derivatives also have more collateral effects, including nausea, disorientation and, in the more severe cases, respiratory failure.

An interventional alternative is locoregional infiltration with analgesic or anti-inflammatory drugs directly at site of major pain. This procedure must be performed only in highly selected patients by clinicians with extensive experience in infiltration. Surgical re-intervention should usually be avoided, as no guarantee is there of a symptoms amelioration.

## 5. Scar Complications

Along with acute wound dehiscence, many late scar complications have been described (Figure 1). They depend primarily on the healing capacity of the individual, but can also be influenced by adjuvant therapies.

For example, radiotherapy may sustain a tissue phlogosis, which usually increases the thickness and pigmentation of the initial scar. On the other hand, chemotherapy may impair healing by braking the activity of the inflammatory cells involved in the healing process, and consequently lead to hypothrophic or hyperthrophic scar.

The treatment of cheloids, hyperthophic scars or radio-induced complications is generally conservative. The patient may self-massage the scar with the help of emollient or soothing creams, possibly containing collagen or other elasticizing substances, from about 2 weeks up to 6-9 months after surgery.

Only in highly selected cases with a very bad aesthetic result or concomitant presence of pain, it is possible to discuss a possible surgical excision of the scar and its revision possibly by the plastic surgeon.

## 6. Medical Complications

Many other conditions can complicate SLNB, as is the case of any surgical procedure performed on oncological patients. In fact, there is a recognized systemic thrombo-embolic risk related to the thrombophilic power of cancer, which can release neoplastic cell aggregates into the bloodstream at any time and stage of the disease. This risk can be usually prevented by perioperative administration of oral or parenteral anticoagulants in high-risk patients.

Thrombo-embolic complications can also be influenced by numerous known or unknown thrombophilic conditions, such as surgical extent and duration, postoperative immobilization, hormone replacement therapies or individual thrombophilic mutations. However, as expected, no difference in the incidence of postoperative pulmonary embolism, deep vein thrombosis or other medical conditions in the case of SLNB has been demonstrated compared with other types of lymph node resection [45].

## 7. Risk Factors for Complications after Sentinel Lymph Node Biopsy

A better understanding of the complications associated with SLNB allows for a better preoperative counseling of patients on their expectations for the postoperative course and can lead clinicians to make intraoperative decisions that could potentially influence the incidence of postoperative complications [46]. Furthermore, several authors have tried to define risk factors for complications, despite their probably underestimated low incidence.

A study involving 339 melanoma patients who have undergone SLNB showed a correlation between the number of removed lymph nodes and the postoperative complications [46]. It is generally preferable to subject only one sentinel node to excision. Most authors describe a mean of about 1.5 excised sentinel nodes. The usual rule is to subject the most radioactive node and all nodes which have more than 10% of radioactivity of the first sentinel node to excision, while in the case of absence of radioactivity or generalized homogeneous radioactivity, a partial or complete lymph node dissection is indicated. However, the number of removed sentinel nodes cannot be controlled by the surgeon, as it depends on numerous technical or anatomical factors. The intentional excision of a single lymph node while not subjecting other nodes that meet the sentinel node criteria to excision leads to an unacceptable rate of false-negatives [47]. Instead, what the surgeon can limit is the involuntary excision of non-sentinel nodes, which may sometimes be included in the sentinel node biopsy, especially in overweight patients.

Another risk factor for complications after SLNB resulted to be the use of closed-suction drains, which are routinely used in soft tissue procedures at risk for seroma [46]. In fact, drainages should reduce wound complications by decreasing skin tension and evacuating fluid collections that may compress lympho-vascular structures or become infected [48, 49]. However, they can also increase wound complications by being a passage for infective pathogens. In addition, the correlation between drainage application and wound complications can also be explained by a systematic selection bias. In fact, patients who have had a drainage placed after SLNB probably also have other variables related to the complications, such as the amount of volume excised.

Furthermore, the biopsy site was also found to affect the complication rate, with an increased incidence for parotid SLNB [46]. It is intuitive that not all anatomical regions are equally easily accessible, in fact the neck is a very delicate region with an increased risk of complications, even in the case of minimally invasive surgery. However, a recent meta-analysis has found the highest incidence of complications for the groin (14.9%), followed by axilla (9.8%) and neck (5.1%) [10].

As for the role of the surgeon, there is a clear inverse relation between the complication incidence and the operator's experience with the procedure [46].

Finally, the coexistence of morbid conditions generally increases the risk of surgical complications [50, 51]. Therefore, patients with known co-morbidities should always be informed of the risks prior to intervention.

# References


[1] Moody J. A., Botham S. J., Dahill K. E., Wallace D. L., Hardwicke J. T., Complications following completion lymphadenectomy versus therapeutic lymphadenectomy for melanoma - A systematic review of the literature. *European journal of surgical oncology : the journal of the European Society of Surgical Oncology and the British Association of Surgical Oncology. 2017*;43:1760–1767. doi:10.1016/j.ejso.2017.07.003.

[2] Read R. L., Pasquali S., Haydu L., Thompson J. F., Stretch J. R., Saw R. P. M., et al. Quality assurance in melanoma surgery: The evolving experience at a large tertiary referral centre. *European journal of surgical oncology: the journal of the European Society of Surgical Oncology and the British Association of Surgical Oncology. 2015*; 41:830–836. doi:10.1016/j.ejso.2014.12.003.

[3] de Vries M., Vonkeman W. G., van Ginkel R. J., Hoekstra H. J., Morbidity after axillary sentinel lymph node biopsy in patients with cutaneous melanoma. *European journal of surgical oncology: the journal of the European Society of Surgical Oncology and the British Association of Surgical Oncology. 2005*;31:778–783. doi: 10.1016/j.ejso.2005.05.003.

[4] Wrightson W. R., Wong S. L., Edwards M. J., Chao C., Reintgen D. S., Ross M. I., et al. Complications associated with sentinel lymph node biopsy for melanoma. *Annals of surgical oncology. 2003*;10:676–680.

[5] Hettiaratchy S. P., Kang N., O'Toole G., Allan R., Cook M. G., Powell B. W. Sentinel lymph node biopsy in malignant melanoma: a series of 100 consecutive patients. *British journal of plastic surgery. 2000*;53:559–562. doi:10.1054/bjps.2000.3409.

[6] Bonenkamp J., Logan D., Suemnig A., Thompson J. The cost of sentinel node biopsy (SNB) for melanoma. *Melanoma Res. 2001*;11:S107.

[7] Jansen L., Nieweg O. E., Peterse J. L., Hoefnagel C. A., Olmos R. A., Kroon B. B. Reliability of sentinel lymph node biopsy for staging melanoma. *The British journal of surgery. 2000*;87:484–489. doi:10.1046/j.1365-2168.2000.01362.x.

[8] Kyrgidis A., Tzellos T., Mocellin S., Apalla Z., Lallas A., Pilati P., et al. Sentinel lymph node biopsy followed by lymph node dissection for localised primary cutaneous melanoma. *The Cochrane database of systematic reviews. 2015*;CD010307. doi:10.1002/14651858.CD010307.pub2.

[9] Wilke L. G,, McCall L. M., Posther K. E., Whitworth P. W., Reintgen D. S., Leitch A. M., et al. Surgical complications associated with sentinel lymph node biopsy: results from a prospective international cooperative group trial. *Annals of surgical oncology. 2006*;13:491–500. doi:10.1245/ASO.2006.05.013.

[10] Moody J. A., Ali R. F., Carbone A. C., Singh S., Hardwicke J. T., Complications of sentinel lymph node biopsy for melanoma - A systematic review of the literature. *European journal of surgical oncology : the journal of the European Society of Surgical Oncology and the British Association of Surgical Oncology. 2017*;43:270–277. doi:10.1016/j.ejso.2016.06.407.

[11] McLaughlin S. A., Bagaria S., Gibson T., Arnold M., Diehl N., Crook J., et al. Trends in risk reduction practices for the prevention of lymphedema in the first 12 months after breast cancer surgery. *Journal of the American College of Surgeons. 2013*; 216:380–9; quiz 511–3. doi:10.1016/j.jamcollsurg.2012.11.004.

[12] Ahmed R. L., Prizment A., Lazovich D., Schmitz K. H., Folsom A. R. Lymphedema and quality of life in breast cancer survivors: the Iowa Women's Health Study. *Journal of clinical oncology : official journal of the American Society of Clinical Oncology. 2008*;26:5689–5696. doi:10.1200/JCO.2008.16.4731.

[13] Kissin M. W., Querci della Rovere G., Easton D., Westbury G. Risk of lymphoedema following the treatment of breast cancer. *The British journal of surgery. 1986*;73:580–584.

[14] Ivens D., Hoe A. L., Podd T. J., Hamilton C. R., Taylor I., Royle G. T. Assessment of morbidity from complete axillary dissection. *British journal of cancer. 1992*;66:136–138.

[15] Veronesi U., Paganelli G., Viale G., Luini A., Zurrida S., Galimberti V., et al. A randomized comparison of sentinel-node biopsy with routine axillary dissection in breast cancer. *The New England journal of medicine. 2003*;349:546–553. doi: 10.1056/NEJMoa012782.

[16] Purushotham A. D., Upponi S., Klevesath M. B., Bobrow L., Millar K., Myles J. P., et al. Morbidity after sentinel lymph node biopsy in primary breast cancer: results from a randomized controlled trial. *Journal of clinical oncology: official journal of the American Society of Clinical Oncology. 2005*;23:4312–4321. doi: 10.1200/JCO.2005.03.228.

[17] Ashikaga T., Krag D. N., Land S. R., Julian T. B., Anderson S. J., Brown A. M., et al. Morbidity results from the NSABP B-32 trial comparing sentinel lymph node dissection versus axillary dissection. *Journal of surgical oncology. 2010*;102:111–118. doi:10.1002/jso.21535.

[18] Norman S. A., Localio A. R., Potashnik S. L., Simoes Torpey H. A., Kallan M. J., Weber A. L., et al. Lymphedema in breast cancer survivors: incidence, degree, time course, treatment, and symptoms. *Journal of clinical oncology : official journal of the American Society of Clinical Oncology. 2009*;27:390–397. doi: 10.1200/JCO.2008.17.9291.

[19] Petrek J. A., Senie R. T., Peters M., Rosen P. P. Lymphedema in a cohort of breast carcinoma survivors 20 years after diagnosis. *Cancer. 2001*;92:1368–1377.

[20] Tsai R. J., Dennis L. K., Lynch C. F., Snetselaar L. G., Zamba G. K. D., Scott-Conner C. The risk of developing arm lymphedema among breast cancer survivors: a meta-analysis of treatment factors. *Annals of surgical oncology. 2009*;16:1959–1972. doi: 10.1245/s10434-009-0452-2.

[21] Ozaslan C., Kuru B. Lymphedema after treatment of breast cancer. *American journal of surgery. 2004*;187:69–72.

[22] Bar Ad V., Dutta P. R., Solin L. J., Hwang W. T., Tan K. S., Both S., et al. Time-course of arm lymphedema and potential risk factors for progression of lymphedema after breast conservation treatment for early stage breast cancer. *The breast journal. 2012*;18:219–225. doi:10.1111/j.1524-4741.2012.01229.x.

[23] Shah C., Wilkinson J. B., Baschnagel A., Ghilezan M., Riutta J., Dekhne N., et al. Factors associated with the development of breast cancer-related lymphedema after whole-breast irradiation. *International journal of radiation oncology, biology, physics. 2012*;83:1095–1100. doi:10.1016/j.ijrobp.2011.09.058.

[24] Shah C., Vicini F. A. Breast cancer-related arm lymphedema: incidence rates, diagnostic techniques, optimal management and risk reduction strategies. *International journal of radiation oncology, biology, physics. 2011*;81:907–914. doi: 10.1016/j.ijrobp.2011.05.043.

[25] Goldberg J. I., Riedel E. R., Morrow M., Van Zee K. J. Morbidity of sentinel node biopsy: relationship between number of excised lymph nodes and patient perceptions of lymphedema. *Annals of surgical oncology. 2011*;18:2866–2872. doi: 10.1245/s10434-011-1688-1.

[26] Torres Lacomba M., Yuste Sanchez M. J., Zapico Goai A., Prieto Merino D., Mayoral del Moral O., Cerezo Tallez E., et al. Effectiveness of early physiotherapy to prevent lymphoedema after surgery for breast cancer: randomised, single blinded, clinical trial. *BMJ (Clinical research ed). 2010*;340:b5396. doi:10.1136/bmj.b5396.

[27] Bar Ad V., Cheville A., Solin L. J., Dutta P., Both S., Harris E. E. R. Time course of mild arm lymphedema after breast conservation treatment for early-stage breast cancer. *International journal of radiation oncology, biology, physics. 2010*;76:85–90. doi:10.1016/j.ijrobp.2009.01.024.

[28] Moskovitz A. H., Anderson B. O., Yeung R. S., Byrd D. R., Lawton T. J., Moe R. E. Axillary web syndrome after axillary dissection. *American journal of surgery. 2001*; 181:434–439.

[29] Yeung W. M., McPhail S. M., Kuys S. S. A systematic review of axillary web syndrome (AWS). *Journal of cancer survivorship: research and practice. 2015*;9:576–598. doi:10.1007/s11764-015-0435-1.

[30] Bergmann A., Mendes V. V., de Almeida Dias R., do Amaral E Silva B., da Costa Leite Ferreira M. G., Fabro E. A. N. Incidence and risk factors for axillary web syndrome after breast cancer surgery. *Breast cancer research and treatment. 2012*; 131:987–992. doi:10.1007/s10549-011-1805-7.

[31] Catania S., Zurrida S., Veronesi P., Galimberti V., Bono A., Pluchinotta A. Mondor's disease and breast cancer. *Cancer. 1992*;69:2267–2270.

[32] Pugh C. M., DeWitty R. L. Mondor's disease. *Journal of the National Medical Association. 1996*;88:359–363.

[33] Tilley A., Thomas-Maclean R., Kwan W. Lymphatic cording or axillary web syndrome after breast cancer surgery. *Canadian journal of surgery Journal canadien de chirurgie. 2009*;52:E105–E106.

[34] Craythorne E., Benton E., Macfarlane S. Axillary web syndrome or cording, a variant of mondor disease, following axillary surgery. *Archives of dermatology. 2009*; 145:1199–1200. doi:10.1001/archdermatol.2009.239.

[35] Johansson K., Ingvar C., Albertsson M., Ekdahl C. Arm Lymphoedema, Shoulder Mobility and Muscle Strength after Breast Cancer Treatment ? A Prospective 2-year Study. *Advances in Physiotherapy. 2001*;3:55–66. doi:10.1080/14038190119371.

[36] Gargya V., Lucas H. D., Wendel Spiczka A. J., Mahabir R. C. Is Routine Pathologic Evaluation of Sebaceous Cysts Necessary?: A 15-Year Retrospective Review of a Single Institution. *Annals of plastic surgery. 2017*;78:e1–e3. doi: 10.1097/SAP.0000000000000826.

[37] Fourie W. J., Robb K. A. Physiotherapy management of axillary web syndrome following breast cancer treatment: discussing the use of soft tissue techniques. *Physiotherapy. 2009*;95:314–320. doi:10.1016/j.physio.2009.05.001.

[38] Wei P., Zhu L., Chen K., Jia W., Hu Y., Su F. Axillary web syndrome following secondary breast-conserving surgery: a case report. *World journal of surgical oncology. 2013*;11:8. doi:10.1186/1477-7819-11-8.

[39] Andersen K. G., Duriaud H. M., Aasvang E. K., Kehlet H. Association between sensory dysfunction and pain 1 week after breast cancer surgery: a psychophysical study. *Acta anaesthesiologica Scandinavica. 2016*;60:259–269. doi:10.1111/aas.12641.

[40] Park S. H., Esquenazi Y., Kline D. G., Kim D. H. Surgical outcomes of 156 spinal accessory nerve injuries caused by lymph node biopsy procedures. *Journal of neurosurgery Spine. 2015*;23:518–525. doi:10.3171/2014.12.SPINE14968.

[41] Leong S. P. L. Role of selective sentinel lymph node dissection in head and neck melanoma. *Journal of surgical oncology. 2011*;104:361–368. doi:10.1002/jso.21964.

[42] Picon A. I., Coit D. G., Shaha A. R., Brady M. S., Boyle J. O., Singh B. B., et al. Sentinel Lymph Node Biopsy for Cutaneous Head and Neck Melanoma: Mapping the Parotid Gland. *Annals of surgical oncology. 2016*;23:9001–9009. doi: 10.1245/ASO.2006.03.051.

[43] Slagelse C., Petersen K. L., Dahl J. B., Finnerup K., Greene K., Leong S. P., et al. Persistent postoperative pain and sensory changes following lymph node excision in melanoma patients: a topical review. *Melanoma research. 2014*;24:93–98. doi: 10.1097/CMR.0000000000000041.

[44] Haimyr H., Rokkones K. A., von Sperling M. L., Finnerup K., Jensen T. S., Finnerup N. B. Persistent pain after lymph node excision in patients with malignant melanoma is neuropathic. *Pain. 2011*;152:2721–2728. doi:10.1016/j.pain.2011.07.009.

[45] Bafford A., Gadd M., Gu X., Lipsitz S., Golshan M. Diminishing morbidity with the increased use of sentinel node biopsy in breast carcinoma. *American journal of surgery. 2010*;200:374–377. doi:10.1016/j.amjsurg.2009.10.012.

[46] Roaten J. B., Pearlman N., Gonzalez R., Gonzalez R., McCarter M. D. Identifying risk factors for complications following sentinel lymph node biopsy for melanoma. *Archives of surgery (Chicago, Ill : 1960). 2005*;140:85–89. doi: 10.1001/archsurg.140.1.85.

[47] McMasters K. M., Reintgen D. S., Ross M. I., Wong S. L., Gershenwald J. E., Krag D. N., et al. Sentinel lymph node biopsy for melanoma: how many radioactive nodes should be removed? *Annals of surgical oncology. 2001*;8:192–197.

[48] Somers R. G., Jablon L. K., Kaplan M. J., Sandler G. L., Rosenblatt N. K. The use of closed suction drainage after lumpectomy and axillary node dissection for breast cancer. A prospective randomized trial. *Annals of surgery. 1992*;215:146–149.

[49] Bafna U. D., Umadevi K., Savitha M. Closed suction drainage versus no drainage following pelvic lymphadenectomy for gynecological malignancies. *International journal of gynecological cancer : official journal of the International Gynecological Cancer Society. 2001*;11:143–146.

[50] Rehman H. U., Mohammed K. Perioperative management of diabetic patients. *Current surgery. 2003*;60:607–611. doi:10.1016/j.cursur.2003.07.002.

[51] Lilienfeld D. E., Vlahov D., Tenney J. H., McLaughlin J. S. Obesity and diabetes as risk factors for postoperative wound infections after cardiac surgery. *American journal of infection control. 1988*;16:3–6.

In: The Sentinel Lymph Node
Editors: A. Londero, S. Bertozzi and C. Cedolini
ISBN: 978-1-53614-557-1


*Chapter 8*

# SENTINEL LYMPH NODE BIOPSY IN THYROID CANCER

***Mattia Portinari*[*] *and Paolo Carcoforo***
Department of Surgery, S. Anna University Hospital of Ferrara,
Ferrara, Italy & Department of Morphology,
Surgery and Experimental Medicine,
University of Ferrara, Ferrara, Italy

**Abstract**

Over the past few decades an upward trend in the incidence of thyroid cancer have been observed due to the increased detection and overdiagnosis of indolent disease. On the other hand, there has been a steady decrease in mortality due to the overdiagnosis of early-stage tumors, as well as changes in the management of the disease. The metastatic rate after sentinel lymph node biopsy for early-stage thyroid cancer is 38.6%. However, its false-negative rate is even 25.4% with a high risk of disease persistence after surgery. Therefore, a new concept of radio-guided surgery for the lymph node staging of patients with papillary thyroid carcinoma has been proposed, based on the use of sentinel lymph node biopsy only as a guide to perform selective lymph node dissection of the sentinel node compartment, regardless of the sentinel node status, and with a very low false-negative rate (1.1%). Sentinel lymph node biopsy can be successfully applied to papillary thyroid carcinoma patients to guide a compartment-oriented lymphadenectomy, increase metastatic yield and intraoperative tumor clearance, and improve disease staging and patient selection for postoperative radio-iodine ablation, which can potentially reduce the persistent disease rate after operative intervention.

**Keywords:** papillary thyroid cancer, sentinel lymph node biopsy, lymph node dissection, radio-guided surgery

## 1. Introduction

Over the past few decades an upward trend in thyroid cancer incidence has been observed due to increased detection and overdiagnosis of indolent disease such as small papillary

[*]Corresponding Author E-mail: mattia.portinari@unife.it.

thyroid carcinoma, which is the most frequent histotype [1, 2]. Interestingly, Rahib and colleagues, in a projection of cancer incidence in the United States for the most common cancer types based on demographic changes and the average annual percentage changes in the incidence rate, showed that thyroid cancer will replace colorectal cancer as the fourth leading cancer diagnosis by 2030 [3].

On the other hand, a steady decrease in mortality has been observed due to the overdiagnosis of early-stage tumors and changes in disease management and treatment [1, 2]. Thyroid cancer, which is generally treated with surgical resection, has an overall 5-year survival rate of 98% [4], and the 2% of cases succumbing to thyroid cancer are mainly rare and highly aggressive subtypes, including diagnoses of anaplastic and medullary thyroid cancer [5]. Currently, the major issue is the increasing overdiagnosis and consequent overtreatment. In light of this, the American Thyroid Association (ATA) 2015 guidelines for the management of adult patients with thyroid nodules and differentiated thyroid cancer recommend increasing the biopsy size threshold of thyroid nodules to reduce overdiagnosis [6]. On the contrary, when a cancer is discovered, even in the case of small tumors, physicians need to face patient's will and expectations regarding the newly diagnosed cancer, that should be taken into account in the treatment of the disease.

Miyauchi and colleagues conducted an observational study to evaluate the safety of non-operative management of papillary thyroid carcinoma ¡1 cm, proposing two options (immediate surgery versus observation followed by surgery for those who showed slight tumor progression) with treatment assignment according to the wishes of the patient. After providing patients with knowledge about papillary carcinoma, such as the high incidence of latent thyroid cancer, the good prognosis of small papillary carcinoma following appropriate surgery, and the good long-term results of their observation trial, many patients chose surgery [2, 7, 8]. This highlights the impact of cancer diagnosis on patient's will. In fact, observation instead of surgery may not be a comfortable option for most patients in the absence of certainty and appropriate psychosocial support [9]. Moreover, there are concerns related to a potential non-compliance or loss of follow-up among patients who agree to undergo surveillance [2].

On the other hand, the overdiagnosis of early-stage tumors may have determined a reduction in the incidence of lymph node metastases at the time of surgery. In fact, a lymph node metastatic rate of 46% was registered by Mazzaferri and colleagues and Jhiang and colleagues [10] in papillary thyroid carcinoma patients treated between 1960 and 1990, almost twice the rate observed (25%) in a study by Durante and colleagues in papillary carcinoma patients consecutively diagnosed between 1990-2008 in 8 Italian hospital centers for thyroid disease [11].

Recently, a systematic review on the sentinel lymph node biopsy (SLNB) for early-stage papillary thyroid carcinoma patients showed that the overall lymph node metastatic rate was 38.6%, showing an illusory increase in the metastatic rate, which was related to the improvement in lymph node staging associated with SLNB, instead of an upward trend in lymph node metastases due to the worse carcinoma stage [12].

In addition, Miyauchi and colleagues in their clinical trial on active surveillance of papillary thyroid carcinoma ¡1 cm without surgery, the percentage of patients whose carcinoma showed novel appearance of lymph node metastases was 3.8% at 10 years of observation. It should be noted that the age under 40 was considered an independent predictive factor of novel lymph node metastases in patients following only active surveillance. The authors highlighted that, for low-risk papillary carcinoma (¡1 cm), the most likely procedure would be hemithyroidectomy with or without central neck dissection. However this procedure is not able to prevent the appearance of nodal metastases in the lateral compartment in most cases. Therefore, such patients would require a second surgery. The authors suggested that observation without immediate surgery would be recommended for low-risk papillary carcinoma, especially in patients 40 years, supported by the fact that patients showing slight progression can always undergo surgery subsequently, with the final conclusion that one surgery is better than two, since the final outcomes appear equally good [8].

The introduction of SLNB and selective lymph node dissection of the sentinel compartment only (i.e., radio-guided selective compartment neck dissection) allowed the identification of occult lymph node metastases in the central, lateral and contralateral neck compartments at the time of the first surgery, reducing both persistent disease and redo surgery [12]. Locoregional recurrence, especially due to persistent disease, has been suggested as a valid endpoint to evaluate the effectiveness of therapy for papillary thyroid carcinoma. Persistent disease within the first 12 months of follow-up after surgical removal of the primary tumor may be due to a lack of dissection of the metastatic lymph node during the first operation that will then cause a recurrence during follow-up [12]. Therefore, in line with the thought that one surgery is better than two, when surgery is considered necessary for patients with papillary carcinoma SLNB and radio-guided selective compartment neck dissection should be considered during the first operation to improve lymph node staging [12].

## 2. Lymph Node Management Guidelines in Differentiated Thyroid Cancer

The ATA 2015 guidelines reported that the basic objectives of the initial therapy for patients with differentiated thyroid cancer are to improve overall and disease-specific survival, reduce the risk of persistent or recurrent disease and associated morbidity, and enable accurate disease staging and risk stratification. The completeness of the surgical resection is an important determinant of the outcome, while residual metastatic lymph nodes represent the most common site of disease persistence or recurrence. Interestingly, it has been highlighted that preoperative ultrasound identifies suspicious lymph node metastases in 20-31% of patients, but no single sonographic feature is adequately sensitive for the detection of metastatic lymph nodes.

However, the ATA guidelines recommend prophylactic central compartment neck dissection to be considered by experienced thyroid surgeons in papillary carcinoma patients with clinically negative lymph nodes (cN0) with advanced primary tumors (cT3 or cT4) or clinically involved lateral neck nodes (cN1b), and low morbidity. On the contrary, for early-stage (cT1 or cT2, cN0) papillary carcinomas, prophylactic central neck dissection is not indicated [6].

Conversely, the National Comprehensive Cancer Network (NCCN) guidelines do not recommend prophylactic central neck dissection if the cervical lymph nodes are clinically negative [13]. This conclusion is based on the results of a randomized controlled trial that showed no difference in outcomes between patients undergoing total thyroidectomy alone and those undergoing total thyroidectomy plus prophylactic central neck dissection. However, in both groups the persistent disease was about 8%, showing a lack of complete tumor clearance during the first operation [14].

Comparable data was shown by Durante and colleagues in an Italian multicenter study reporting a persistent disease of 7.1%, although the decision on prophylactic central neck dissection and postoperative radio-iodine ablation was based on institutional guidelines and therefore quite variable across the study population [11]. In contrast, the largest prospective study conducted by Carcoforo and colleagues, where papillary thyroid carcinoma patients were treated with SLNB and radio-guided selective lymph node dissection of the sentinel node compartment showed a persistent disease of 0.6% [15]. Thus, the type of surgery may play a role in reducing the risk of persistent disease in patients with papillary carcinoma and, according to the ATA and NCCN guidelines, a persistent disease may be expected.

Postoperative staging for thyroid cancer is recommended for all patients with differentiated thyroid carcinoma, with the following intents: prognostic value; risk stratification; patient management and adjuvant therapy planning; follow-up schedule [6]. As reported in the ATA guidelines, pathological reports should contain useful information for risk assessment such as the status of resection margins, the presence of vascular invasion and the number of invaded vessels, the number of lymph nodes examined and involved with tumor, the size of the largest metastatic focus to the lymph node and the presence or absence of extra-nodal extension of the metastatic tumor [6].

However, according to the ATA and NCCN guidelines, papillary carcinoma patients who have not undergone prophylactic lymph node dissection are classified as pNx because their regional lymph nodes cannot be histologically assessed. In partucular, the ATA guideline underline that the removal of cN0 level VI lymph nodes detects a substantial number of patients with pN1 disease. However, doubts have been expressed as to the direct effect of this on long-term outcomes [6]. It is clear that the use of lymph node staging information may change the planning of adjuvant therapy. However, the ATA guidelines have shown that microscopic nodal upstaging may lead to excessive use of radio-iodine ablation and patient follow-up. On the other hand, demonstration of uninvolved lymph nodes by prophylactic dissection may decrease the use of radio-iodine ablation for some patients [6].

## 3. Sentinel Lymph Node Biopsy in Differentiated Thyroid Cancer and Its Clinical Implications

In a meta-analysis on sentinel lymph node detection in patients with thyroid cancer, Raijmakers and colleagues showed that the radio-guided technique yielded a sentinel node detection rate approximately 13% higher than the dye technique [16]. This data was reinforced by a more recent meta-analysis. [17]. Furthermore, the radiotracer injection for radio-guided surgery is performed preoperatively, therefore eliminating the potential disruption of the lymphatic channel during the initial dissection, which normally occurs since the intraoperative dye injection may reduce the SLNB detection rate [12]. These findings support the use of the radio-guided technique instead of the dye method in thyroid cancer patients.

The preoperative intratumoral injection of the radiotracer (i.e., technetium-99) allow to obtain a high intraoperative identification rate (median 100%; range 95.8-100%) of the sentinel node [12], but the SLNB learning curve is an important parameter in the success of the sentinel node mapping [12]. However, the role of SLNB in the treatment of papillary thyroid carcinoma patients remains open to debate.

In some cases, a radio-guided SLNB with frozen section sentinel node evaluation has been used to identify patients with sentinel node metastases in whom lymph node dissection of the neck compartments should be performed and patients with negative sentinel node in whom the neck dissection can be avoided [18]. Among studies in which frozen section sentinel node evaluation was performed, the median value of the false-negative rate of intraoperative pathological examination was 9.5% (range, 8.3%-17.2%). Therefore, this procedure is not recommended to avoid complete lymph node dissection during surgery for papillary thyroid carcinoma patients [12].

Carcoforo and colleagues instead proposed a new concept of radio-guided selective compartment surgery for the lymph node staging of papillary thyroid carcinoma patients, based on the use of SLNB only as a guide to perform a selective lymph node dissection of the sentinel node compartment (i.e., central or lateral neck compartments), regardless of the sentinel node status, due to the high SLNB false-negative rate when performed alone (40.8%) [15].

As shown by a recent systematic review that included 12 studies and 800 patients, the overall false-negative rate of SLNB was 25.4%, underlining that a negative SLNB does not definitively exclude the presence of metastatic lymph nodes [12]. In addition, lymph node metastases were found in the central (23%) and lateral (10.6%) compartments, highlighting that the central neck compartment is considered the preferential lymph node metastasization pathway of papillary thyroid carcinoma. However, the lateral neck compartments were involved by tumor cells in a relevant percentage of papillary carcinomas, which were discovered through SLNB [12].

Considering the false-negative rate as the single most important quality element for the SLNB technique, the high false-negative rate of this procedure may influence the persistent disease during follow-up as a result of the lack of tumor clearance in the first operation [12]. It should be noted that the false-negative rate of radio-guided selective compartment neck dissection, based on persistent disease during the first 12 months of follow-up, is very low (1.1%), suggesting the safety of the procedure [15]. This new approach can safely increase the identification of patients with lymph node metastases and possibly reduce persistent disease, and may avoid unnecessary central neck lymph node dissection in selected patients thanks to the lymphatic drainage in the lateral compartment [12].

In conclusion, given its high false-negative rate, SLNB alone should be abandoned and converted into a technique that guides lymphadenectomy through radioactivity in a specific neck compartment (i.e., central or lateral), regardless of the sentinel node status.

### 3.1. Radio-Guided Selective Compartment Neck Dissection: Preoperative Nuclear Medicine Protocol and Operative Procedure

On the day before the operation, patients with papillary thyroid carcinoma confirmed by fine needle aspiration cytology (FNAC), with or without the presence of V600E BRAF gene mutation and with clinically negative lymph nodes (cN0), are submitted to an ultrasound-guided injection near the tumor of about 84 MBq of technetium-99 nanocolloidal albumin

(Nanocoll, GE Healthcare S.r.l., Milano, Italy), with an average particle size of <80 nm.

Lymphoscintigraphy is completed by planar observation in the anterior projection (Figure 1), associated with single photon emission computed tomography (SPECT) combined with computed tomography (CT) for both attenuation correction and improved morphologic localization of the sentinel lymph node compartment (Figure 2). At the end of both planar CT and SPECT/CT image acquisition, the skin is marked on the cutaneous projection of the sentinel node compartment to direct the radio-guided selective compartment neck dissection on the following day.

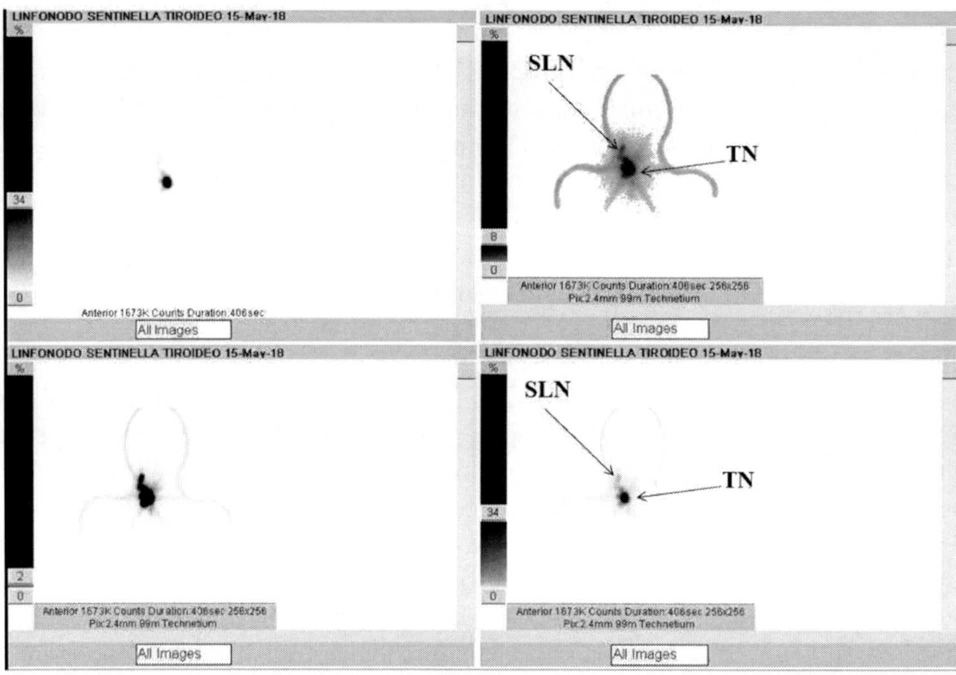


Figure 1. Preoperative lymphoscintigraphy showing the radioactive thyroid nodule (TN) and the sentinel lymph node (SLN) in the lateral neck compartment (i.e., level II).

On the day of the operation, the patient is brought to the operating room and subjected to total thyroidectomy through a standard Kocher incision before radio-guided selective compartment neck dissection to remove the radioactivity of the thyroid nodule and facilitate the identification of the sentinel node compartment. After thyroid removal, a handheld gamma detection probe (Europrobe, Eurorad S. A.) is used to identify the sentinel node compartment and to scan all the compartments of the neck.

The tracer activity in the lymph nodes is measured as counts per second. The "hottest" lymph node (i.e., 3-10 times greater than the basic uptake) is considered the sentinel lymph node, and a radio-guided selective compartment neck dissection of the sentinel node compartment is performed. The sentinel node is sent to the pathologist and analyzed separately by being sectioned every 200 μm. The sentinel lymph node and all nodes resected in the same neck compartment are stained with hematoxylin-eosin and cytokeratin.

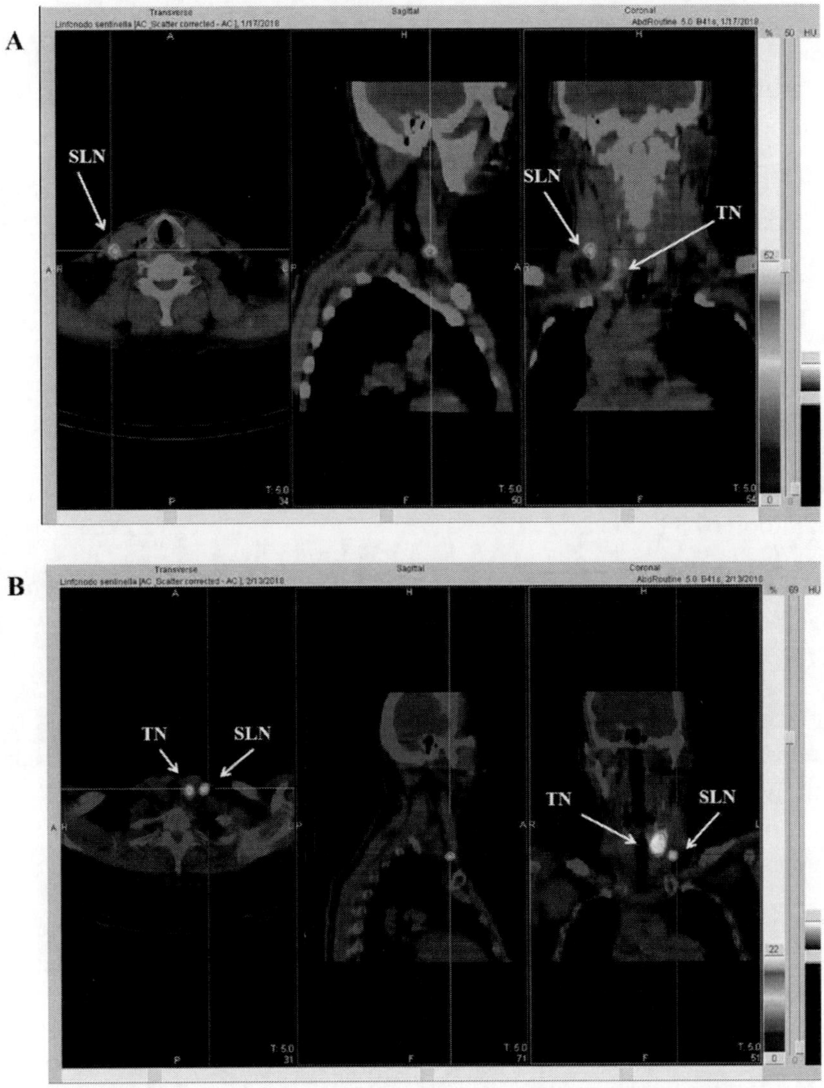


Figure 2. Preoperative single photon emission tomography (SPECT) combined with computed tomography (CT) showing the radioactive thyroid nodule (TN) and the sentinel lymph node (SLN) in the lateral neck compartments (i.e., Panel A - level III; Panel B - level IV).

# Conclusion

The SLNB may be successfully applied to papillary thyroid carcinoma patients to guide the compartment-oriented lymphadenectomy through radio-guided selective compartment neck dissection to increase the metastatic yield and the intraoperative tumor clearance, as well as to improve disease staging and patient selection for postoperative radio-iodine ablation, which may potentially reduce the persistent disease rate after operative intervention.

## References

[1] La Vecchia C., Malvezzi M., Bosetti C., Garavello W., Bertuccio P., Levi F., et al. Thyroid cancer mortality and incidence: a global overview. *Int J Cancer. 2015*;136:2187–2195. doi:10.1002/ijc.29251.

[2] Lubitz C. C., Sosa J. A. The changing landscape of papillary thyroid cancer: Epidemiology, management, and the implications for patients. *Cancer. 2016*;122:3754–3759. doi:10.1002/cncr.30201.

[3] Rahib L., Smith B. D., Aizenberg R., Rosenzweig A. B., Fleshman J. M., Matrisian L. M. Projecting cancer incidence and deaths to 2030: the unexpected burden of thyroid, liver, and pancreas cancers in the United States. *Cancer Res. 2014*;74:2913–2921. doi:10.1158/0008-5472.CAN-14-0155.

[4] Siegel R., Ma J., Zou Z., Jemal A. Cancer statistics, 2014. *CA Cancer J Clin. 2014*; 64:9–29. doi:10.3322/caac.21208.

[5] Heller K. S. Do all cancers need to be treated? The role of thyroglobulin in the management of thyroid cancer: the 2006 Hayes Martin lecture. *Arch Otolaryngol Head Neck Surg. 2007*;133:639–643. doi:10.1001/archotol.133.7.639.

[6] Haugen B. R., Alexander E. K., Bible K. C., Doherty G. M., Mandel S. J., Nikiforov Y. E., et al. 2015 American Thyroid Association Management Guidelines for Adult Patients with Thyroid Nodules and Differentiated Thyroid Cancer: The American Thyroid Association Guidelines Task Force on Thyroid Nodules and Differentiated Thyroid Cancer. *Thyroid. 2016*;26:1–133. doi:10.1089/thy.2015.0020.

[7] Ito Y, Miyauchi A., Inoue H., Fukushima M., Kihara M., Higashiyama T., et al. An observational trial for papillary thyroid microcarcinoma in Japanese patients. *World J Surg. 2010*;34:28–35. doi:10.1007/s00268-009-0303-0.

[8] Miyauchi A., Clinical Trials of Active Surveillance of Papillary Microcarcinoma of the Thyroid. *World J Surg. 2016*;40:516–522. doi:10.1007/s00268-015-3392-y.

[9] Tufano R. P., Noureldine S. I., Angelos P. Incidental thyroid nodules and thyroid cancer: considerations before determining management. *JAMA Otolaryngol Head Neck Surg. 2015*;141:566–572. doi:10.1001/jamaoto.2015.0647.

[10] Mazzaferri E. L., Jhiang S. M. Long-term impact of initial surgical and medical therapy on papillary and follicular thyroid cancer. *Am J Med. 1994*;97:418–428.

[11] Durante C., Montesano T., Torlontano M., Attard M., Monzani F., Tumino S., et al. Papillary thyroid cancer: time course of recurrences during postsurgery surveillance. *J Clin Endocrinol Metab. 2013*;98:636–642. doi:10.1210/jc.2012-3401.

[12] Portinari M., Carcoforo P. Radioguided sentinel lymph node biopsy in patients with papillary thyroid carcinoma. *Gland surgery. 2016*;5:591–602. doi: 10.21037/gs.2016.11.08.

[13] NCCN Clinical Preactice Guidelines in Oncology. *Thyroid Carcinoma* [Version 1. 2018 - May 22, 2018]. Available from: https://www.nccn.org/professionals/physician_gls/pdf/thyroid.pdf, accessed on 18.04.2018.

[14] Viola D., Materazzi G., Valerio L., Molinaro E., Agate L., Faviana P., et al. Prophylactic central compartment lymph node dissection in papillary thyroid carcinoma: clinical implications derived from the first prospective randomized controlled single institution study. *J Clin Endocrinol Metab. 2015*;100:1316–1324. doi:10.1210/jc.2014-3825.

[15] Carcoforo P., Portinari M., Feggi L., Panareo S., De Troia A., Zatelli M. C., et al. Radio-guided selective compartment neck dissection improves staging in papillary thyroid carcinoma: a prospective study on 345 patients with a 3-year follow-up. *Surgery. 2014*;156:147–157. doi:10.1016/j.surg.2014.03.045.

[16] Raijmakers P. G. H. M., Paul M. A., Lips P. Sentinel node detection in patients with thyroid carcinoma: a meta-analysis. *World J Surg. 2008*;32:1961–1967. doi: 10.1007/s00268-008-9657-y.

[17] Balasubramanian S. P., Harrison B. J. Systematic review and meta-analysis of sentinel node biopsy in thyroid cancer. *Br J Surg. 2011*;98:334–344. doi:10.1002/bjs.7425.

[18] Pelizzo M. R., Toniato A., Sorgato N., Losi A., Torresan F., Merante Boschin I. 99Tc nanocolloid sentinel node procedure in papillary thyroid carcinoma: our mono-institutional experience on a large series of patients. *Acta Otorhinolaryngol Ital. 2009*; 29:321–325.

In: The Sentinel Lymph Node
Editors: A. Londero, S. Bertozzi and C. Cedolini
ISBN: 978-1-53614-557-1


*Chapter 9*

# SENTINEL LYMPH NODE BIOPSY IN VULVAR CANCER

***Ambrogio P. Londero***[1,*]***, Eva Wilhelmer***[2]***, Serena Bertozzi***[3]***, Arrigo Fruscalzo***[4] ***and Ralph J. Lellé***[5]
[1]Clinic of Obstetrics and Gynecology, University Hospital of Udine, Italy
[2]IHR Klinikum Osnabrück, Osnabrück, Germany
[3]Breast Unit, University Hospital of Udine, Italy
[4]Klinik für Gynäkologie und Geburtshilfe, St. Franziskus-Hospital Ahlen, Germany
[5]Klinik für Frauenheilkunde und Geburtshilfe, Universitätsklinikum Münster, Westfälische Wilhelms-Universität Münster, Germany

**Abstract**

Although vulvar cancer is a rare disease, among Central and Western European countries, such as Germany and the Netherlands, the incidence of the disease has increased significantly during the last decades. Usual treatment of early-stage disease consists of extended local surgery and complete inguino-femoral lymph node dissection, leading to a high curability of the disease. However, morbidity correlated with complete inguino-femoral lymph node dissection is extremely high. Therefore, new conservative techniques have been developed to maintain high standards of curability, while reducing morbidity, such as the sentinel lymph node biopsy, which has a false-negative rate of 6.4% (CI 95% 4.4-8.7%) and a groin recurrence rate in node-negative cases of 4% (CI 95% 2-6%), while the inguino-femoral lymph node dissection has a groin recurrence rate in node-negative cases of 1% (CI 95% 0-3%). Mortality among groin recurrences is still extremely high (72%; CI 95% 60-82%). In order to reduce the false-negative rate of sentinel lymph node biopsy, the technique must be performed by highly-trained medical specialists in gynecological oncological departments. New technical improvements should be assessed in experimental settings to reduce the false-negative rate as well as morbidity correlated with extended surgical treatment, while maintaining a high curability of early-stage disease.

*Corresponding Author E-mail: ambrogio.londero@gmail.com.

**Keywords:** vulvar cancer, sentinel lymph node bipsy, false negative rate, groin recurrence rate, groin recurrence mortality

# 1. Introduction

In Europe the annual incidence of invasive carcinoma of the vulva ranges between 1.8 and 4.0 cases per 100,000 women [1]. In particular, in Germany the incidence of vulvar cancer has nearly doubled over the past decade, exceeding the rates observed in other European countries [1]. Moreover, in Hamburg and Saarland the incidence rate of vulvar cancer has reached six cases per 100,000 women [1]. In the Netherlands, as well, the incidence rate has significantly increased between 1989 and 2010 in women aged less than 60 [2].

This typically rare malignancy has a high curability at early stages. However, outcomes are still poor for patients with advanced and recurrent disease. Squamous cell carcinoma (81%) is the most common histological type of vulvar cancer, followed by basal cell carcinoma (6%) [2].

Vulvar cancer is associated with either human papilloma virus (HPV) related dysplasia (more common among young women) or with vulvar dermatoses (i.e. lichen sclerosis, more common among older women). In fact, preinvasive lesions of the vulva are since 2014 classified as HPV positive usual type vulvar intra-epitelial neoplasia (VIN) and HPV negative differentiated VIN (dVIN) [3]. According to its severity, usual type VIN is actually classified into VIN 1 (or low-grade squamous intraepithelial lesion LSIL), and VIN 2-3 (or high-grade squamous intraepithelial lesion HSIL) [3]. In particular, the risk of progression from HSIL and dVIN to invasive cancer is significant and dVIN tends to progress faster [3]. Other risk factors associated with the development of vulvar cancer are smoking habit, sexually transmitted diseases, immunosupression, hypertension, diabetes mellitus, and obesity [4].

The most common clinical presentations of vulvar cancer are vulvar pruritus and a self-palpable lesion. The actual staging of vulvar cancer is performed according to the 2017 TNM classification and the 2009 FIGO classification [5, 6]. In particular, the staining system updated in 2017 is shown in Table 1.

Since lymph nodes positivity plays a crucial prognostic role in staging the disease, the concepts of lymph-node isolated tumor cells (ITCs) and micrometastases have been introduced also for vulvar cancer. In particular, ITCs and micrometastases are detected by subjecting sentinel lymph nodes to pathologic ultrastaging.

Early-stage vulvar cancer is traditionally treated with radical surgery and complete inguinal lymphadenectomy. In any case, this type of surgery is correlated with high morbidity due to lower limb lymphedema. For this reason, there has been a search for alternative interventions to be as effective as the classical intervention, while associated with less morbidity. Initially, superficial inguinal lymphadenectomy was suggested, as well as sentinel lymph node biopsy (SLNB) prior to classical radical inguinal lymphadenectomy.

The main questions on this subject are the following. Can SLNB be a standard technique for vulvar pathology? What is the prevalence of failure of this technique in finding the sentinel lymph node? What is the prevalence of false negatives? What is the prevalence of recurrences in patients who do not undergo lymphadenectomy after negative sentinel node biopsy? The next sections will answer these questions.

**Table 1. FIGO/TNM staging, update 2017 [5, 6]. In N0 staging are included also isolated tumor cells (ITCs) ($N0_{(i+)}$)**

| Stage | FIGO/TNM 2017 |
|---|---|
| | Pathologic staging |
| I | Vulva/perineum (N0)<br>I-a) Lesion $\leq 2cm$ and stromal invasiona $\leq 1.0mm$ - (T1a)<br>I-b) Lesion ¿2cm or any size with stromal invasiona ¿ 1.0 mm - (T1b) |
| II | Vulva/perineum any size (N0) with extension to: (1) lower/distal third of the urethra; (2) lower/distal third of the vagina; (3) anal involvement - (T2) |
| III | T1/T2 AND:<br>III-a) ¡3 lymph node metastases each ¡5 mm (also micro-metastases) - (N1a) OR ¡2 lymph node metastasis $\geq 5mm$ (N1b)<br>III-b) $\geq$ 3 lymph node metastases each less than 5 mm (also micro-metastases) - (N2a) OR two OR $\geq$ 2 lymph node metastases $\geq 5mm$ (N2b)<br>III-c) Lymph node(s) with extranodal extension (N2c) |
| IV | IV-a) Tumor of any size with extension to any of the following: (1) upper/proximal 2/3 of the urethra; (2) upper/proximal 2/3 of the vagina; (3) bladder mucosa, or rectal mucosa, or fixed to the pelvic bone - (T3) AND/OR fixed or ulcerated regional lymph-node metastasis - (N3)<br>IV-b) Distant metastasis (including pelvic lymph node metastasis) (M1) |

## 2. The Rationale of Sentinel Lymph Node Biopsy in Vulvar Cancer

Since the 1990s, many studies on SLNB in vulvar cancer have been published. The GROINSS-V (GROningen INational Study on Sentinel nodes in Vulvar cancer) is a prospective observational study that analyzed a female cohort where dissection was performed only in the case of a positive sentinel lymph node. This study was carried out by the Netherlands in collaboration with some international institutes, such as the IEO of Milan [7, 8]. Data from this study has been published in two articles. The first article, published in 2008, presented data from patients with a negative sentinel lymph node, while the second article, published in 2010, reviewed data from patients with a positive sentinel lymph node and subsequent radical dissection [7, 8].

A second major prospective observational study was conducted by the German working group AGO (Arbeitsgemeinschaft Gynäkologische Onkologie) [9]. In this multicenter study, the sentinel lymph node was first identified and, subsequently, complete inguinal lymphadenectomy was in any case performed.

A third multicenter prospective study conducted by the American group GOG (Gynecologic Oncology Group) was presented at the annual congress ASCO (American Society of Clinical Oncology) in 2009 and published in 2013 [10, 11]. As in the German study, also in this case the sentinel lymph node was identified before performing routine inguino-femoral lymph node dissection.

However, many other studies have considered SLNB in vulvar cancer [12, 13, 14, 15, 16, 17, 18, 19, 9, 20, 21, 22, 8, 23, 24, 25, 26, 27, 28, 29, 30, 31, 32, 33, 34, 35]. In addition, there is also a series of retrospective studies that have reported the outcome of patients with early-stage disease who did not undergo inguinal dissection or who underwent it only partially (superficial inguinal lymphadenectomy) [8, 36, 37, 38, 39, 40, 41, 42].

As in all the methods that require surgical skills, there is an unquestionable operator-to-operator variability in sentinel lymph node biopsy. This is even more evident in multicentric studies. Since vulvar carcinoma is a rare pathology, studies to obtain adequate numbers must involve many centers. Therefore, one of the limitations of the studies on SLNB in vulvar cancer is the technical variability between different surgeons and the difficulty of gathering an adequate experience, given the few cases per type of surgery for the surgeon [12].

## 2.1. Recurrences and Outcome

In Figure 1 the prevalence of recurrences in the different studies considered is shown. Through these studies it has been possible to compare the recurrence rate between cases that have undergone classical complete inguino-femoral lymph node dissection and cases where no lymphadenectomy has been performed or a non-standard surgical technique has been applied (i.e. superficial lymphadenectomy or SLNB). In detail, it can be noted that local recurrence in groins of patients with initial malignancies affected about 17% (CI.95 8-28%) of cases not treated with lymphadenectomy and only 8% (CI.95 6-11%) of cases treated with superficial negative lymphadenectomy alone. In addition, the locoregional recurrence rate was 4% (CI.95 2-6%) in patients with negative SLNB without subsequent dissection and only 1% (CI.95 0-3.0%) in patients who underwent complete dissection after negative SLNB. In a recent meta-analysis, recurrence rates were 2.8% (CI.95 1.5-4.4%) after performing SLNB alone, while decreased to even 1.4% (CI.95 0.5-2.6%) after complete dissection [43]. Probably, the difference between data reported in Figure 1 and data of Covens and colleagues is due to the inclusion in the meta-analysis of only node-negative patients, and consequently of adequate complete dissections only after negative SLNB.

Although these prevalences are difficult to compare, as data derives from different studies conducted at different time periods when the knowledge and techniques applied were clearly different, they do provide an interesting overview of how the chosen technique and the risk of recurrence correlate. Furthermore, Figure 2 shows that in the case of any non-standard technique, the appearance of a groin recurrence is associated with a very high prevalence of mortality of up to 72% (CI.95 60-82%) that, as can be seen, has only slightly decreased in recent years.

## 2.2. True-Positive Rate

In order to understand the reasons for the success of the sentinel lymph node concept, even in the case of vulvar neoplasms it is important to analyze the prevalence of lymph node positivity in patients who undergo inguinal lymphadenectomy. In fact, if this prevalence is very high, SLNB would probably not succeed in reducing morbidity by sparing the node-negative population from unnecessary dissections.

In this perspective, Figure 3A clearly shows that positive lymph nodes are usually found only in 32% (CI.95 26-38%) of patients with vulvar neoplasia. Therefore, most interventions are useless from a therapeutic and staging perspective, and even harmful due to the major complications they are associated with. However, without this type of intervention it

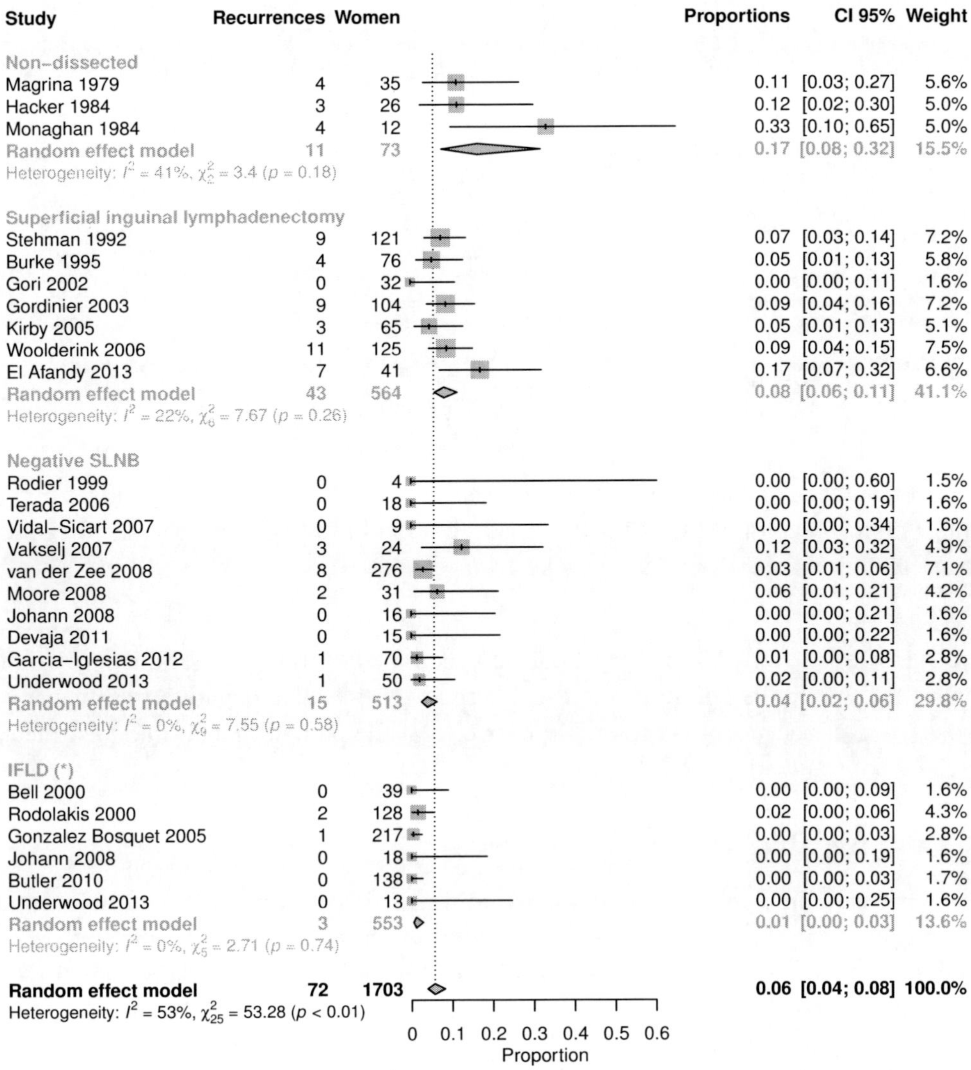


Figure 1. Recurrence prevalence in non-standard techniques for groin lymph-node treatment and in inguino-femoral lymph-node dissection (IFLND; (*) included only FIGO stage I or II or negative nodes) among vulvar cancer affected women [41, 38, 39, 44, 36, 45, 46, 47, 48, 49, 27, 8, 22, 50, 26, 51, 52, 53, 21, 54, 55, 51, 56, 57, 58, 21]. Updated data from an unpublished meta-analysis performed in 2010.

is not possible to distinguish between groins with subclinical metastases and groins that are actually free from the disease.

In Figure 3B the denominator is the number of dissected groins, instead of the number of women. It is thus possible to see that the true positive rate is around 22% (CI.95 16-29%). Therefore, most of the groins that have been dissected are definitely negative for the presence of metastases, meaning that the morbidity is probably not correlated with higher

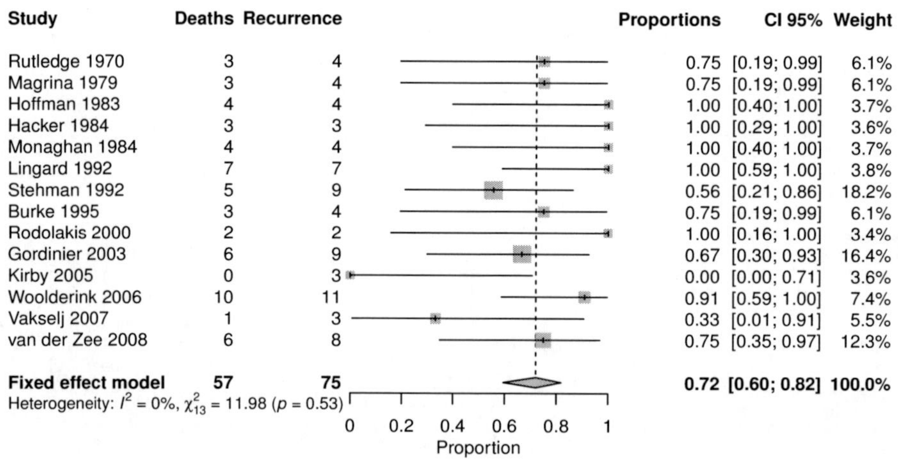


Figure 2. Prevalence of death in inguinal recurrences, in patients with non-standard inguino-femoral lymphadenectomy [42, 41, 40, 38, 39, 37, 45, 44, 57, 47, 48, 36, 53, 8]. Updated data from an unpublished meta-analysis performed in 2010.

survival. However, from a more practical perspective and giving importance to women's survival, the clinician is certainly more concerned by the false-negative rate than by the true positive rate, because it is preferable to overtreat the patient than to underestimate the disease and consequently undertreat it.

## 2.3. False-Negative Rate

In fact, what the clinician really wants to avoid in the field of oncology are false-negative cases, and therefore the administration of suboptimal treatments to patients with a false-negative result. In the literature, considering at least one false-negative groin, the false-negative rate is about 12% of women (CI.95 7-21%) (Figure 4A, unpublished data from a meta-analysis carried out in 2010). In other studies, however, the false-negative rate reached up to 27-31% (Figure 4A).

Thus, if the number of groins treated is taken into account, the prevalence of false-negative cases is around 8% (CI.95 4-14%) (Figure 4B). To calculate the false-negative rate in the studies shown in Figures 4A and 4B, SLNB has always been followed by complete inguino-femoral lymphadenectomy. Moreover, in a recent meta-analysis, the false-negative rate after SLNB was 6.4% (CI.95 4.4-8.7%) [43].

The standard therapy currently available for vulvar carcinoma is still surgical treatment, whose demolition intent has undergone essential modifications, starting with the Way incision. Over the years, in fact, we have witnessed a reduction in the demolitive surgical intent by maintaining surgical radicality. Examples of this are the resection of the neoplasm with adequate disease-free margins and the completion of the surgery with inguino-femoral lymphadenectomy with two separate incisions (also known as the three incision technique). All these changes have been made with the aim of improving the quality of life of women who survive the disease.

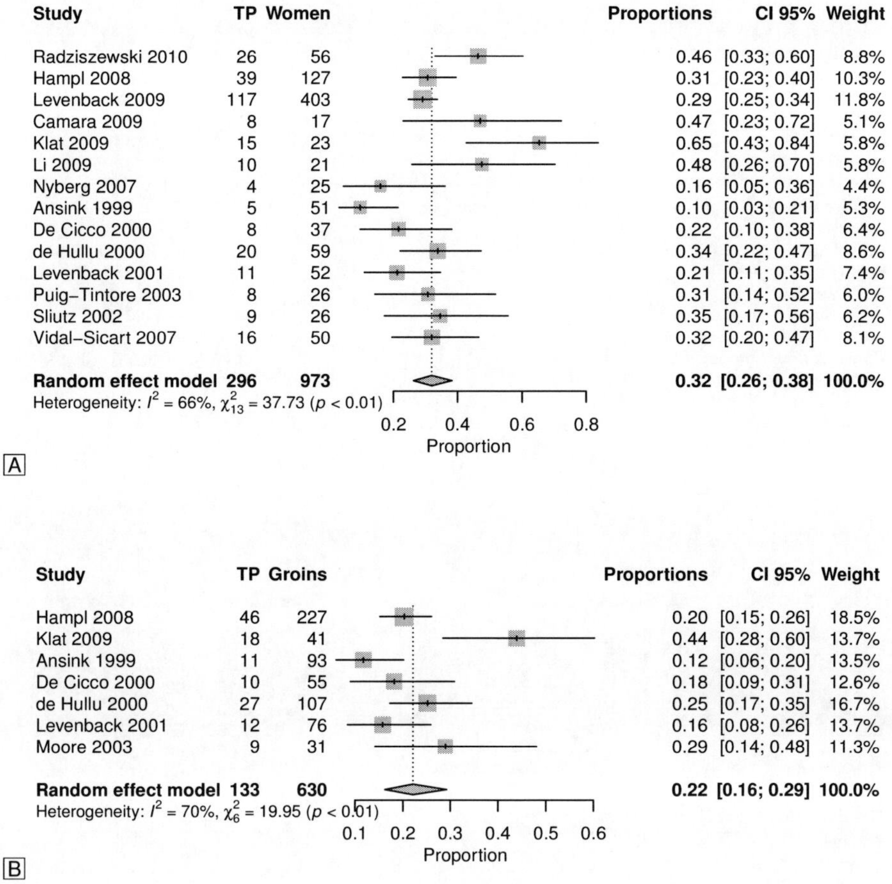


Figure 3. (Panel A) Prevalence of positive lymph nodes in dissected patients [12, 9, 10, 15, 16, 17, 25, 34, 32, 33, 31, 29, 30, 26]. (Panel B) Prevalence of positive lymph nodes in dissected patients, analysis by groin [9, 16, 34, 32, 33, 31, 28]. Data from an unpublished meta-analysis performed in 2010.

Among the side effects of complete inguino-femoral lymphadenectomy, lower limb lymphedema remains the most common long-term sequela, affecting about 50% of women who have undergone complete inguino-femoral lymphadenectomy. Van der Zee and colleagues have pointed out that complications associated with SLNB alone compared with complications associated with complete inguino-femoral lymphadenectomy are significantly lower both in the short and long term [8]. In fact, the group that underwent inguino-femoral lymphadenectomy reported a significantly higher incidence of surgical wound complications and cellulitis (surgical wound infection) in the short term and a higher prevalence of recurrent erysipelas and lower limb lymphedema in the long term [8].

The high prevalence of complications after lymph node dissection, together with the consideration that only 22% of groins are certainly affected by metastases, led clinicians to

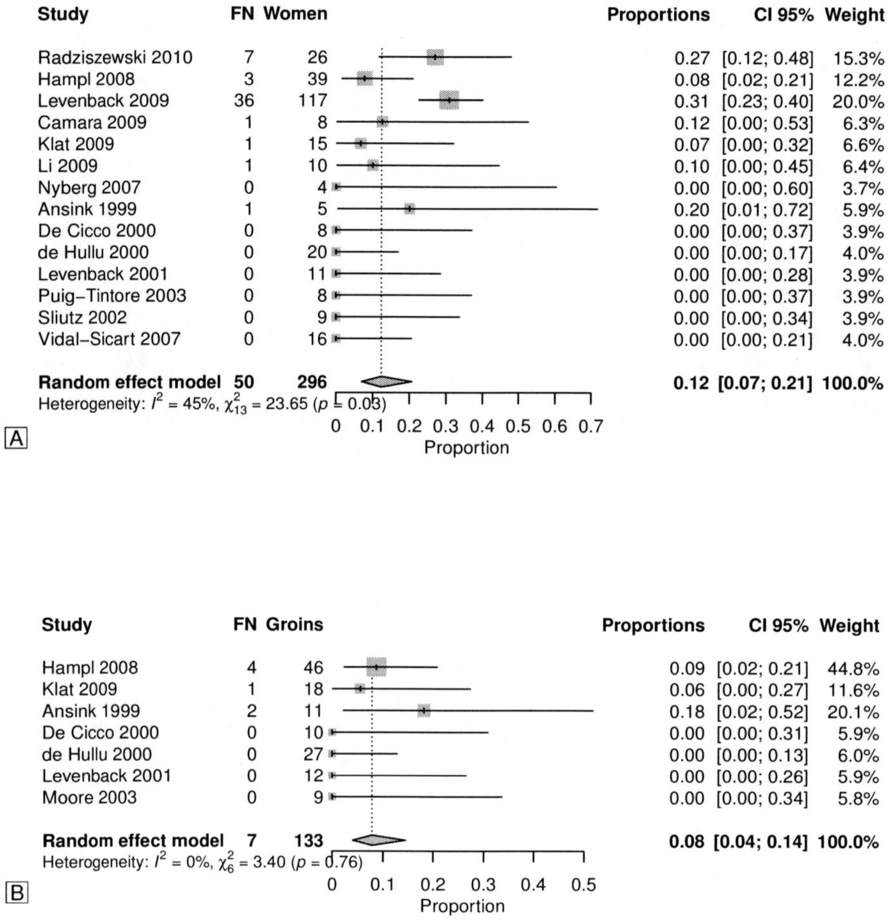


Figure 4. (Panel A) False-negative rate (FNR) [12, 9, 10, 15, 16, 17, 25, 34, 32, 33, 31, 29, 30, 26]. (Panel B) FNR, analysis by groin [9, 16, 34, 32, 33, 31, 28]. Data from an unpublished meta-analysis performed in 2010.

explore new therapies, such as the superficial inguinal lymphadenectomy and the SLNB, to decide whether or not to perform complete lymphadenectomy. However, these less invasive techniques have to deal with the possibility of false-negative cases and the possible presence of inguinal metastases or future recurrences. Both metastases and recurrences have a particularly important predictive and prognostic role in decision-making for vulvar cancer. In fact, the presence of inguinal metastases will guide the adjuvant therapy, while inguinal recurrences are life-threatening and correlated with high mortality in patients with vulvar neoplastic pathology (Figure 2).

The mortality rate is particularly high because there is no sufficiently effective chemotherapy nor radiotherapy to treat distant vulvar disease yet. For this reason, local surgical procedure is still the gold standard of treatment in patients with vulvar cancer. It is clear, however, that there is much room for improvement and there are many clinicians who are seeking to make this improvement possible through their theories, such as Levenback, who introduced SLNB in squamous cell carcinoma of the vulva for the first time [59]. Current expectations for sentinel lymph node techniques in vulvar cancer are characterized both by radicality in the case of node-positive disease and the attempt to safeguard patients' quality of life without increasing the risk of unfortunate events.

Now, we will take a look at the process that leads the clinician to choose whether or not to perform SLNB. It is essential to discuss with the patient the possible complications, risks and benefits of different surgical techniques. In a study conducted by Dr. Rhonda Farrell and colleagues, from Prof. Hacker's group, one of the most distinguished names in the field of vulvar cancer surgery, the trade-off between quality of life and survival duration was measured using a questionnaire. In particular, the trade-off was assessed between the risk of missing lymph node metastases after negative SLNB versus finding all the possible metastases by inguino-femoral lymph node dissection. In the first case, missing possible metastases of the lymph nodes will almost certainly lead to death, but in the second case, performing a complete dissection even in unnecessary cases will lead to a 60% probability of developing chronic lower limb lymphedema [60]. Therefore, the study consisted of informing 60 patients about the risks and benefits, and subsequently asking them which risk they were willing to take in order to obtain minor complications from the current standard intervention. 5% of women were undecided, 15% would have accepted a risk of 1:2/1:100; 17% of 1:200/1:1000; 10% of 1:1,000,000. However, up to 53% would not accept any risk [60]. It is therefore clear from this study that there are patients who would prefer to opt for an intervention that has fewer side effects but a higher risk of recurrences; in any case, most patients do not want to take this risk. For this reason, adequate information is essential to enable patients to choose how to proceed.

In any case, current medicine has never given up, and the best strategy to guarantee the best possible treatment in the future with the least side effects is to carry out randomized clinical trials concerning SLNB, with a multicentric observational design and a longer follow-up. In addition, new techniques for the execution of SLNB have been explored, as well as the effectiveness of multimodal treatment, such as the combination of SLNB and subsequent radiation therapy. The goal is still to reduce surgical invasiveness and complications by maintaining its effectiveness in terms of oncological radicality.

Another possible approach is to develop predictive models for the presence of inguinal positive nodes, not only on the basis of classical, pathological and clinical results, but also of molecular biology to better classify the prognosis of vulvar cancer [61]. For example, a possible innovative system to spare the axillary lymph nodes that are certainly not affected by the disease is the axillary reverse mapping, that makes use of a preoperative injection of patent blue to visualize the lymph nodes draining exclusively the ipsilateral limb [62]. Using this approach, in the case of sentinel lymph node positivity, it would be possible to perform selective regional lymphadenectomy of lymph nodes draining the tumor, while saving the lymph nodes draining the limb. At the moment, this technique has been tested only for breast cancer, but it cannot be excluded that in the future it will also be applied to vulvar carcinoma to spare the lymph nodes involved exclusively in the drainage of the lower limb.

Finally, in order to better treat early-stage invasive vulvar carcinoma, the aforementioned advancements in surgical technique could probably be surpassed by new effective medical therapies, as occured for Imiquimod in the therapy of the vulvar neoplasm in stage FIGO 0, i.e. the VIN III [63] or Paget disease of the vulva [64].

# 3. Technical Aspects

## 3.1. Patient Selection

A recent meta-analysis and current guidelines recommend that SLNB should be performed in a selected group of women with unifocal tumors smaller than 4 cm and in the absence of clinically or imaging suspicious inguinal nodes or previous vulvar surgery, which may have altered lymphatic flow in the inguinal region [43, 65, 66, 8]. In fact, there is not enough evidence in the literature to recommend SLNB in women with tumors of 4 cm or greater in size, or multifocal disease [43, 65]. In any case, this procedure is not recommended in the presence of clinically suspicious inguinal nodes [43, 65].

## 3.2. Surgeon Learning Curve

The introduction of sentinel lymph node biopsy for vulvar cancer clearly showed that it was a challenging technique, as the cases to be tested and gain experience from are extremely few, especially because of the rarity of this condition. Recent guidelines have suggested an appropriate surgical training of the surgeon, which consists of supervised experience with SLNB procedure followed by complete inguino-femoral lymphadenectomy without any false-negative case [43]. At the end of the training period, on-going annual experience with this procedure is recommended to maintain the competence [43].

Therefore, in order to optimize patient's safety and outcome, SLNB should ideally be performed by a high-volume surgeon in specialized Gynecologic Oncology Centers [43, 65]. It is also suggested that the learning curve for a successful training should include at least ten patients undergoing supervised SLNB followed by complete inguino-femoral dissection without any false-negative case [43]. Furthermore, the annual experience needed to maintain the competence is estimated in about ten cases per center or, better still, per surgeon [43]. In low-volume centers, a multidisciplinary management should be the ideal choice, using the help of surgeons with experience in this technique, such as breast surgeons or surgeons performing SLNB for melanomas [43].

## 3.3. Sentinel Lymph Node Detection Techniques

Due to its high sensitivity, in the literature the preferred method for sentinel lymph node detection is the combined use of radiocolloid tracers and blue dye [67, 68, 69, 43, 65]. Radiocolloid tracers are also frequently used alone, but in the case of a suspicious lymphoscintigraphy that does not show any evident sentinel node in the groin of interest, the use of blue dye is an essential addition. In contrast, the use of blue dye alone should be discouraged due to its low sentinel lymph node detection rate (63% with blue dye alone vs 85% with radioactive technetium alone) [43]. Despite the growing interest in near-infrared tracers, such as indocyanine green, there is still not enough evidence to make recommendations for or against the use of these tracers. For this reason they should be only used in experimental and controlled settings [43, 65].

Technetium-99 sulfur colloid is the most common tracer injected into vulvar cancer to find the sentinel lymph node. Technetium-99 sulfur colloid tracer is typically injected 2-4 hours prior to surgery (for vulvectomy and lymphadenectomy procedures). Although there is not sufficient data to produce recommendations based on evidence regarding pre-operative lymphoscintigraphy, it can be useful to anatomically locate the sentinel node and identify the number of radioactive sentinel nodes. It should also be noted that the timing of radiocolloid injection may in general vary between 30 minutes to 24 hours before surgery, and this time interval depends mainly on the size of the radiocolloid used. For this reason, manufacturer's instructions must be followed scrupulously [43, 65].

The most commonly used vital dye is isosulfan blue 1%. 3-4 cc of dye is usually injected around the tumor site into normal tissue with a four-quadrant pattern intradermal injection. Blue dye is usually injected in the operating room about 15-30 minutes before surgery start time. In addition, blue dye localization can be made for only 30-60 minutes in the first group of nodes, which correspond to the real sentinel nodes of vulvar cancer. This means that the procedure must be promptly performed after the induction of anaesthesia. In any case, a four-point injection method is used in both blue dye and radiocolloid techniques, which includes injections at 2, 5, 7, and 10 o'clock position around the lesion site. In order to identify the sentinel lymph node it is necessary to consider a threshold of 5 times the background radioactivity, while to find the blue lymph nodes it is necessary to follow the blue lymphatic channels [43, 65].

Prior to the surgical inguinal incision, the detection of the hottest radiocolloid point within the inguino-femoral region by means of the gamma probe is recommended to better tailor the location and size of the incision itself [65]. In addition, it is also recommended to perform SLNB procedure prior to the surgical excision of the vulvar cancer in order to avoid disrupting the lymphatic network between the primary tumor and lymph nodes.

Obviously, if no ipsilateral sentinel lymph node is found, complete inguino-femoral lymphadenectomy is recommended.

## 3.4. Sentinel Lymph Node Detection Failure

Figure 5 shows that the prevalence of failure of sentinel lymph node detection is around 4% (CI.95 2-7%), and thus very low. This prevalence appears to be higher in studies where the blue patent was used alone than in those where it was combined with the use of a radioactive tracer. In fact, the inguinal SLNB detection rate using blue dye together with radiocolloid tracer was 87% (CI.95 82-92%) [43]. In the literature, the combination of blue dye and radiocolloid tracer is the most commonly used technique. In addition, other tracer agents, such as near-infrared fluorescent indocyanine green, may further improve the sentinel lymph node detection rate. However, at the moment, there is not enough data regarding SLNB procedure in patients with vulvar cancer [70, 71].

## 3.5. Pathological Considerations

Sufficient evidence is not available for the use of intraoperative frozen section in the case of sentinel lymph node biopsy for vulvar cancer. However, it is known from other medical fields that the accuracy of the frozen section is inferior to that of definitive histological examination or new molecular biology-based technologies, such as the OSNA method.

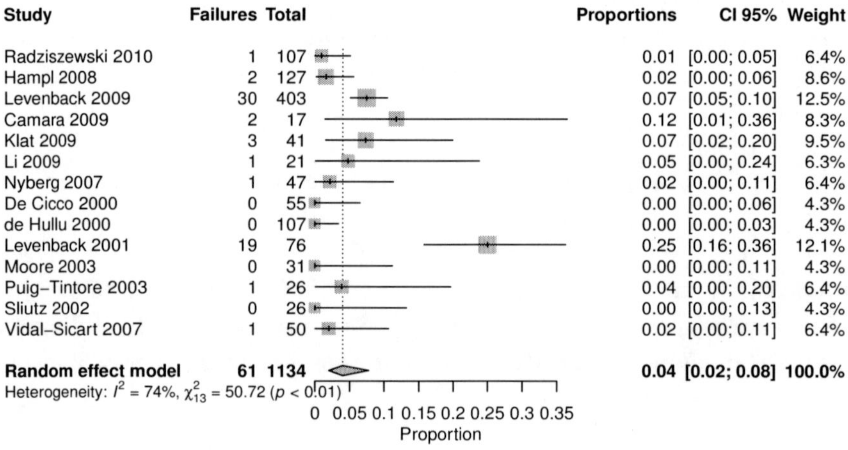


Figure 5. Failure of detection of sentinel lymph node [12, 9, 10, 15, 16, 17, 25, 32, 33, 31, 28, 29, 30, 26]. Data from an unpublished meta-analysis performed in 2010.

In any case, for the evaluation of sentinel lymph node in vulvar cancer it is recommended to use the ultrastaging technique, which consists of the serial sectioning of the lymph node in 3 mm blocks. At least two sections 40 m apart from each other should be taken for each block. The first section shall be examined by routine hematoxylin-eosin staining and, if negative for metastatic disease, the second section shall be examined after immunohistochemical staining for cytokeratin.

## 4. Lymph Node and Non-Sentinel Lymph-Node Involvement Prediction

There are currently no clinically validated algorithms for predicting non-sentinel lymph node involvement for vulvar cancer. However, selection criteria for SLNB in patients with vulvar cancer exclude high risk patients. In particular, patients with multifocal disease were excluded from a study conducted by Van der Zee and colleagues, as two patients with multiple lesions and a negative sentinel node suffered from an inguinal recurrence within a short period of time [8].

Moreover, inguinal lymph node treatment may be omitted in vulvar cancer with a stromal invasion of 1 mm or less, as it is a strong predictive factor for negative inguinal nodes [72, 61]. However, even in this case, there is a probability of missing positive nodes, although it is extremely low. As a matter of fact, in the literature, inguinal recurrences in T1a vulvar cancer cases have also been described [72].

# 5. Management of the Positive or Negative Sentinel Lymph Node Biopsy

There is still uncertainty about the management of a positive sentinel lymph node. In fact, studies are still ongoing to evaluate the best management between complete inguino-femoral lymphadenectomy and adjuvant radiation therapy for the affected groin or both.

There is uncertainty also about the contralateral groin management in the case of a positive ipsilateral sentinel lymph node. In the absence of different evidence, the contralateral groin should be evaluated surgically and treated with adjuvant irradiation if needed. Therefore, in the case of a negative contralateral SLNB, it may be reasonable to omit complete inguino-femoral lymphadenectomy in the contralateral groin, even when detecting a positive node in the ipsilateral groin. Despite the lack of evidence on this subject, considering the expected low incidence of metastases on the contralateral groin and the high incidence of surgical complications by performing complete lymphadenectomy, current literature suggests to spare the contralateral groin in the presence of a negative sentinel node.

# Conclusion

At the present state of our knowledge, SLNB in early-stage vulvar cancer is routinely applied as the gold standard treatment only in specialized centers. In fact, the possible benefits are counterbalanced by the possibility of inguinal recurrences in the case of a false negativity, since inguinal recurrences are often fatal.

An important factor to keep in mind is that the SLNB false-negative rate is highly operator-dependent and that, due to the rarity of vulvar cancer, it is often difficult to accumulate an adequate experience, given the few cases that each center is able to collect. Also, even in large multicenter studies, there are only limited number of cases reported for each center. For this reason, it would be desirable in the future to collect all cases in super-specialized centers, which would then be able to develop the experience needed to give women optimal treatment, with the least number of side effects that could compromise their quality of life.

The hope for the future is that new techniques with greater accuracy will improve early-stage vulvar carcinoma surgery. In particular, the concept of reverse mapping proposed for axillary lymphadenectomy could lead to new advancements in vulvar carcinoma, as it would be able to identify the lymph nodes draining exclusively the lower limb and not the vulva, thus sparing the disease-free lymph nodes and reducing the side effects of complete inguinal lymphadenectomy.

# References

[1] Buttmann-Schweiger N., Klug S. J., Luyten A., Holleczek B., Heitz F., du Bois A., et al. Incidence patterns and temporal trends of invasive nonmelanotic vulvar tumors in Germany 1999-2011. A population-based cancer registry analysis. *PLoS ONE. 2015*;10:e0128073. doi:10.1371/journal.pone.0128073.

[2] Schuurman M. S., van den Einden L. C. G., Massuger L. F. A. G., Kiemeney L. A., van der Aa M. A., de Hullu J. A. Trends in incidence and survival of Dutch women with vulvar squamous cell carcinoma. *Eur J Cancer. 2013*;49:3872–3880. doi:10.1016/j.ejca.2013.08.003.

[3] Reich O., Regauer S., Marth C., Schmidt D., Horn L. C., Dannecker C., et al. Precancerous Lesions of the Cervix, Vulva and Vagina According to the 2014 WHO Classification of Tumors of the Female Genital Tract. *Geburtshilfe Frauenheilkd. 2015*; 75:1018–1020. doi:10.1055/s-0035-1558052.

[4] Dellinger T. H., Hakim A. A., Lee S. J., Wakabayashi M. T., Morgan R. J., Han E. S. Surgical Management of Vulvar Cancer. *J Natl Compr Canc Netw. 2017*;15:121–128.

[5] Pecorelli S. Revised FIGO staging for carcinoma of the vulva, cervix, and endometrium. *Int J Gynaecol Obstet. 2009*;105:103–104.

[6] American College of Surgeons. *AJCC Cancer Staging Manual (Eighth Edition).* Springer. 2017.

[7] Oonk M. H., van Hemel B. M., Hollema H., de Hullu J. A., Ansink A. C., Vergote I., et al. Size of sentinel-node metastasis and chances of non-sentinel-node involvement and survival in early stage vulvar cancer: results from GROINSS-V, a multicentre observational study. *Lancet Oncol. 2010*;11:646–652. doi:10.1016/S1470-2045(10)70104-2.

[8] Van der Zee A. G. J., Oonk M. H., Hullu J. A. D., Ansink A. C., Vergote I., Verheijen R. H., et al. Sentinel node dissection is safe in the treatment of early-stage vulvar cancer. *J Clin Oncol. 2008*;26:884–889. doi:10.1200/JCO.2007.14.0566.

[9] Hampl M., Hantschmann P., Michels W., Hillemanns P., Group G. M. S. Validation of the accuracy of the sentinel lymph node procedure in patients with vulvar cancer: results of a multicenter study in Germany. *Gynecol Oncol. 2008*;111:282–288.

[10] Levenback C. F., Tian C., Coleman R. L., Gold M. A., Fowler J. M., Judson P. L. Sentinel node (SN) biopsy in patients with vulvar cancer: A Gynecologic Oncology Group (GOG) study. *J Clin Oncol (Meeting Abstracts). 2009*;27:5505–.

[11] Coleman R. L., Ali S., Levenback C. F., Gold M. A., Fowler J. M., Judson P. L., et al. Is bilateral lymphadenectomy for midline squamous carcinoma of the vulva always necessary? An analysis from Gynecologic Oncology Group (GOG) 173. *Gynecol Oncol. 2013*;128:155–159. doi:10.1016/j.ygyno.2012.11.034.

[12] Radziszewski J., Kowalewska M., Jedrzejczak T., Kozlowicz-Gudzinska I., Nasierowska-Guttmejer A., Bidzinski M., et al. The accuracy of the sentinel lymph node concept in early stage squamous cell vulvar carcinoma. *Gynecol Oncol. 2010*; 116:473–477. doi:10.1016/j.ygyno.2009.10.072.

[13] Trifirò G., Travaini L. L., Sanvito F., Pacifici M., Mallia A., Ferrari M. E., et al. Sentinel node detection by lymphoscintigraphy and sentinel lymph node biopsy in vulvar

melanoma. *Eur J Nucl Med Mol Imaging. 2010*;37:736–741. doi:10.1007/s00259-009-1358-8.

[14] Achimas-Cadariu P., Harter P., Fisseler-Eckhoff A., Beutel B., Traut A., Bois A. D. Assessment of the sentinel lymph node in patients with invasive squamous carcinoma of the vulva. *Acta Obstet Gynecol Scand. 2009*;88:1209–1214. doi: 10.3109/00016340903317982.

[15] Camara O., Gonnert H., Herrmann J., Egbe A., Diebolder H., Gajda M., et al. Sentinel lymph node biopsy in vulvar cancer: a pilot study. *Eur J Gynaecol Oncol. 2009*; 30:622–624.

[16] Klát J., Sevcík L., Simetka O., Gráf P., Waloschek T., Kraft O., et al. Characteristics of sentinel lymph nodes' metastatic involvement in early stage of vulvar cancer. *Aust N Z J Obstet Gynaecol. 2009*;49:672–676. doi:10.1111/j.1479-828X.2009.01073.x.

[17] Li B., ying Wu L., Liu L., Zhang R., yi Zhang G., zhi Yu G. [An initial experience of the use of sentinel lymph node biopsy in squamous cell cancer of the vulva]. *Zhonghua Fu Chan Ke Za Zhi. 2009*;44:364–368.

[18] Pazin V., Dragojevi c S., Mikovi c Z., Duki c M., Raki c S., Marinkovi c J., et al. The value of sentinel lymphadenectomy in radical operative treatment of cervical cancer. *Vojnosanit Pregl. 2009*;66:539–543.

[19] Brunner A. H., Polterauer S., Tempfer C., Joura E., Reinthaller A., Horvat R., et al. The accuracy of intraoperative frozen section of the inguinal sentinel lymph node in vulvar cancer. *Anticancer Res. 2008*;28:4091–4094.

[20] Hefler L. A., Grimm C., Six L., Seebacher V., Polterauer S., Joura E., et al. Inguinal sentinel lymph node dissection vs. complete inguinal lymph node dissection in patients with vulvar cancer. *Anticancer Res. 2008*;28:515–517.

[21] Johann S., Klaeser B., Krause T., Mueller M. D. Comparison of outcome and recurrence-free survival after sentinel lymph node biopsy and lymphadenectomy in vulvar cancer. *Gynecol Oncol. 2008*;110:324–328. doi:10.1016/j.ygyno.2008.04.004.

[22] Moore R. G., Robison K., Brown A. K., DiSilvestro P., Steinhoff M., Noto R., et al. Isolated sentinel lymph node dissection with conservative management in patients with squamous cell carcinoma of the vulva: a prospective trial. *Gynecol Oncol. 2008*; 109:65–70. doi:10.1016/j.ygyno.2007.12.027.

[23] Martínez-Palones J. M., Pérez-Benavente M. A., Gil-Moreno A., Díaz-Feijoo B., Roca I., García-Jiménez A., et al. Comparison of recurrence after vulvectomy and lymphadenectomy with and without sentinel node biopsy in early stage vulvar cancer. *Gynecol Oncol. 2006*;103:865–870. doi:10.1016/j.ygyno.2006.05.024.

[24] Robison K., Steinhoff M. M., Granai C. O., Brard L., Gajewski W., Moore R. G. Inguinal sentinel node dissection versus standard inguinal node dissection in patients with vulvar cancer: A comparison of the size of metastasis detected in inguinal lymph nodes. *Gynecol Oncol. 2006*;101:24–27. doi:10.1016/j.ygyno.2005.08.052.

[25] Nyberg R. H., Iivonen M., Parkkinen J., Kuoppala T, Mäenpää JU. Sentinel node and vulvar cancer: a series of 47 patients. *Acta Obstet Gynecol Scand. 2007*;86:615–619. doi:10.1080/00016340701286793.

[26] Vidal-Sicart S., Puig-Tintoré L. M., Lejárcegui J. A., Paredes P., Ortega M. L., Muñoz A., et al. Validation and application of the sentinel lymph node concept in malignant vulvar tumours. *Eur J Nucl Med Mol Imaging. 2007*;34:384–391. doi: 10.1007/s00259-006-0237-9.

[27] Terada K. Y., Shimizu D. M., Jiang C. S., Wong J. H. Outcomes for patients with T1 squamous cell cancer of the vulva undergoing sentinel node biopsy. *Gynecol Oncol. 2006*;102:200–203. doi:10.1016/j.ygyno.2005.11.042.

[28] Moore R. G., DePasquale S. E., Steinhoff M. M., Gajewski W., Steller M., Noto R., et al. Sentinel node identification and the ability to detect metastatic tumor to inguinal lymph nodes in squamous cell cancer of the vulva. *Gynecol Oncol. 2003*;89:475–479.

[29] Puig-Tintoré L. M., Ordi J., Vidal-Sicart S., Lejárcegui J. A., Torné A., Pahisa J., et al. Further data on the usefulness of sentinel lymph node identification and ultrastaging in vulvar squamous cell carcinoma. *Gynecol Oncol. 2003*;88:29–34.

[30] Sliutz G., Reinthaller A., Lantzsch T., Mende T., Sinzinger H., Kainz C., et al. Lymphatic mapping of sentinel nodes in early vulvar cancer. *Gynecol Oncol. 2002*;84:449–452. doi:10.1006/gyno.2001.6572.

[31] Levenback C., Coleman R. L., Burke T. W., Bodurka-Bevers D., Wolf J. K., Gershenson D. M. Intraoperative lymphatic mapping and sentinel node identification with blue dye in patients with vulvar cancer. *Gynecol Oncol. 2001*;83:276–281. doi: 10.1006/gyno.2001.6374.

[32] De Cicco C., Sideri M., Bartolomei M., Grana C., Cremonesi M., Fiorenza M., et al. Sentinel node biopsy in early vulvar cancer. *Br J Cancer. 2000*;82:295–299. doi: 10.1054/bjoc.1999.0918.

[33] de Hullu J. A., Hollema H., Piers D. A., Verheijen R. H., van Diest P. J., Mourits M. J., et al. Sentinel lymph node procedure is highly accurate in squamous cell carcinoma of the vulva. *J Clin Oncol. 2000*;18:2811–2816.

[34] Ansink A. C., Sie-Go D. M., van der Velden J., Sijmons E. A., de Barros Lopes A., Monaghan J. M., et al. Identification of sentinel lymph nodes in vulvar carcinoma patients with the aid of a patent blue V injection: a multicenter study. *Cancer. 1999*; 86:652–656.

[35] de Hullu J. A., Doting E., Piers D. A., Hollema H., Aalders J. G., Koops H. S., et al. Sentinel lymph node identification with technetium-99m-labeled nanocolloid in squamous cell cancer of the vulva. *J Nucl Med. 1998*;39:1381–1385.

[36] Woolderink J. M., de Bock G. H., de Hullu J. A., Davy M. J., van der Zee A. G. J., Mourits M. J. E. Patterns and frequency of recurrences of squamous cell carcinoma of the vulva. *Gynecol Oncol. 2006*;103:293–299. doi:10.1016/j.ygyno.2006.03.010.

[37] Lingard D., Free K., Wright R. G., Battistutta D. Invasive squamous cell carcinoma of the vulva: behaviour and results in the light of changing management regimens. A review of clinicohistological features predictive of regional lymph node involvement and local recurrence. *Aust N Z J Obstet Gynaecol. 1992*;32:137–145.

[38] Hacker N. F., Berek J. S., Lagasse L. D., Nieberg R. K., Leuchter R. S. Individualization of treatment for stage I squamous cell vulvar carcinoma. *Obstet Gynecol. 1984*; 63:155–162.

[39] Monaghan J. M., Hammond I. G. Pelvic node dissection in the treatment of vulval carcinoma–is it necessary? *Br J Obstet Gynaecol. 1984*;91:270–274.

[40] Hoffman J. S., Kumar N. B., Morley G. W. Microinvasive squamous carcinoma of the vulva: search for a definition. *Obstet Gynecol. 1983*;61:615–618.

[41] Magrina J. F., Webb M. J., Gaffey T. A., Symmonds R. E. Stage I squamous cell cancer of the vulva. *Am J Obstet Gynecol. 1979*;134:453–459.

[42] Rutledge F., Smith J. P., Franklin E. W. Carcinoma of the vulva. *Am J Obstet Gynecol. 1970*;106:1117–1130.

[43] Covens A., Vella E. T., Kennedy E. B., Reade C. J., Jimenez W., Le T. Sentinel lymph node biopsy in vulvar cancer: Systematic review, meta-analysis and guideline recommendations. *Gynecol Oncol. 2015*;137:351–361. doi:10.1016/j.ygyno.2015.02.014.

[44] Burke T. W., Levenback C., Coleman R. L., Morris M., Silva E. G., Gershenson D. M. Surgical therapy of T1 and T2 vulvar carcinoma: further experience with radical wide excision and selective inguinal lymphadenectomy. *Gynecol Oncol. 1995*;57:215–220. doi:10.1006/gyno.1995.1128.

[45] Stehman F. B., Bundy B. N., Dvoretsky P. M., Creasman W. T. Early stage I carcinoma of the vulva treated with ipsilateral superficial inguinal lymphadenectomy and modified radical hemivulvectomy: a prospective study of the Gynecologic Oncology Group. *Obstet Gynecol. 1992*;79:490–497.

[46] Gori J. R., Fritsches H. W., Castaño R., Toziano M., Habich D. Ipsilateral superficial inguinal lymphadenectomy for the treatment of early cancer of the vulva. *J Low Genit Tract Dis. 2002*;6:150–154.

[47] Gordinier M. E., Malpica A., Burke T. W., Bodurka D. C., Wolf J. K., Jhingran A., et al. Groin recurrence in patients with vulvar cancer with negative nodes on superficial inguinal lymphadenectomy. *Gynecol Oncol. 2003*;90:625–628.

[48] Kirby T. O., Rocconi R. P., Numnum T. M., Kendrick J. E., Wright J., Fowler W., et al. Outcomes of Stage I/II vulvar cancer patients after negative superficial inguinal lymphadenectomy. *Gynecol Oncol. 2005*;98:309–312. doi:10.1016/j.ygyno.2005.05.011.

[49] El Afandy A., Soliman H., El Sherbiny M., Abo Elkasem H. Groin recurrence in patients with early vulvar cancer following superficial inguinal node dissection. *J Egypt Natl Canc Inst. 2013*;25:121–124. doi:10.1016/j.jnci.2013.05.001.

[50] García-Iglesias A., Rodríguez-Martín M. O., Ruano R., Beltrán D., Peñalosa L., Hernández-Barreiro B., et al. Sentinel node disection in the treatment of early stages of vulvar cancer. *Eur J Gynaecol Oncol. 2012*;33:151–154.

[51] Underwood M., Yap J. K. W., Elattar A., Ganesan R., Notghi A., Crockett C., et al. The use of sentinel node sampling in vulval cancer. *J Obstet Gynaecol. 2013*;33:892–897. doi:10.3109/01443615.2013.834301.

[52] Rodier J. F., Janser J. C., Routiot T., David E., Ott G., Schneegans O., et al. Sentinel node biopsy in vulvar malignancies: a preliminary feasibility study. *Oncol Rep. 1999*; 6:1249–1252.

[53] Vakselj A., Bebar S. The role of sentinel lymph node detection in vulvar carcinoma and the experiences at the Institute of Oncology Ljubljana. *Radiology and Oncology. 2007*;41. doi:10.2478/v10019-007-0027-4.

[54] Devaja O., Mehra G., Coutts M., Adamson S., Montalto S. A., Donaldson J., et al. A prospective study of sentinel lymph node detection in vulval carcinoma: is it time for a change in clinical practice? *Int J Gynecol Cancer. 2011*;21:559–564. doi: 10.1097/IGC.0b013e3182119d8d.

[55] Butler J. S. B., Milliken D. A., Dina R., Eccles S. A., Maghami S. G., Jameson C., et al. Isolated groin recurrence in vulval squamous cell cancer (VSCC). The importance of node count. *Eur J Gynaecol Oncol. 2010*;31:510–513.

[56] Bell J. G., Lea J. S., Reid G. C. Complete groin lymphadenectomy with preservation of the fascia lata in the treatment of vulvar carcinoma. *Gynecol Oncol. 2000*;77:314–318. doi:10.1006/gyno.2000.5790.

[57] Rodolakis A., Diakomanolis E., Voulgaris Z., Akrivos T., Vlachos G., Michalas S. Squamous vulvar cancer: a clinically based individualization of treatment. *Gynecol Oncol. 2000*;78:346–351. doi:10.1006/gyno.2000.5882.

[58] Gonzalez Bosquet J., Magrina J. F., Gaffey T. A., Hernandez J. L., Webb M. J., Cliby W. A., et al. Long-term survival and disease recurrence in patients with primary squamous cell carcinoma of the vulva. *Gynecol Oncol. 2005*;97:828–833. doi: 10.1016/j.ygyno.2005.03.006.

[59] Levenback C., Burke T. W., Gershenson D. M., Morris M., Malpica A., Ross M. I. Intraoperative lymphatic mapping for vulvar cancer. *Obstet Gynecol. 1994*;84:163–167.

[60] Farrell R., Gebski V., Hacker N. F. Quality of life after complete lymphadenectomy for vulvar cancer: do women prefer sentinel lymph node biopsy? *Int J Gynecol Cancer. 2014*;24:813–819. doi:10.1097/IGC.0000000000000101.

[61] Homesley H. D., Bundy B. N., Sedlis A., Yordan E., Berek J. S., Jahshan A., et al. Prognostic factors for groin node metastasis in squamous cell carcinoma of the vulva (a Gynecologic Oncology Group study). *Gynecol Oncol. 1993*;49:279–283. doi: 10.1006/gyno.1993.1127.

[62] Thompson M., Korourian S., Henry-Tillman R., Adkins L., Mumford S., Westbrook K. C., et al. Axillary reverse mapping (ARM): a new concept to identify and enhance lymphatic preservation. *Ann Surg Oncol. 2007*;14:1890–1895. doi:10.1245/s10434-007-9412-x.

[63] van Seters M., van Beurden M., ten Kate F. J. W., Beckmann I., Ewing P. C., Eijkemans M. J. C., et al. Treatment of vulvar intraepithelial neoplasia with topical imiquimod. *N Engl J Med. 2008*;358:1465–1473. doi:10.1056/NEJMoa072685.

[64] Bertozzi S., Londero A. P., Fruscalzo A., Marchesoni D., Lellé R. J. [Paget disease of the vulva: resolution after local treatment with imiquimod–report of a case and review of the literature]. *Gynakol Geburtshilfliche Rundsch. 2009*;49:326–330. doi: 10.1159/000301110.

[65] Koh W. J., Greer B. E., Abu-Rustum N. R., Campos S. M., Cho K. R., Chon H. S., et al. Vulvar Cancer, Version 1.2017, NCCN Clinical Practice Guidelines in Oncology. *J Natl Compr Canc Netw. 2017*;15:92–120.

[66] PDQ Adult Treatment Editorial Board. Vulvar Cancer Treatment (PDQ). *PDQ Cancer Information Summaries. 2018*;.

[67] Wills A., Obermair A. A review of complications associated with the surgical treatment of vulvar cancer. *Gynecol Oncol. 2013*;131:467–479. doi: 10.1016/j.ygyno.2013.07.082.

[68] Reade C. J., Eiriksson L. R., Mackay H. Systemic therapy in squamous cell carcinoma of the vulva: current status and future directions. *Gynecol Oncol. 2014*;132:780–789. doi:10.1016/j.ygyno.2013.11.025.

[69] van Doorn H. C., Ansink A., Verhaar-Langereis M., Stalpers L. Neoadjuvant chemoradiation for advanced primary vulvar cancer. *The Cochrane database of systematic reviews. 2006*;CD003752. doi:10.1002/14651858.CD003752.pub2.

[70] Cibula D., Oonk M. H. M., Abu-Rustum N. R. Sentinel lymph node biopsy in the management of gynecologic cancer. *Current opinion in obstetrics & gynecology. 2015*; 27:66–72. doi:10.1097/GCO.0000000000000133.

[71] Lawrie T. A., Patel A., Martin-Hirsch P. P. L., Bryant A., Ratnavelu N. D. G., Naik R., et al. Sentinel node assessment for diagnosis of groin lymph node involvement in vulval cancer. *The Cochrane database of systematic reviews. 2014*;CD010409. doi: 10.1002/14651858.CD010409.pub2.

[72] Sidor J., Diallo-Danebrock R., Eltze E., Lellé R. J. Challenging the concept of microinvasive carcinoma of the vulva: report of a case with regional lymph node recurrence and review of the literature. *BMC Cancer. 2006*;6:157. doi:10.1186/1471-2407-6-157.

In: The Sentinel Lymph Node
Editors: A. Londero, S. Bertozzi and C. Cedolini
ISBN: 978-1-53614-557-1


*Chapter 10*

# SENTINEL LYMPH NODE BIOPSY IN CERVICAL CANCER

***Anna Biasioli,* Giulia Trombetta, Ambrogio P. Londero and Angelo Cagnacci***
Clinic of Obstetrics and Gynecology, DAME,
University of Udine, University Hospital of Udine, Italy

**Abstract**

As with other cancers, there is sufficient data to suggest that sentinel lymph node biopsy should become the standard of care in modern cervical cancer management, and recently, the technique has been included in the NCCN Guideline for Cervical Cancer as an option to be considered. Sentinel lymph node biopsy should be offered to patients with cervical cancers below stage IB1, with no evidence of metastatic disease at preoperative or intraoperative assessment. To increase procedural sensitivity, sentinel nodes must be identified bilaterally, and side-specific lymphadenectomy must be performed in the case of side-specific lymph node detection failure. The sensitivity of frozen section analysis to detect micrometastases intraoperatively is not optimal. Ultrastaging and immunohistochemistry protocols must be adopted to identify small volume disease. Since it would be very complicated to subject patients to two general anesthesiae and two surgical procedures, sentinel node evaluation and primary cancer surgery should be preferably performed at one setting. However, for micrometastases identified only at final pathology, surgeons must choose either to complete the lymph node staging surgically or offer adjuvant treatments to patients. In conclusion, in the setting of surgical treatment of early cervical cancer, sentinel node mapping with additional side-specific concept for unilateral sentinel node detection and ultrastaging in the case of negative nodes at traditional hematoxylin-eosin staining is a safe and accurate technique.

**Keywords:** cervix cancer, sentinel lymph node biopsy, frozen section, ultrastaging

*Corresponding Author E-mail: biasioli.anna@gmail.com.

# 1. Introduction

Thanks to improved screening programs, cervical cancer is diagnosed more frequently in its early stage and in approximately 50% of cases the disease is clinically located in the cervix [1]. Although the International Federation of Gynecology and Obstetrics (FIGO) staging system does not include the lymph node status [2], the presence of nodal metastases is considered the most important prognostic factor in cervical cancer patients [3].

The current standard of care (NCCN 2017) for most women with early-stage cervical cancer (FIGO IA1-IB1) includes radical hysterectomy or trachelectomy and bilateral pelvic lymphadenectomy. However, the majority of these patients (80%) do not have lymph node metastases [4]. Furthermore, pelvic (and para-aortic) lymphadenectomy is associated with short and long term morbidity, such as prolonged duration of surgery, increased blood loss, infection, nerve and vascular injury, venous thromboembolism, lymphocysts and lower extremity lymphedema [5].

With the goal of reducing morbidity while maintaining a reliable assessment of the nodal status, there is significant interest in validating lymphatic mapping and sentinel lymph node biopsy (SLNB) for cervical carcinoma as well. The technique has been developed and studied by several groups with encouraging data in term of sensitivity and negative predictive value.

The sentinel lymph node is the first lymph node to receive drainage from the primary tumor. Therefore, if the sentinel node is negative for metastases, the remaining lymph nodes of the same basin should also be tumor-free. The use of lymphatic mapping and SLNB was first described by Cabanas in 1977 for penile carcinoma [6]. Since then, it has become the standard of care for the management of various malignancies, such as melanoma and breast cancer. Some authors [7] now consider the technique as a standard of care, with definitive studies allowing the adoption of SLNB in the treatment of early cervical cancer as well.

# 2. Sentinel Lymph Node Detection Techniques

Blue dye (isosulfan blue, methylene blue or patent blue) was the first described technique for the identification of the sentinel node in 1999 [8]. Immediately following general anesthesia, 1 ml of blue dye is injected in each quadrant of the cervix or at 3 and 9 o'clock position, 5 mm or more (10-15 mm) into the cervical stroma. The dye is visualized intraoperatively with the naked eye, the pelvic retroperitoneum is then meticulously dissected, blue capillaries and nodes are searched for, identified and selectively removed.

With this technique, it is important to identify the sentinel node quickly because in 5-10 minutes the stain is adsorbed by the lymphatics and reaches lymph nodes other than the sentinel node. Moreover, in patients who have undergone a prior cone biopsy, the injection is given directly into the conization site. In any case, blue dye should be applied peritumorally and not directly to the tumor, because intratumoral injection decreases the sentinel node detection rate.

Some adverse effects are described in relation to this procedure, such as transient discoloration of the skin and urine or decrease in pulse oximetry measurement, and rarely severe reactions, such as anaphylaxis [9, 10].

A second technique is based on the intracervical injection of radioisotopes, technetium-99 being the most widely used. The radiation dose is variable, but the overall exposure is anyway minimal. No significant reaction to radiocolloids has been described. There are different injecting timing protocols: a "long" and a "short" protocol are described in the current literature. In the first case, the tracer is injected the day before the surgery, while in the second case only a few hours prior to the surgery (Table 1). Radiocolloids have a half-life of 6 hours and tend to remain in the sentinel nodes longer than blue dyes.

The detection of radioactive nodes depends preoperatively on lymphoscintigraphy or single photon emission computed tomography (SPECT) (which are not used in the ultra-short protocol) and intraoperatively on a gamma probe [11]. Nodes showing radioactivity are considered "hot nodes" when they exceed by five times the baseline activity. When more than one "hot node" is identified, the nodes can be classified by the level of radioactivity [12]. After removal of the sentinel nodes, the gamma probe is reintroduced to verify the expected absence of residual radioactivity in the pelvis and para-aortic region.

Some authors believe that lymphatic mapping with lymphoscintigraphy or SPECT is useful because it allows the localization of sentinel nodes to be known before surgery. In addition, uncommon draining pathways can be identified, and the removal of their nodes can reduce the risk of possible recurrence [12]. In any case, this opinion is not shared by some authors, who think that preoperative procedures do not add value to the intra-operative mapping of sentinel nodes, due to the poor concordance between preoperative lymphoscintigraphy and intraoperative lymphatic mapping [13].

Unlike lymphoscintigraphy, SPECT is an imaging method that uses gamma-rays to provide three-dimensional imaging information. Its utility for lymphatic mapping in cervical cancer patients is promising. In particular, some studies report a high concordance rate between images and anatomic nodes location (95-100%) and an improved detection rate compared to lymphoscintigraphy [14, 15, 16, 17].

Recently, great efforts have been made all over the world to find a more efficient and reliable tracer. Indocyanine green, for example, is a fluorescent dye that has been used in a variety of medical applications since the 1950s and has been evaluated for the sentinel node mapping of several solid tumors. Like other tracers, indocyanine green is injected intracervically in the operating room at a concentration of 1.25 mg/ml. A total of 4 ml of the solution is injected at 3 and 9 o'clock position (1 ml deeply [1-2 cm], 1 ml superficially [1-3 mm]) [15]. The detection of positive nodes is then performed using a fluorescence-detecting camera 40 minutes after injection. No significant adverse events have been reported with this kind of tracer.

**Table 1. Radioisotope protocols**

| | **Injection** | **Lymphoscintigraphy** | **Dose (mCi)** |
|---|---|---|---|
| Long | 24 h before | 1-3 h after injection | 2-4 |
| Short | 2-4 h before | 30 min after injection | 0.2-1 |
| Ultrashort | Immediately before | no | 0.4-0.55 |

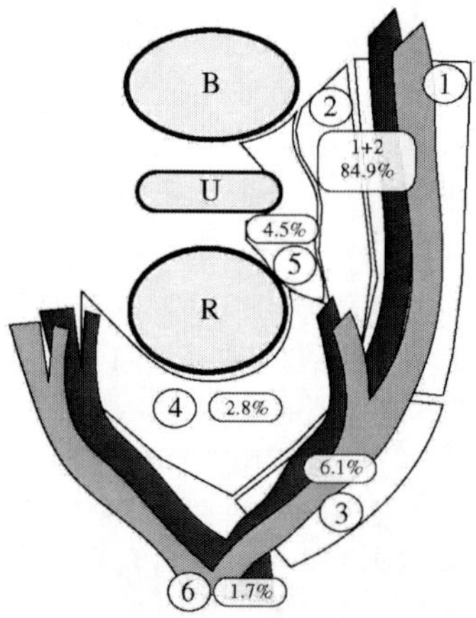


Figure 1. Sentinel nodes distribution modified from Lukas and colleagues [11] (drawing by APL): 1. External iliac artery region; 2. Obturator region; 3. Common internal iliac artery region; 4. Presacral region; 5. Paracervical region; 6. Low para-aortic region.

## 2.1. Distribution of Sentinel Lymph Nodes

In a systematic review of 12 papers with ¿50 cases, Lukas and colleagues [11] showed that the most frequent and usual localizations of the sentinel nodes are the external iliac, the obturator and the internal iliac or interiliac area in the 84.9% of cases (Figure 1). Less frequent or unusual localizations are the parametrial (4.5%), the common iliac (6%), the presacral (2.8%) and the low para-aortic area (1.7%). Later, in a retrospective evaluation of 151 women, Marnitz and colleagues found that 71% of sentinel nodes are located in the interiliac region [16]. In the SENTICOL trial, 85% of all sentinel nodes were external, internal and common iliac nodes [17].

An important finding from these mapping studies is that about 10-15% of sentinel nodes are located in less common regions (presacral, parametrial, above aortic bifurcation), which are not universally approached during systematic lymphadenectomy. Therefore, a theoretical advantage of the SLNB is the increased reliability of surgical node staging [18].

## 2.2. Sentinel Lymph Node Detection Failure

Because the cervix is a midline structure, the detection rate per patient is less accurate than the detection rate per hemipelvis. Optimal management involves the identification of at least one sentinel node at each side. The detection rate in the literature varies between 55% and 100% [19]. In individuals with early-stage cervical cancer, SLNB has similar outcomes when performed by laparoscopy, laparotomy, or robotic techniques.

Among the factors that can influence sentinel node detection, the applied technique plays surely an important role. In fact, the sentinel node detection rate when using blue dye alone is between 70% and 100% [4], and is comparable to the radioisotope technique detection rate. On the other hand, when the two techniques are combined, the sentinel node detection rate is higher. In the French prospective multicenter study SENTICOL the majority of patients (133 out of 139) received the combined technique, and at least one sentinel node was detected in 98% of cases, while bilateral detection was achieved in 77% of cases [20].

Excluding studies with blue dye and including only studies with at least 50 patient (15% of the studies), in 2013 Lukas and colleagues [11] found a sentinel node detection rate of 92.3% among 1811 patients. In 2015, Tax and colleagues included 47 studies with at least 40 patients in an overview of the literature. They reported that, in 44 studies that included 3931 patients, the detection rate was 91% for at least one sentinel node, 74% for more than one ipsilateral node, and 60% for bilateral sentinel nodes, respectively. In the case of a single sentinel node, the detection rate was 85% for the blue dye, 89% for the radioisotope and 94% for their combination. In the case of bilateral sentinel nodes, these rates were 56%, 52% and 72%, respectively. Correspondingly, the combined technique detected 20% more sentinel nodes, which might not have been detected by the use of a single technique. Blue dye is very useful when the sentinel node is located in the parametrium, which is a rare finding in early-stage disease. In that area, in fact, the gamma-probe count is contaminated by the proximity to the cervix, and therefore not always reliable [12].

Recently, the detection rate of the sentinel node appears to have increased using indocyanine green, although the studies on this subject are more limited than for the techniques described previously. In 227 cases collected in the United States at the Memorial Sloan Kettering Cancer Center [21], the side-specific sentinel node detection rate was 95%, while the bilateral detection rate was 79%. This seems to be an improvement over the detection rates reported for blue dye alone and comparable to the combined blue dye and technetium-99 method.

Similar results are confirmed by other authors in smaller series. A recent study performed on 65 patients with previous conization, reported a superior sentinel node detection rate for at least one sentinel node (100% vs 95.7% p=0.354) and for bilateral sentinel nodes (95.2% vs 69.6% p=0.016) using indocyanine green injection versus combined radiotracer and blue dye technique [22]. Table 2 summarizes data retrieved from available studies about indocyanine green. As a result, the fluorescence imaging appears to provide a much simpler technique for securely recognizing and identifying sentinel nodes, without the additional cost and inconvenience of technetium-99 or blue dye [23].

In addition to the technique used (appropriate volume, site, injection depth and timing), the detection rate is also determined by the size of the tumor [18]. In a recent review review [24], a subgroup analysis of tumor size among patients with bilateral sentinel nodes showed that bilateral sentinel node detection was the highest (87%) when a combined tracer was used in early-stage patients with a tumor size ¡20 mm (Figure 2). It has been hypothesized that the lymphatic channels of larger tumors may be occluded by metastases. In addition, larger tumors may have necrosis and exophytic growth, preventing a proper dye injection. For these cases, a modified technique has been described, which consists in injecting the tracer (combined blue dye dilution 2:1 and radiocolloid) into the residual stroma with a spinal needle and controlling the stroma injection by its leakage in the vagina and the resistance during application (high in the stroma, low in the tumor). However, the group found no significant differences in sentinel node detection rates for tumor volume ¡ or ¿ 2 cm [25] (Figure 3).

In large tumors IB1 ¿2 cm a higher sentinel node detection rate was achieved with indocyanine green compared to radiotracer alone or combined with blue dye (100% vs 91.5% p¡0.025). The technique of injection of indocyanine green is the same as described for small tumors, but 1 ml of the solution was injected with penetration at a depth of 1 cm into the stroma and 1 ml into the submucous layer on the left and right side of the cervix [26].

The sentinel node detection rate seems to be influenced also by the surgical approach (it is higher for laparoscopy and robotic surgery than for laparotomy) [27, 28], any previous conization, the neoadjuvant therapy, the surgeon's skill and experience in the application of the technique [27] and a high BMI due to the difficulty of directly identifying nodes in the adipose tissue. In obese women, indocyanine green may increase the sentinel node detection rate, but near infrared imaging can reach a penetration depth of no more than 1 cm [29].

**Table 2. Summary of data about indocyanine green**

| | Years | Surgery | Tracer | Cases | DR (%) |
|---|---|---|---|---|---|
| Imboden et al [30] | 2015 | laparoscopy | ICG | 22 | 95.5 |
| Rossi et al [31] | 2012 | Robotic | ICG | 4 | 88 |
| Schaafsma [32] | 2012 | Lapartotomy | ICG | 18 | 78 |
| Buda et al [33] | 2016 | Laparoscopt | ICG | 68 | 100 |
| Jewell et al [21] | 2014 | Robotic | ICG | 18 | 95 |
| Van der vorst [34] | 2011 | Laparoscopy | ICG | 9 | 100 |
| Buda et al [35] | 2016 | Laparoscopy | ICG | 9 | 100 |
| Crane et al [36] | 2011 | Laparotomy | ICG | 10 | 60 |
| Furukava et al [37] | 2010 | Laparotomy | ICG | 12 | 100 |
| Buda et al [15] | 2016 | Laparoscopy | ICG | 21 | 100 |
| Beavis et al [38] | 2016 | Robotic | ICG | 27 | 93.3 |
| Tanaka et al [39] | 2017 | Laparoscopic | ICG | 43 | 61.6 |

# 3. Sentinel Node Histopathological Evaluation

Sentinel nodes are usually 2 to 4 per patient, and their number does not seem to increase the accuracy of sentinel node mapping [40]. Moreover, the protocols for pathological evaluation are not standardized. Usually, the node is embedded in paraffin, sectioned once along longitudinal axis and stained by hematoxylin-eosin. This procedure allows the identification of macrometastases ($\geq$2 mm). On the other hand, serial sectioning is required for the identification of micrometastases (¡2 mm and ¿0.2 mm) or isolated tumor cells (ITCs) (¡0.2mm), as described previously for breast cancer [41].

This practice, called ultrastaging, is strongly recommended to improve the sensitivity of the procedure. It consists in slicing the sentinel node sections in more serial sections of

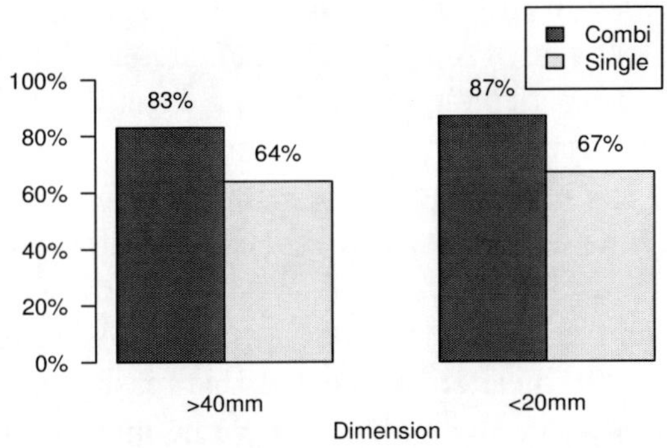


Figure 2. Bilateral detection rate in early stage cervical cancer per technique and tumor size [24] (drawing by APL).

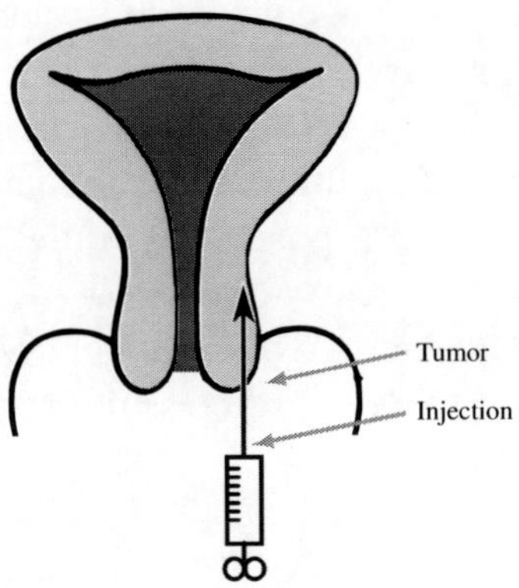


Figure 3. Modified technique in large tumor modified by Dostalek and colleagues [25] (drawing by APL).

4-5 m thick, cut at 40 to 250 m intervals. This operation, followed by immunohistochemistry, allows the detection of small volume disease, such as micrometastases and ITCs. The largest retrospective SLNB series for cervical cancer showed a high sensitivity of the sentinel node ultrastaging for micrometastases (sensibility 91%; 95%CI 86-95), which was further increased if bilateral sentinel nodes were detected and removed (97%; 95%CI 91-99%) [19].

Unlike other primary cancers, in cervical cancer micrometastases have the same prognostic impact as macrometastases [42, 19]. No prognostic significance was instead found for ITCs. In 2012, Cibula reported that overall survival is significantly reduced in patients with macro- and micrometastases (HR 6.85 and 6.86 respectively CI 95% 2.59-18.05 and 2.09-22.61) [19]. In a multivariate model, micrometastases are an independent prognostic factor for overall survival [42]. On the other hand, the clinical significance of ITCs is still unknown, but most authors classify ITCs as tumor-free.

A major controversy concerns the role of frozen section. In fact, its accuracy is significantly limited by the inability to detect small volume metastases, with a sensitivity for the detection of micrometastases reported by some authors of only 8% [43]. Despite the theoretical benefits for the patient and intraoperative triage, this technique has several limitations, such as prolongation of the operative time, low accuracy, and tissue loss for postoperative evaluation [11]. On the other hand, serial sectioning combined with immunohistochemistry is difficult, time-consuming and expensive, even when limited to the sentinel nodes.

The one-step nucleic acid amplification (OSNA) assay was initially developed for the intraoperative assessment of sentinel node metastases in breast cancer. This assay measures the cytokeratin 19 (CK19) mRNA copy number, an epithelial marker, not normally present in lymph nodes. It is currently in clinical use for the diagnosis of nodal metastases in breast cancer and is being explored for potential use in the detection of nodal metastases in gastric and colorectal cancers, and can be applied to assess lymph node metastases in a variety of cancers expressing CK19.

Considering the time needed to transport the samples to the laboratory, prepare the sample and extract mRNA by homogenizing and centrifuging the material, followed by 16 minutes of amplification, the average total time needed to complete the OSNA assay is approximately 40 minutes. The cut-off for the mRNA copies number was determined by Tsujimoto and colleagues, based on thorough examination of the axillary lymph nodes of breast cancer patients, where OSNA-positive is equivalent to metastases equal or greater than 0.2mm [44].

However, despite its advantages in reducing operative time and improving the detection of small sized metastases, the OSNA method is not currently used in the case of cervical cancer.

## 4. Sentinel Lymph Node Biopsy Sensitivity

Sensitivity is a key feature of SLNB reliability, as it measures the risk of involvement of any other pelvic node if the sentinel nodes are negative. Several single-institution studies have reported on their experience with SLNB in cervical cancer with good results in terms of negative predictive values and a sensitivity varying from 94% to 100% [4].

In an attempt to validate these studies, in 2008 Altagassen and colleagues [45] published the AGO Study, a multicenter trial on 507 women with cervical cancer who underwent SLNB with blue dye, radioisotope or both, and then were subjected to conventional lymphadenectomy. The overall sensitivity was low (77%), and the main problems with the study were the following: the study protocol did not include ultrastaging and immunoistochemical analysis for the detection of micrometastases; there was no information on the surgeon's experience; more than 20% of the cases included were large tumors. When the analysis was restricted to tumors ¡2 cm the sensitivity was 91%.

In the SENTICOL study, the largest multi-institutional prospective trial including 139 SLNB procedures for early-stage cervical cancer, the overall sensitivity with blue dye, radiocolloid or both was 92% and increased to 100% in the subset of patients with bilateral sentinel nodes. In fact, there were only two false-negative cases, of which in one the positive node was found in the unmapped hemipelvis [20].

Similar data was obtained from a large retrospective study on 645 patients [27] with IA1-IIB cervical cancer subjected to SLNB and ultrastaging. In the study, the false-negative rate of SLNB ultrastaging was low (¡3% of cases). Moreover, in two thirds of these false-negative cases (n=12), sentinel nodes were detected only unilaterally. If we consider only the subset of patients with optimally bilateral sentinel nodes detected (n=463), the false-negative rate would decrease to 1.3% and the ultrastaging sensitivity would increase to 97%. Bilateral sentinel nodes detection and pathological ultrastaging increased the detection of micrometastases. Sentinel nodes ultrastaging allowed the identification of lymph node metastases in 11% of patients with only low-volume disease of the sentinel nodes that would have been missed by standard pathological processing.

In his review of 43 studies, Tax and colleagues [24] reported a pooled sensitivity of 81% (47-59%) reaching 94% (80-99%) with ultrastaging. This is due to the correct identification of metastases in 74 out of 94 false-negative patients at frozen section or at hematoxylin-eosin analysis. With ultrastaging, false-negative sentinel nodes were found in 19 out of 1275 patients with a risk of undertreatment of 1.5%. In any case, excluding from the latter patients with tumor sizes ¿40 mm (1/18), unilateral detection (9/18), advanced FIGO stages (6/18), and suspicious pre- or intraoperative lymph nodes (2/18), only one case out of 1275 remained false-negative, with the risk of undertreatment dropping to 0.08%.

In a recent study by the MD Anderson Cancer Center [29], 188 patients with early cervical cancer were retrospectively evaluated, who have been subjected to SLNB with blue dye, technetium-99 or indocyanine green, and subsequent complete pelvic lymphadenectomy. Excluding false-negative cases related to side-specific detection, there was only one false-negative patient, with a sensitivity of 96.4% and a negative predictive value of 99.3%.

Finally, one study was conducted by Okamoto and colleagues [28] to examine the usefulness of OSNA in detecting sentinel node metastases in cervical cancer patients. In the OSNA method, 250 copies/L of KRT19 mRNA seemed to be an optimal cut-off value. OSNA exhibited a 96.2% agreement with a 2 mm interval histopathological examination. Therefore, the author concluded that OSNA testing is useful in cervical cancer patients, but further validation studies are needed.

In conclusion, the literature shows in substance that a high SLNB sensitivity can be achieved when sentinel nodes are detected bilaterally and ultrastaging is performed.

## 5. Complications of the Sentinel Lymph Node Biopsy

The clinical benefits of SLNB include a reduced risk of intraoperative complications, such as nerve, great vessel, ureteral injuries and blood loss, or postoperative sequelae, such as lymphedema and sensory loss. In addition, the SLNB allows a reduction in overall operative time and hospital stay.

However, unlike other cancers (i.e. breast cancer and melanoma), for which SLNB can be performed under local anesthesia before planning the definitive surgery, the situation is more complex in cervical cancer. The cervix is a central organ whose lymphatic drainage is bilateral and located deep in the pelvis, thus requiring general anesthesia. This obviously let to an increase in the surgical complication incidence.

Lymphedema is the most disabling long-term morbidity associated with pelvic node removal. The incidence of lymphedema is between 10-15% [5], and up to 40% [46]. Lymphedema can negatively affect quality of life and lead to significant healthcare expenditure.

A model-based economic evaluation on SLNB cost-effectiveness, reported in 2017 by Brar and colleagues [47], concluded that the most effective strategy in terms of progression free-survival and morbidity free-survival is the one based on the use of technetium-99 and blue dye (and potentially indocyanine green) and ultrastaging. Some complications caused by blue dye have been reported, such as transient discoloration of the skin and urine, an imbalanced pulse oximetry measurement, and rarely severe reactions, such as anaphylaxis [9, 10].

# 6. Management of Positive and Negative Sentinel Lymph Node Biopsy

An algorithm was proposed by Comier and collegues of the Memorial Sloan Kettering Cancer Center to guide the management of metastases for SLNB in cervical cancer [48]:

- Sentinel nodes are removed and, if negative on routine hematoxylin-eosin staining, they are submitted to ultrastaging. If metastases are detected by the traditional hematoxylin-eosin staining, no further pathological ultrastaging is needed.
- Any suspicious nodes are removed regardless of the mapping, as fully infiltrated lymph nodes may have lower radioactivity and may not appear blue, as the blue dye and radiotracer could have bypassed these nodes.
- If there is no mapping of the hemi-pelvis, then a side-specific lymph node dissection including interiliac or subaortic nodes is performed. Presacral nodes can be a site of metastases, as they are located at the midline and receive afferent lymphatics from deep trunks draining form the parametria from both sides, and should be included in a side-specific lymphadenectomy when ipsilateral mapping has failed.
- Parametrectomy is performed with an en-bloc resection of the cervical tumor. Parametrial nodes are difficult to identify as sentinel nodes because they are located in close proximity to the cervix. With a radiocolloid tracer, their proximity to the injection site makes it impossible to search for a hot node. A better performance may be achieved using blue dye, but sometimes parametria are stained, making it more difficult to isolate the sentinel nodes. Parametrectomy is usually not necessary in microinvasive (IA1) tumors due to a documented low rate of parametrial metastases. For stage IA2 and selected stage IB1 patients, some teams have proposed omitting parametrectomy in those patients with favorable prognostic factors, such as tumor size ¡2cm, absence of lympho-vascular invasion and of pelvic nodal metastases, or in the case in which the sentinel node is negative for metastases [38, 39, 23, 25]. In these cases the parametrium was the only site of metastases in 3 out of 25 metastatic patients.

By applying this protocol the author reported a patient-based sensitivity of 87.5% and a side-specific sensitivity of 92.6%. With the addition of parametrectomy, sensitivity increased to 100% without any false-negative results. They concluded that, in the setting of the surgical treatment of early stage cervical cancer, the sentinel node mapping with additional side-specific concept in the case of unilateral sentinel nodes detection and ultrastaging in the case of negative nodes at traditional hematoxylin-eosin staining, is a safe and accurate technique that increases metastatic nodal detection rates by 3.5%. In experienced hands this protocol could spare approximately 75% of patients from a complete bilateral pelvic lymphadenectomy while maintaining the diagnostic performance of SLNB.

If the sentinel nodes are negative at ultrastaging, the patient does not need lymphadenectomy or adjuvant therapy. On the other hand, if ultrastaging is positive for micrometastases, the surgeon must choose whether to resume surgery and complete the lymph node staging or to offer the patient adjuvant treatments.

At this point the main concern remains whether adjuvant radiotherapy will be successful in the treatment of positive nodes that have not been removed by surgery [18]. Furthermore, it is not clear whether patients with only one isolated micrometastasis can be followed conservatively [12].

If sentinel lymph nodes or gross nodes are positive at frozen section, this may actually lead to an intraoperative triage of the patients. In particular, it would allow the abandonment of radical hysterectomy or fertility sparing procedures in favour of exclusive chemoradiotherapy. Such management would help to reduce post-treatment morbidity [18]. To perform a complete lymphadenectomy in these patients, the surgeon may encounter multiple complications, which do not have an impact on survival even when several nodes are removed. Furthermore, there are also controversies on the therapeutic value of completion pelvic lymph node dissection [48].

Fertility sparing surgery is another possible application of sentinel node mapping that cannot be performed if nodes or parametria are involved. Although the sensitivity of the sentinel node mapping in fertility sparing surgery is high in several studies, larger studies are needed before recommending routine use to tailor the radicality of cervical cancer surgery in this setting of patients, due to the low accuracy of frozen section and the difficulty of identifying parametrial nodes [49].

Recently, data from women with FIGO stages IA1-IIA1 cervical cancer have been collected retrospectively by six Italian institutions for a total of 368 patients. Among these, 333 (90.5%) showed no enlarged nodes suspected of involvement at preoperative magnetic resonance imaging (MRI). None of the 106 patients with negative MRI, tumor size ¡20 mm and squamous or adenosquamous histotype had nodal metastases because in this subset tumor size ¡20 mm was the only independent predictor of lymph node status (p¡0.005) [50]. On this basis, a more tailored algorithm has been proposed in order to bypass the difficulty of an "optimal mapping" involving a bilateral SLNB and a hemipelvis side-specific lymphadenectomy in the case of no side-specific detection. In order to spare patients from unnecessary pelvic lymphadenectomy, a subgroup of low-risk cervical cancer patients has been identified in which even SLNB can be avoided (negative MRI nodal assessment, tumor size ¡20 mm, squamous and adenosquamous histotype). This approach can reduce operative time and costs, but can also reduce the chances of correctly classifying risk categories by omitting the ultrastaging procedure.

Finally, it can be argued that there is a scarcity of data on the long-term outcomes for patients undergoing SLNB without subsequent lymphadenectomy. Lennox and colleagues [51] evaluated the recurrence free-survival in the SLNB group (110) compared to the bilateral pelvic lymphadenectomy group (1188) and found no difference except for a reduced short-term morbidity in the SLNB group.

## Conclusion

There is sufficient data to suggest that SLNB should become the standard of care in the modern management of cervical cancer [7]. In recent years, the technique has been included into the NCCN Guideline for Cervical Cancer as an option to be considered.

The incorporation of SLNB into routine clinical practice will require time and planning. Some suggestions for its success are as follows:

- The surgeon must complete a learning curve before performing SLNB alone;
- Patients must be appropriately selected and SLNB should be offered to patients with cervical cancers at below stage IB1 with no evidence of metastatic disease at preoperative or intraoperative assessment;
- Sentinel nodes should be identified bilaterally and surgeons should strive to improve their technique to achieve this;
- The sensitivity of frozen section analysis for detecting micrometastases intraoperatively is not optimal. It is hoped that new techniques will emerge in the near future to improve the detection of micrometastases at frozen section. Ultrastaging and immunohistochemistry protocols must be adopted to identify small volume disease. In cases where a micrometastasis is identified only at final pathology, surgeons must choose to surgically complete the lymph node staging or offer adjuvant treatments to patients.

## References

[1] Siegel R. L., Miller K. D., Jemal A. Cancer statistics, 2018. *CA Cancer J Clin. 2018*; 68:7–30. doi:10.3322/caac.21442.

[2] Pecorelli S., Zigliani L., Odicino F. Revised FIGO staging for carcinoma of the cervix. *Int J Gynaecol Obstet. 2009*;105:107–108. doi:10.1016/j.ijgo.2009.02.009.

[3] Biewenga P., van der Velden J., Mol B. W. J., Stalpers L. J. A., Schilthuis M. S., van der Steeg J. W., et al. Prognostic model for survival in patients with early stage cervical cancer. *Cancer. 2011*;117:768–776. doi:10.1002/cncr.25658.

[4] Holman L. L., Levenback C. F., Frumovitz M. Sentinel lymph node evaluation in women with cervical cancer. *J Minim Invasive Gynecol. 2014*;21:540–545. doi:10.1016/j.jmig.2013.12.095.

[5] Matsuura Y., Kawagoe T., Toki N., Tanaka M., Kashimura M. Long-standing complications after treatment for cancer of the uterine cervix–clinical significance of medical examination at 5 years after treatment. *Int J Gynecol Cancer. 2006*;16:294–297. doi:10.1111/j.1525-1438.2006.00354.x.

[6] Cabanas R. M. An approach for the treatment of penile carcinoma. *Cancer. 1977*; 39:456–466.

[7] Frumovitz M. Sentinel Lymph Node Biopsy for Cervical Cancer Patients - What's It Gonna Take? *Gynecol Oncol. 2017*;144:3–4. doi:10.1016/j.ygyno.2016.12.009.

[8] Echt M. L., Finan M. A., Hoffman M. S., Kline R. C., Roberts W. S., Fiorica J. V. Detection of sentinel lymph nodes with lymphazurin in cervical, uterine, and vulvar malignancies. *South Med J. 1999*;92:204–208.

[9] Vieira S. C., Sousa R. B., Tavares M. B. A. C., de Abreu B. A. L., Ibiapina J. O., de Sousa Oliveira A. K., et al. Changes in pulse oximetry after patent blue dye injection into the uterine cervix. *Ann Surg Oncol. 2008*;15:2862–2866. doi: 10.1245/s10434-008-0089-6.

[10] Bricou A., Barranger E., Uzan S., Darai E. Anaphylactic shock during the sentinel lymph node procedure for cervical cancer. *Gynecol Oncol. 2009*;114:375–376. doi: 10.1016/j.ygyno.2009.04.027.

[11] Lukas R., Robova H., Halaska M. J., Hruda M., Skapa P. Current status of sentinel lymph node mapping in the management of cervical cancer. *Expert Rev Anticancer Ther. 2013*;13:861–870. doi:10.1586/14737140.2013.811147.

[12] Roy M., Bouchard-Fortier G., Popa I., Grégoire J., Renaud M. C., Têtu B., et al. Value of sentinel node mapping in cancer of the cervix. *Gynecol Oncol. 2011*;122:269–274. doi:10.1016/j.ygyno.2011.04.002.

[13] Frumovitz M., Coleman R. L., Gayed I. W., Ramirez P. T., Wolf J. K., Gershenson D. M., et al. Usefulness of preoperative lymphoscintigraphy in patients who undergo radical hysterectomy and pelvic lymphadenectomy for cervical cancer. *Am J Obstet Gynecol. 2006*;194:1186–93; discussion 1193–5. doi:10.1016/j.ajog.2005.12.018.

[14] Belhocine T. Z., Prefontaine M., Lanvin D., Bertrand M., Rachinsky I., Ettler H., et al. Added-value of SPECT/CT to lymphatic mapping and sentinel lymphadenectomy in gynaecological cancers. *Am J Nucl Med Mol Imaging. 2013*;3:182–193.

[15] Buda A., Bussi B., Di Martino G., Di Lorenzo P., Palazzi S., Grassi T., et al. Sentinel Lymph Node Mapping With Near-Infrared Fluorescent Imaging Using Indocyanine Green: A New Tool for Laparoscopic Platform in Patients With Endometrial and Cervical Cancer. *J Minim Invasive Gynecol. 2016*;23:265–269. doi: 10.1016/j.jmig.2015.09.022.

[16] Marnitz S., Kuhler C., Bongardt S., Braig U., Hertel H., Schneider A., et al. Topographic distribution of sentinel lymph nodes in patients with cervical cancer. *Gynecol Oncol. 2006*;103:35–44. doi:10.1016/j.ygyno.2006.01.061.

[17] Bats A. S., Mathevet P., Buenerd A., Orliaguet I., Mery E., Zerdoud S., et al. The sentinel node technique detects unexpected drainage pathways and allows nodal ultrastaging in early cervical cancer: insights from the multicenter prospective SENTICOL study. *Ann Surg Oncol. 2013*;20:413–422. doi:10.1245/s10434-012-2597-7.

[18] Cibula D., Oonk M. H. M., Abu-Rustum N. R. Sentinel lymph node biopsy in the management of gynecologic cancer. *Curr Opin Obstet Gynecol. 2015*;27:66–72. doi: 10.1097/GCO.0000000000000133.

[19] van de Lande J., Torrenga B., Raijmakers P. G. H. M., Hoekstra O. S., van Baal M. W., Brölmann HAM, et al. Sentinel lymph node detection in early stage uterine cervix carcinoma: a systematic review. *Gynecol Oncol. 2007*;106:604–613. doi:10.1016/j.ygyno.2007.05.010.

[20] Lécuru F., Mathevet P., Querleu D., Leblanc E., Morice P., Daraï E., et al. Bilateral negative sentinel nodes accurately predict absence of lymph node metastasis in early cervical cancer: results of the SENTICOL study. *J Clin Oncol. 2011*;29:1686–1691. doi:10.1200/JCO.2010.32.0432.

[21] Jewell E. L., Huang J. J., Abu-Rustum N. R., Gardner G. J., Brown C. L., Sonoda Y., et al. Detection of sentinel lymph nodes in minimally invasive surgery using indocyanine green and near-infrared fluorescence imaging for uterine and cervical malignancies. *Gynecol Oncol. 2014*;133:274–277. doi:10.1016/j.ygyno.2014.02.028.

[22] Buda A., Papadia A., Di Martino G., Imboden S., Bussi B., Guerra L., et al. Real-Time Fluorescent Sentinel Lymph Node Mapping with Indocyanine Green in Women with Previous Conization Undergoing Laparoscopic Surgery for Early Invasive Cervical Cancer: Comparison with RadiotracerBlue Dye. *J Minim Invasive Gynecol. 2018*; 25:455–460. doi:10.1016/j.jmig.2017.10.002.

[23] Rocha A., Domínguez A. M., Lécuru F., Bourdel N. Indocyanine green and infrared fluorescence in detection of sentinel lymph nodes in endometrial and cervical cancer staging - a systematic review. *Eur J Obstet Gynecol Reprod Biol. 2016*;206:213–219. doi:10.1016/j.ejogrb.2016.09.027.

[24] Tax C., Rovers M. M., de Graaf C., Zusterzeel P. L. M., Bekkers R. L. M. The sentinel node procedure in early stage cervical cancer, taking the next step; a diagnostic review. *Gynecol Oncol. 2015*;139:559–567. doi:10.1016/j.ygyno.2015.09.076.

[25] Dostálek L., Zikan M., Fischerova D., Kocian R., Germanova A., Frühauf F., et al. SLN biopsy in cervical cancer patients with tumors larger than 2cm and 4cm. *Gynecol Oncol. 2018*;148:456–460. doi:10.1016/j.ygyno.2018.01.001.

[26] Di Martino G., Crivellaro C., De Ponti E., Bussi B., Papadia A., Zapardiel I., et al. Indocyanine Green versus Radiotracer with or without Blue Dye for Sentinel Lymph Node Mapping in Stage ¿IB1 Cervical Cancer (¿2cm). *J Minim Invasive Gynecol. 2017*;24:954–959. doi:10.1016/j.jmig.2017.05.011.

[27] Cibula D., Abu-Rustum N. R., Dusek L., Slama J., Zikán M., Zaal A., et al. Bilateral ultrastaging of sentinel lymph node in cervical cancer: Lowering the false-negative rate and improving the detection of micrometastasis. *Gynecol Oncol. 2012*;127:462–466. doi:10.1016/j.ygyno.2012.08.035.

[28] Okamoto S., Niikura H., Nakabayashi K., Hiyama K., Matoda M., Takeshima N., et al. Detection of sentinel lymph node metastases in cervical cancer: assessment of KRT19 mRNA in the one-step nucleic acid amplification (OSNA) method. *Gynecol Oncol. 2013*;130:530–536. doi:10.1016/j.ygyno.2013.06.027.

[29] Salvo G., Ramirez P. T., Levenback C. F., Munsell M. F., Euscher E. D., Soliman P. T., et al. Sensitivity and negative predictive value for sentinel lymph node biopsy in women with early-stage cervical cancer. *Gynecol Oncol. 2017*;145:96–101. doi: 10.1016/j.ygyno.2017.02.005.

[30] Imboden S., Papadia A., Nauwerk M., McKinnon B., Kollmann Z., Mohr S., et al. A Comparison of Radiocolloid and Indocyanine Green Fluorescence Imaging, Sentinel Lymph Node Mapping in Patients with Cervical Cancer Undergoing Laparoscopic Surgery. *Ann Surg Oncol. 2015*;22:4198–4203. doi:10.1245/s10434-015-4701-2.

[31] Rossi E. C., Ivanova A., Boggess J. F. Robotically assisted fluorescence-guided lymph node mapping with ICG for gynecologic malignancies: a feasibility study. *Gynecol Oncol. 2012*;124:78–82. doi:10.1016/j.ygyno.2011.09.025.

[32] Schaafsma B. E., van der Vorst J. R., Gaarenstroom K. N., Peters A. A. W., Verbeek F. P. R., de Kroon C. D., et al. Randomized comparison of near-infrared fluorescence lymphatic tracers for sentinel lymph node mapping of cervical cancer. *Gynecol Oncol. 2012*;127:126–130. doi:10.1016/j.ygyno.2012.07.002.

[33] Buda A., Papadia A., Zapardiel I., Vizza E., Ghezzi F., De Ponti E., et al. From Conventional Radiotracer Tc-99(m) with Blue Dye to Indocyanine Green Fluorescence: A Comparison of Methods Towards Optimization of Sentinel Lymph Node Mapping in Early Stage Cervical Cancer for a Laparoscopic Approach. *Ann Surg Oncol. 2016*; 23:2959–2965. doi:10.1245/s10434-016-5227-y.

[34] van der Vorst J. R., Hutteman M., Gaarenstroom K. N., Peters A. A. W., Mieog J. S. D., Schaafsma B. E., et al. Optimization of near-infrared fluorescent sentinel lymph node mapping in cervical cancer patients. *Int J Gynecol Cancer. 2011*;21:1472–1478. doi:10.1097/IGC.0b013e31822b451d.

[35] Buda A., Crivellaro C., Elisei F., Di Martino G., Guerra L., De Ponti E., et al. Impact of Indocyanine Green for Sentinel Lymph Node Mapping in Early Stage Endometrial and Cervical Cancer: Comparison with Conventional Radiotracer (99m)Tc and/or Blue Dye. *Ann Surg Oncol. 2016*;23:2183–2191. doi:10.1245/s10434-015-5022-1.

[36] Crane L. M. A., Themelis G., Pleijhuis R. G., Harlaar N. J., Sarantopoulos A., Arts H. J. G., et al. Intraoperative multispectral fluorescence imaging for the detection of the sentinel lymph node in cervical cancer: a novel concept. *Mol Imaging Biol. 2011*; 13:1043–1049. doi:10.1007/s11307-010-0425-7.

[37] Furukawa N., Oi H., Yoshida S., Shigetomi H., Kanayama S., Kobayashi H. The usefulness of photodynamic eye for sentinel lymph node identification in patients with cervical cancer. *Tumori*. 2010;96:936–940.

[38] Beavis A. L., Salazar-Marioni S., Sinno A. K., Stone R. L., Fader A. N., Santillan-Gomez A., et al. Sentinel lymph node detection rates using indocyanine green in women with early-stage cervical cancer. *Gynecol Oncol. 2016*;143:302–306. doi: 10.1016/j.ygyno.2016.08.236.

[39] Tanaka T., Terai Y., Ashihara K., Tsunetoh S., Akagi H., Yamada T., et al. The detection of sentinel lymph nodes in laparoscopic surgery for uterine cervical cancer using 99m-technetium-tin colloid, indocyanine green, and blue dye. *J Gynecol Oncol. 2017*; 28:e13. doi:10.3802/jgo.2017.28.e13.

[40] Papadia A., Imboden S., Gasparri M. L., Siegenthaler F., Fink A., Mueller M. D. Endometrial and cervical cancer patients with multiple sentinel lymph nodes at laparoscopic ICG mapping: How many are enough? *J Cancer Res Clin Oncol. 2016*; 142:1831–1836. doi:10.1007/s00432-016-2193-5.

[41] American College of Surgeons. *AJCC Cancer Staging Manual (Eighth Edition).* Springer. 2017.

[42] Cibula D., Abu-Rustum N. R., Dusek L., Zikán M., Zaal A., Sevcik L., et al. Prognostic significance of low volume sentinel lymph node disease in early-stage cervical cancer. *Gynecol Oncol. 2012*;124:496–501. doi:10.1016/j.ygyno.2011.11.037.

[43] Slama J., Dundr P., Dusek L., Cibula D. High false negative rate of frozen section examination of sentinel lymph nodes in patients with cervical cancer. *Gynecol Oncol. 2013*;129:384–388. doi:10.1016/j.ygyno.2013.02.001.

[44] Tamaki Y. One-step nucleic acid amplification (OSNA): where do we go with it? *Int J Clin Oncol. 2017*;22:3–10. doi:10.1007/s10147-016-1030-9.

[45] Altgassen C., Hertel H., Brandstädt A., Köhler C., Dürst M., Schneider A., et al. Multicenter validation study of the sentinel lymph node concept in cervical cancer: AGO Study Group. *J Clin Oncol. 2008*;26:2943–2951. doi:10.1200/JCO.2007.13.8933.

[46] Biglia N., Librino A., Ottino M. C., Panuccio E., Daniele A., Chahin A. Lower limb lymphedema and neurological complications after lymphadenectomy for gynecological cancer. *Int J Gynecol Cancer. 2015*;25:521–525. doi:10.1097/IGC.0000000000000341.

[47] Brar H., Hogen L., Covens A. Cost-effectiveness of sentinel node biopsy and pathological ultrastaging in patients with early-stage cervical cancer. *Cancer. 2017*; 123:1751–1759. doi:10.1002/cncr.30509.

[48] Cormier B., Diaz J. P., Shih K., Sampson R. M., Sonoda Y., Park K. J., et al. Establishing a sentinel lymph node mapping algorithm for the treatment of early cervical cancer. *Gynecol Oncol. 2011*;122:275–280. doi:10.1016/j.ygyno.2011.04.023.

[49] Kadkhodayan S., Hasanzadeh M., Treglia G., Azad A., Yousefi Z., Zarifmahmoudi L., et al. Sentinel node biopsy for lymph nodal staging of uterine cervix cancer: a

systematic review and meta-analysis of the pertinent literature. *Eur J Surg Oncol. 2015*;41:1–20. doi:10.1016/j.ejso.2014.09.010.

[50] Fagotti A., Pedone Anchora L., Conte C., Chiantera V., Vizza E., Tortorella L., et al. Beyond sentinel node algorithm. Toward a more tailored surgery for cervical cancer patients. *Cancer medicine. 2016*;5:1725–1730. doi:10.1002/cam4.722.

[51] Lennox G. K., Covens A. Can sentinel lymph node biopsy replace pelvic lymphadenectomy for early cervical cancer? *Gynecol Oncol. 2017*;144:16–20. doi: 10.1016/j.ygyno.2016.08.337.

In: The Sentinel Lymph Node
Editors: A. Londero, S. Bertozzi and C. Cedolini
ISBN: 978-1-53614-557-1


*Chapter 11*

# SENTINEL LYMPH NODE BIOPSY IN ENDOMETRIAL CANCER

***Monica Della Martina**, *Martina Venier, Ambrogio P. Londero and Angelo Cagnacci***
Clinic of Obstetrics and Gynecology, DAME, University of Udine,
University Hospital of Udine, Italy

**Abstract**

Endometrial cancer is the most common gynecological malignancy in industrialized countries and in 4% of cases affects women under 40 years of age. In endometrial cancer, surgical staging with lymphadenectomy defines patients at high risk of recurrence, enabling decision-making on adjuvant treatments. However, complete lymph node dissection is a surgical procedure with many perioperative complications. Sentinel lymph node biopsy has been shown to be feasible in endometrial cancer patients, especially in intermediate- and high-risk patients, to obtain adequate lymph node assessment while reducing lymphatic complications associated with complete lymphadenectomy. Furthermore, the in vivo lymph node mapping is contributing to our knowledge on the lymphatic drainage of endometrial cancer. Recently, a decrease in the incidence of pelvic sidewall recurrences among women undergoing sentinel lymph node biopsy has been reported. This recurrence reduction is attributed to the ability of this procedure to find and remove lymph nodes in unusual locations, which are not routinely sampled in the standard lymphadenectomy, such as the presacral, parametrial and internal iliac vein areas. However, further studies are needed to better understand the potential of the sentinel lymph node biopsy procedure in endometrial cancer and to confirm its utility in terms of staging and survival.

**Keywords:** endometrial cancer, sentinel lymph node biopsy, lymph node pathologic ultrastaging, pelvic lymph node dissection, para-aortic lymph node dissection

## 1. Introduction

Endometrial cancer is the most common gynecological malignancy in industrialized countries. Its prognosis depends on the histotype and stage. The age-standardized incidence of

*Corresponding Author E-mail: m.dellamartina@libero.it.

endometrial cancer in Europe is 13.6 cases per 100'000 women and the cumulative lifetime risk for endometrial cancer diagnosis is of 1.71% [1]. It usually affects post-menopausal women, but about 4% of cases are under 40 years of age [1].

The National Comprehensive Cancer Network (NCCN) guidelines recommend managing endometrial cancer with total hysterectomy and bilateral salpingo-oophorectomy [2]. Surgical staging with lymphadenectomy defines the recurrence risk, and thus helps clinical decision-making in selecting high-risk patients for adjuvant treatments. However, systematic lymphadenectomy increases perioperative morbidity and lymphatic complications such as lymphedema, lymphocyst formation and genito-femoral nerve injury. The indications for lymphadenectomy and the therapeutic role of this procedure have been controversial since its first use [2].

Lymphadenectomy is not performed worldwide. It has been widely used in North America and Australia [3, 4]. In Europe, the standard of care for stage I endometrial cancer was surgery combined with radiotherapy in cases with risk factors for nodal metastases or recurrence. In stage I endometrial cancer the rate of pelvic node metastases is about 10%, but it is only 3-5% in well-differentiated endometrial cancer with ¡50% of myometrial invasion [4]. Lymph node involvement increases to 20% if endometrial cancer is poorly differentiated or with $\geq$ 50% of myometrial invasion [4]. Two large prospective trials showed that pelvic lymphadenectomy has no therapeutic effect [5, 6]. Benedetti-Panici and colleagues randomized 514 women with stage I endometrial cancer to systematic pelvic lymphadenectomy or no lymphadenectomy. The study showed no improvement in disease-free or overall survival in the lymphadenectomy group. The ASTEC study randomized 1408 women to standard surgery with and without lymphadenectomy. The results demonstrated no benefit of systematic lymphadenectomy on overall, disease-specific or recurrence-free survivals.

The extent of lymphadenectomy is also a subject of debate. Pelvic lymphadenectomy can be associated with para-aortic lymphadenectomy up to the inferior mesenteric artery or the renal vessels. In fact, the para-aortic nodes may be positive in the absence of positive pelvic nodes [6, 7, 8]. Data from the Mayo Clinic showed a nodal metastases rate of 22% in high-risk endometrial cancer patients: 51% of these women had both positive pelvic and para-aortic nodes, 33% had only positive pelvic nodes and 3% had positive para-aortic lymph nodes with negative pelvic lymph nodes [9]. 67-77% of the para-aortic nodal metastases were above the inferior mesenteric artery, supporting the need of a para-aortic lymphadenectomy up to the renal vessels [9, 10]. The SEPAL study [11] showed a longer overall survival in intermediate- or high-risk endometrial cancer patients treated with pelvic and para-aortic lymphadenectomy than in patients treated with pelvic lymphadenectomy alone.

Recently, the ESMO Guidelines [1] have identified the risk of recurrence as low in grade 1-2 endometrioid endometrial cancer with ¡50% of myometrial invasion and no lymphovascular space invasion. The risk results intermediate in grade 1-2 endometrioid endometrial cancer with $\geq$ 50% of myometrial invasion and and no lymphovascular invasion. The risk is high-intermediate in grade 3 endometrioid endometrial cancer with ¡50% of myometrial invasion, regardless of the lymphovascular invasion status and in grade 1-2 endometrioid endometrial cancer with lymphovascular invasion, regardless of the depth of invasion. Finally, the risk is high in grade 3 endometrioid endometrial cancer with $\geq$ 50% of myometrial invasion, regardless of the lymphovascular invasion status or in all non-endometrioid endometrial cancers.

Surgical treatment must be tailored based to the prognostic factor risk. The ESMO Guidelines 2017 recommend lymphadenectomy (including pelvic and para-aortic nodes up to the level of the renal veins) in high-risk endometrioid endometrial cancer or in serous carcinoma, clear-cell carcinoma and clinical stage I carcinosarcoma. No lymph node resection is recommended in low-risk endometrioid endometrial cancer. Sentinel lymph node biopsy (SLNB) is an option to target lymph nodes that are most likely involved with metastatic cancer as it limits surgical extension and may also represent a good compromise between non-dissection and complete dissection to reduce morbidity in intermediate- and high-intermediate-risk endometrial cancer.

## 2. Lymphatic Pathways

The purpose of lymphatic mapping is to identify one or more sentinel nodes representative of the rest of the lymph nodes that drain the tumor. Burke and colleagues first described lymphatic mapping in endometrial cancer in 1996 using an injection of isosulfan blue into the uterine fundus [12]. Preliminary observations indicated that the lymphatic network draining the uterus is complex and involves both para-aortic and pelvic lymph nodes.

In recent years, three consistent lymphatic pathways of uterine drainage have been identified [13]: an upper para-cervical pathway, which develops along the uterine artery and drains the external iliac and/or obturator lymph nodes; a lower para-cervical pathway, which extends along the uterine vein to the hypogastric and/or pre-sacral lymph nodes, and an infundibolo-pelvic pathway which develops along the infundibolo-pelvic ligament to the para-aortic lymph nodes (Figure 1). However, there is no agreement on which nodes are most commonly involved in endometrial cancer. In fact, some authors describe the external iliac nodes, while others describe the nodes of the obturator fossa as the most involved [14].

The growing experience in lymphatic mapping from different medical groups seems to indicate that once a certain level of competency is reached, a very high rate of mapping can be achieved. However, the mapping of the aortic area has been less successful. The sentinel node detection rate in the aortic area after a cervical injection is approximately 5% [15]. If para-aortic sentinel node mapping fails, pelvic sentinel node mapping is likely to be sufficient in most patients, given the low likelihood of isolated para-aortic metastases in this setting.

Since metastatic nodes, when present, are most commonly encountered above the inferior mesenteric artery when the pelvic nodes are negative [9], the sampling of the lower aortic nodes (below the inferior mesenteric artery) increases operative time and complications, with minimal clinical benefit. It is important to note that an aortic node can be considered a sentinel node only in the absence of other hot nodes in the infra-mesenteric area. Otherwise, it may be a secondary lymph node. In the absence of sentinel lymph nodes in the high aortic area, the surgeon can still perform an aortic lymph node dissection regardless of the results of the pelvic lymph node mapping.

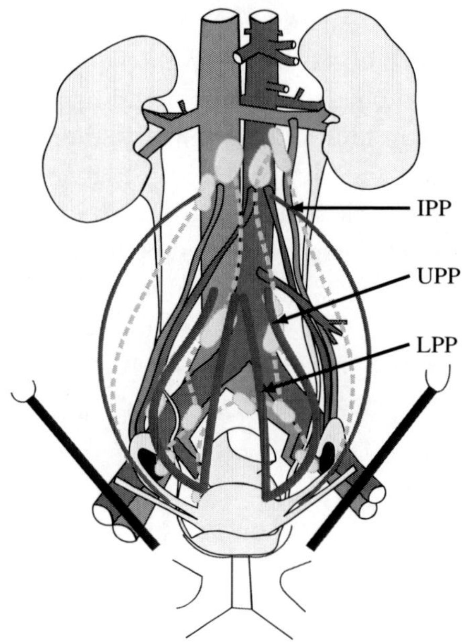


Figure 1. Lymph node pathways modified from Geppert and colleagues [13]. IPP: infundibolo-pelvic pathway; LPP: lower paracervical pathway; UPP upper paracervical pathway (drawing by APL).

## 3. Technical Aspects

The two technical aspects to be accurately evaluated are the determination of the most appropriate injection site to better follow the route of the potential metastatic spread and the marker to be injected to obtain the highest detection rate.

### 3.1. Injection Site

The main advantage of the cervix uteri as an injection site is its accessibility, since the cervix is almost always clearly visualized and accessible, despite the major distortion of the uterine corpus. However, concerns have been raised as to whether the lymphatic drainage of the cervix represents the actual lymphatic drainage of the tumor situated in the corpus uteri, both within the pelvis and in the para-aortic area. The cervical injection approach has a high detection rate, especially for the lower and upper paracervical pathways.

On the contrary, the proposed advantages of the fundus uteri as the injection site is its proximity to the tumor. The hysteroscopic approach is associated with high detection rates of both pelvic and aortic nodal areas and allows a direct visualization of the tumor. The radioactive technetium-99 colloid was used as a tracer due to the lower sensitivity obtained with blue-dye [16]. However, this technique has not been widely adopted because often the hysteroscopic visualization of the tumor is not easy, particularly when the tumor is either too large occupying the whole cavity, too small, or when the uterus is distorted by the presence of leiomyomas [17]. In addition, this technique requires a separate procedure performed two hours prior to the major surgery and, possibly an associated lymphoscintigraphy 15-30 minutes after the radiotracer injection. Vagal symptoms during hysteroscopy may also occur [18].

A meta-analysis reported improved sentinel node detection rates with the cervical injection compared with other injection sites [19]. The same results were confirmed in a recent study where cervical injection was associated with a higher technical success rate and an easier use compared with the fundal injection [13]. In the study, the overall detection rate of at least one sentinel node was 100% after a cervical injection and 93% after a fundal injection, while the bilateral detection rate was 98% and 80%, respectively.

Recent anatomic studies demonstrated a deep injection into the stroma of the cervix to have excellent penetration into the uterine vessels, parametria, lower uterine segment and cornual region [20, 21]. The most common cervical injection method involves the superficial (1-3 mm) and deep injection (1-2 cm) into the cervix at 3 and 9 o'clock positions. This method have a detection rate of 89%, 65%, and 3% for the overall, bilateral and para-aortic sentinel nodes, respectively [22].

### 3.2. Injected Tracers

Three tracers have been used for the identification of sentinel nodes: technetium-99, blue dye, and, more recently, indocyanine green. Pelvic lymphatic mapping using blue dyes and/or technetium-99 has been largely described [23], with detection rates ranging between 80-85% for each tracer alone and 89-95% when using blue dye and technetium-99 combined [24].

The use of technetium-99 is associated with a higher cost and complexity. It requires a preoperative injection, lymphoscintigraphy before surgery and an intraoperative gamma probe to identify the hot nodes. The blue dye injection is the simplest method because it does not require any special equipment, but seems to be associated with a lower rate of bilateral mapping when compared to the other techniques [15]. More recently, the feasibility of a new near-infrared fluorescence imaging system using indocyanine green has been described for sentinel node mapping.

Indocyanine green has been demonstrated to be superior to blue dye and comparable or superior to technetium-99 for sentinel node mapping [25]. Additionally, its use has several advantages over technetium-99, such as reduced pain at injection, lower cost, fewer adverse effects and quick real-time visualization [26]. A recent meta-analysis showed that the use of indocyanine green is associated with a higher rate of bilateral SLNB than the use of blue dye or technetium-99 [27].

Recent anatomic studies [28, 29] demonstrated that a deep injection into the cervical stroma towards the lower uterine segment results in excellent diffusion throughout the uterus, including the fundal region. Another recent study showed that both cervical and fundal indocyanine green injections offer good overall detection rates and improve the mapping of the aortic area versus cervical injection alone [30]. In addition, indocyanine green also appears to improve success rate of sentinel node mapping in obese patients [31].

### 3.3. Surgical Algorithm

An algorithm for sentinel node mapping has recently been published. In summary, the surgical algorithm includes: peritoneal and serosal evaluations and washings; retroperitoneal evaluation, including removal of all sentinel nodes and any suspicious nodes; and side-specific pelvic, common iliac, and interiliac lymph node dissections if there is no mapping on the hemi-pelvis. Para-aortic lymphadenectomy is left to the discretion of the clinician. (Figure 2).

The application of the algorithm reduced the false-negative rate from 15% to 2% and only one patient with an isolated para-aortic lymph node metastasis was missed [32].

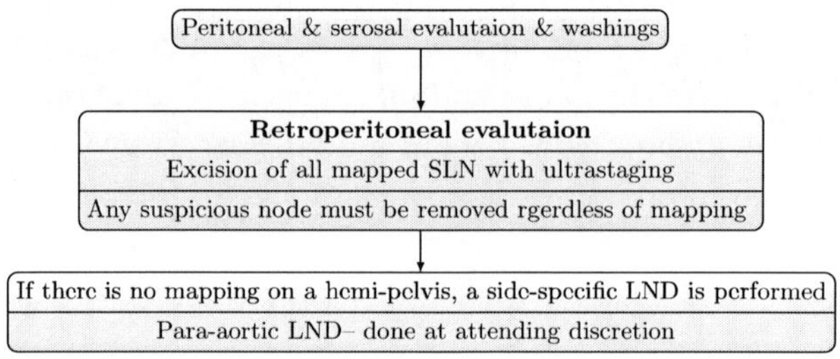


Figure 2. Sentinel lymph node algorithm for surgical staging of endometrial cancer from Barlin JN et al. [32]. SLN: sentinel lymph node; LND: lymph node dissection.

## 4. Advantages of Sentinel Lymph Node Biopsy in Endometrial Cancer

Surgical staging with lymphadenectomy defines recurrence risk and helps clinicians in their decision-making regarding the administration of adjuvant treatment. However, complete pelvic and para-aortic lymphadenectomy is associated with major comorbidities including lymphedema, lymphocyst formation, genitofemoral nerve injury [33] and is technically difficult to achieve in obese populations. SLNB is considered for patients with apparent uterine-confined endometrial cancer to assess whether they have metastatic pelvic lymph nodes. With this new technique patients may be able to avoid the morbidity of a standard complete lymphadenectomy.

A recent multicenter prospective cohort study conducted by Rossi and colleagues by performing SLNB followed by complete pelvic (with or without para-aortic) lymphadenectomy confirmed that SLNB alone would have missed only one positive node (false-negative rate of 3%), with the advantage of exposing fewer patients to the morbidity of a complete lymphadenectomy [34].

Lower extremity lymphedema is the most common lymphatic complication following complete lymphadenectomy. Its incidence is about 14-18%, but it is significantly reduced to 1.3% following SLNB alone. Thus, SLNB reduces by 93% the risk of developing lower extremity lymphedema compared with complete pelvic and infrarenal lymphadenectomy. The second most common lymphatic complication following lymphadenectomy is lymphocele development. The incidence of lymphocele decreased to 2.6% after SLNB alone [35], which is significantly lower than the incidence of 13.3% occurring after infrarenal, para-aortic and pelvic lymphadenectomy.

In addition, sentinel lymph node ultrastaging detects micrometastases otherwise undiagnosed with conventional histology, even in patients classified at low-risk based on the grade and depth of myometrial invasion [36]. In a retrospective analysis of patients with early-stage endometrial cancer who underwent SLNB with lymphadenectomy versus lymphadenectomy alone, sentinel node mapping led to the detection of a wider number of metastases and was associated with a greater use of adjuvant therapy [37].

The results of a multicenter prospective study, the FIRES trial, suggest that the sentinel node algorithm might be better than traditional complete lymphadenectomy for a series of reasons: the sentinel node being more likely to contain metastatic disease, the pathologists being required to ultrastage a smaller number of more relevant nodes, and the sentinel node mapping identifying positive nodes that may be located outside traditional surgical boundaries [34]. In particular, sentinel node ultrastaging results in the detection of micrometastases and isolated tumor cells (ITCs), and therefore may reveal lymph node metastases undetected by conventional histology, leading to possible upstaging from 5% to 15% of patients [2, 38, 39].

Additionally, How and colleagues [40] demonstrated that sentinel node mapping decreased pelvic sidewall recurrences and attributed this to the detection of sentinel nodes at unusual locations. In a follow-up study, they reported that these atypical regions, which are not routinely sampled in a "complete" lymphadenectomy, included the presacral, parametrial and internal iliac vein areas.

As an alternative to ultrastaging a new diagnostic method, the one-step nucleic acid amplification (OSNA), has been proposed [41, 42]. For the OSNA analysis of the sentinel node, an optimal mRNA marker (cytokeratin 19) is selected: the OSNA assay can determine mRNA copy numbers using reverse transcription loop-mediated isothermal amplification reactions. Nagai and colleagues demonstrated that when the cut-off value was set at 250 copies (using CK19 mRNA) the OSNA assay had a sensitivity of 93.3% and a specificity of 99.5%. Moreover, the results of this study suggested that the OSNA assay had the same diagnostic capability as conventional frozen-section histology with 2-mm intervals [41]. The advantage of the OSNA assay is that it requires less time for analysis than conventional molecular biology techniques.

## 5. Management of Positive Sentinel Lymph Node

Standard lymph node assessment involves sectioning the node once along the longitudinal axis and staining it with hematoxylin-eosin to determine if it contains metastatic tumor cells. If this initial test is negative, ultrastaging of the sentinel node is performed. At ultrastaging low-volume metastases can be detected, including micrometastases and ITCs. The American Joint Committee on Cancer (AJCC) defined micrometastases as a focus of metastatic tumor cells larger than 0.2 mm and smaller than 2 mm, while ITCs are described as microscopic clusters and single cells of size less than or equal to 0.2 mm. [43]. The use of a sentinel node algorithm with pathologic ultrastaging for endometrial cancer led to increased detection of low-volume lymph node metastases in the form of ITCs and micrometastases [44, 45]. However, the clinical significance of these findings in endometrial cancer is still unknown.

There is a lack of data on clinical outcomes in the setting of low-volume lymph node metastases in endometrial cancer. Two retrospective studies analyzed patients with negative lymph nodes with the immunohistochemistry technique. Erklani and colleagues examined 47 patients and found that the presence of micrometastases in the sentinel lymph nodes correlated with a worse 36-months progression-free survival [46].

The only study that specifically addresses the outcome issue and adjuvant treatment in patients with micrometastases detected by sentinel node mapping is the study of St. Clair and colleagues, a large prospectively collected series of 844 patients with endometrial cancer [39]. In the study 47 patients had macrometastases (5.6%), 21 had micrometastases (2.5%), and 23 had ITCs (2.7%). Patients with ITCs or micrometastases had a better 3-year recurrence-free survival than patients with macrometastases, but all patients were considered to have stage IIIC disease and received adjuvant treatment. The natural history of untreated low-volume metastases is unclear.

In another recent study conducted by Plante and colleagues, patients with low-risk endometrial cancer and ITCs in the sentinel node showed a progression-free survival at 3 years of 100%, which was independent from receiving either vault brachytherapy only or no adjuvant treatment. On this basis, the authors suggest that patients with ITCs are likely to receive very little benefit from receiving additional adjuvant treatment [46].

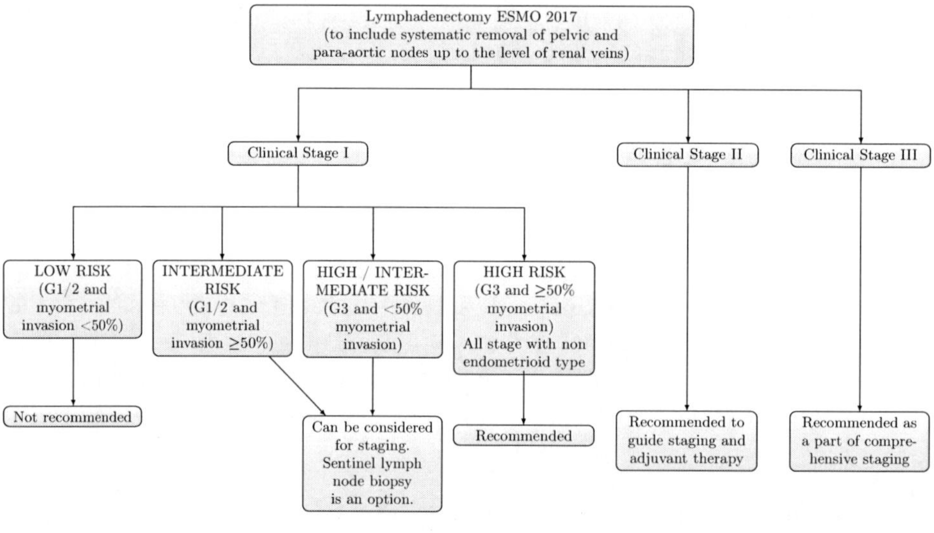


Figure 3. Surgical management algorithm modified by Colombo and colleagues [1].

In order to define this patient population, more data with a larger number of patients and a longer follow-up are needed. At the moment, post-surgical management of patients with ITCs is unsettled and should be individualized. Probably the decision for adjuvant treatment should not be based only on the presence of ITCs, but also take into account all the other elements of the pathology report, the uterine factors and the patient's overall condition.

## 6. Management of Negative Sentinel Lymph Node

SLNB is important for the identification of patients with lymphatic dissemination. Like lymph node dissection, SLNB as well identifies patients requiring adjuvant treatment. If the sentinel node is negative, it is reasonable to think that endometrial cancer is confined to the uterus. In this case, no further lymph node dissection is required.

## Conclusion

The use of sentinel node mapping has become more widespread and is now considered an option for the surgical staging of endometrial cancer [2, 1] (Figure 3) in intermediate-risk and high-intermediate-risk patients to reduce lymphadenectomy morbidity and tailor adjuvant therapy. Further studies are needed to confirm the utility of ultrastaging in improving progression-free survival.

## References

[1] Colombo N., Creutzberg C., Amant F., Bosse T., González-Martín A., Ledermann J., et al. ESMO-ESGO-ESTRO Consensus Conference on Endometrial Cancer: diagnosis, treatment and follow-up. *Ann Oncol. 2016*;27:16–41. doi:10.1093/annonc/mdv484.

[2] Koh W. J., Abu-Rustum N. R., Bean S., Bradley K., Campos S. M., Cho K. R., et al. Uterine Neoplasms, Version 1.2018, NCCN Clinical Practice Guidelines in Oncology. *J Natl Compr Canc Netw. 2018*;16:170–199. doi:10.6004/jnccn.2018.0006.

[3] Kilgore L. C., Partridge E. E., Alvarez R. D., Austin J. M., Shingleton H. M., Noojin F., et al. Adenocarcinoma of the endometrium: survival comparisons of patients with and without pelvic node sampling. *Gynecol Oncol. 1995*;56:29–33. doi:10.1006/gyno.1995.1005.

[4] Creasman W. T., Morrow C. P., Bundy B. N., Homesley H. D., Graham J. E., Heller P. B. Surgical pathologic spread patterns of endometrial cancer. A Gynecologic Oncology Group Study. *Cancer. 1987*;60:2035–2041.

[5] Benedetti Panici P., Basile S., Maneschi F., Alberto Lissoni A., Signorelli M., Scambia G, et al. Systematic pelvic lymphadenectomy vs. no lymphadenectomy in early-stage endometrial carcinoma: randomized clinical trial. *J Natl Cancer Inst. 2008*;100:1707–1716. doi:10.1093/jnci/djn397.

[6] ASTEC study group, Kitchener H., Swart A. M. C., Qian Q., Amos C., Parmar M. K. B. Efficacy of systematic pelvic lymphadenectomy in endometrial cancer (MRC ASTEC trial): a randomised study. *Lancet. 2009*;373:125–136. doi:10.1016/S0140-6736(08)61766-3.

[7] Abu-Rustum N. R., Gomez J. D., Alektiar K. M., Soslow R. A., Hensley M. L., Leitao M. M., et al. The incidence of isolated paraaortic nodal metastasis in surgically staged

endometrial cancer patients with negative pelvic lymph nodes. *Gynecol Oncol. 2009*; 115:236–238. doi:10.1016/j.ygyno.2009.07.016.

[8] Dowdy S. C., Aletti G., Cliby W. A., Podratz K. C., Mariani A. Extra-peritoneal laparoscopic para-aortic lymphadenectomy–a prospective cohort study of 293 patients with endometrial cancer. *Gynecol Oncol. 2008*;111:418–424. doi:10.1016/j.ygyno.2008.08.021.

[9] Kumar S., Podratz K. C., Bakkum-Gamez J. N., Dowdy S. C., Weaver A. L., McGree M. E., et al. Prospective assessment of the prevalence of pelvic, paraaortic and high paraaortic lymph node metastasis in endometrial cancer. *Gynecol Oncol. 2014*; 132:38–43. doi:10.1016/j.ygyno.2013.10.002.

[10] Mariani A., Dowdy S. C., Cliby W. A., Gostout B. S., Jones M. B., Wilson T. O., et al. Prospective assessment of lymphatic dissemination in endometrial cancer: a paradigm shift in surgical staging. *Gynecol Oncol. 2008*;109:11–18. doi:10.1016/j.ygyno.2008.01.023.

[11] Todo Y., Kato H., Kaneuchi M., Watari H., Takeda M., Sakuragi N. Survival effect of para-aortic lymphadenectomy in endometrial cancer (SEPAL study): a retrospective cohort analysis. *Lancet. 2010*;375:1165–1172. doi:10.1016/S0140-6736(09)62002-X.

[12] Burke T. W., Levenback C., Tornos C., Morris M., Wharton J. T., Gershenson D. M. Intraabdominal lymphatic mapping to direct selective pelvic and paraaortic lymphadenectomy in women with high-risk endometrial cancer: results of a pilot study. *Gynecol Oncol. 1996*;62:169–173. doi:10.1006/gyno.1996.0211.

[13] Geppert B., Lönnerfors C., Bollino M., Arechvo A., Persson J. A study on uterine lymphatic anatomy for standardization of pelvic sentinel lymph node detection in endometrial cancer. *Gynecol Oncol. 2017*;145:256–261. doi:10.1016/j.ygyno.2017.02.018.

[14] Mariani A., Webb M. J., Keeney G. L., Podratz K. C. Routes of lymphatic spread: a study of 112 consecutive patients with endometrial cancer. *Gynecol Oncol. 2001*; 81:100–104. doi:10.1006/gyno.2000.6111.

[15] Cormier B., Rozenholc A. T., Gotlieb W., Plante M., Giede C., of Practice (CoP) Group of Society of Gynecologic Oncology of Canada (GOC) C. Sentinel lymph node procedure in endometrial cancer: A systematic review and proposal for standardization of future research. *Gynecol Oncol. 2015*;138:478–485. doi:10.1016/j.ygyno.2015.05.039.

[16] Raspagliesi F., Ditto A., Kusamura S., Fontanelli R., Vecchione F., Maccauro M., et al. Hysteroscopic injection of tracers in sentinel node detection of endometrial cancer: a feasibility study. *Am J Obstet Gynecol. 2004*;191:435–439. doi:10.1016/j.ajog.2004.03.008.

[17] Frumovitz M., Bodurka D. C., Broaddus R. R., Coleman R. L., Sood A. K., Gershenson D. M., et al. Lymphatic mapping and sentinel node biopsy in women with high-risk endometrial cancer. *Gynecol Oncol. 2007*;104:100–103. doi:10.1016/j.ygyno.2006.07.033.

[18] Maccauro M., Lucignani G., Aliberti G., Villano C., Castellani M. R., Solima E., et al. Sentinel lymph node detection following the hysteroscopic peritumoural injection of 99mTc-labelled albumin nanocolloid in endometrial cancer. *Eur J Nucl Med Mol Imaging. 2005*;32:569–574. doi:10.1007/s00259-004-1709-4.

[19] Kang S., Yoo H. J., Hwang J. H., Lim M. C., Seo S. S., Park S. Y. Sentinel lymph node biopsy in endometrial cancer: meta-analysis of 26 studies. *Gynecol Oncol. 2011*; 123:522–527. doi:10.1016/j.ygyno.2011.08.034.

[20] Leitao M. M., Khoury-Collado F., Gardner G., Sonoda Y., Brown C. L., Alektiar K. M., et al. Impact of incorporating an algorithm that utilizes sentinel lymph node mapping during minimally invasive procedures on the detection of stage IIIC endometrial cancer. *Gynecol Oncol. 2013*;129:38–41. doi:10.1016/j.ygyno.2013.01.002.

[21] Abu-Rustum N. R., Khoury-Collado F., Gemignani M. L. Techniques of sentinel lymph node identification for early-stage cervical and uterine cancer. *Gynecol Oncol. 2008*;111:S44–S50. doi:10.1016/j.ygyno.2008.07.027.

[22] How J. A., O'Farrell P., Amajoud Z., Lau S., Salvador S., How E., et al. Sentinel lymph node mapping in endometrial cancer: a systematic review and meta-analysis. *Minerva Ginecol. 2018*;70:194–214. doi:10.23736/S0026-4784.17.04179-X.

[23] Khoury-Collado F., Murray M. P., Hensley M. L., Sonoda Y., Alektiar K. M., Levine D. A., et al. Sentinel lymph node mapping for endometrial cancer improves the detection of metastatic disease to regional lymph nodes. *Gynecol Oncol. 2011*;122:251–254. doi:10.1016/j.ygyno.2011.04.030.

[24] Rossi E. C., Jackson A., Ivanova A., Boggess J. F. Detection of sentinel nodes for endometrial cancer with robotic assisted fluorescence imaging: cervical versus hysteroscopic injection. *Int J Gynecol Cancer. 2013*;23:1704–1711. doi:10.1097/IGC.0b013e3182a616f6.

[25] How J., Gotlieb W. H., Press J. Z., Abitbol J., Pelmus M., Ferenczy A., et al. Comparing indocyanine green, technetium, and blue dye for sentinel lymph node mapping in endometrial cancer. *Gynecol Oncol. 2015*;137:436–442. doi:10.1016/j.ygyno.2015.04.004.

[26] Ruscito I., Gasparri M. L., Braicu E. I., Bellati F., Raio L., Sehouli J., et al. Sentinel Node Mapping in Cervical and Endometrial Cancer: Indocyanine Green Versus Other Conventional Dyes-A Meta-Analysis. *Ann Surg Oncol. 2016*;23:3749–3756. doi:10.1245/s10434-016-5236-x.

[27] Bodurtha Smith A. J., Fader A. N., Tanner E. J. Sentinel lymph node assessment in endometrial cancer: a systematic review and meta-analysis. *Am J Obstet Gynecol. 2017*;216:459–476.e10. doi:10.1016/j.ajog.2016.11.1033.

[28] Abu-Rustum N. R., Khoury-Collado F., Pandit-Taskar N., Soslow R. A., Dao F., Sonoda Y., et al. Sentinel lymph node mapping for grade 1 endometrial cancer: is it the answer to the surgical staging dilemma? *Gynecol Oncol. 2009*;113:163–169. doi: 10.1016/j.ygyno.2009.01.003.

[29] Khoury-Collado F., Abu-Rustum N. R. Lymphatic mapping in endometrial cancer: a literature review of current techniques and results. *Int J Gynecol Cancer. 2008*; 18:1163–1168. doi:10.1111/j.1525-1438.2007.01188.x.

[30] Ruiz R., Gorostidi M., Jaunarena I., Goiri C., Aguerre J., Lekuona A. Sentinel Node Biopsy in Endometrial Cancer With Dual Cervical and Fundal Indocyanine Green Injection. *Int J Gynecol Cancer. 2018*;28:139–144. doi:10.1097/IGC. 0000000000001151.

[31] Eriksson A. G. Z., Montovano M., Beavis A., Soslow R. A., Zhou Q., Abu-Rustum N. R., et al. Impact of Obesity on Sentinel Lymph Node Mapping in Patients with Newly Diagnosed Uterine Cancer Undergoing Robotic Surgery. *Ann Surg Oncol. 2016*;23:2522–2528. doi:10.1245/s10434-016-5134-2.

[32] Barlin J. N., Khoury-Collado F., Kim C. H., Leitao M. M., Chi D. S., Sonoda Y., et al. The importance of applying a sentinel lymph node mapping algorithm in endometrial cancer staging: beyond removal of blue nodes. *Gynecol Oncol. 2012*;125:531–535. doi:10.1016/j.ygyno.2012.02.021.

[33] Abu-Rustum N. R., Alektiar K., Iasonos A., Lev G., Sonoda Y., Aghajanian C., et al. The incidence of symptomatic lower-extremity lymphedema following treatment of uterine corpus malignancies: a 12-year experience at Memorial Sloan-Kettering Cancer Center. *Gynecol Oncol. 2006*;103:714–718. doi:10.1016/j.ygyno.2006.03.055.

[34] Rossi E. C., Kowalski L. D., Scalici J., Cantrell L., Schuler K., Hanna R. K., et al. A comparison of sentinel lymph node biopsy to lymphadenectomy for endometrial cancer staging (FIRES trial): a multicentre, prospective, cohort study. *Lancet Oncol. 2017*;18:384–392. doi:10.1016/S1470-2045(17)30068-2.

[35] Tada H., Teramukai S., Fukushima M., Sasaki H. Risk factors for lower limb lymphedema after lymph node dissection in patients with ovarian and uterine carcinoma. *BMC Cancer. 2009*;9:47. doi:10.1186/1471-2407-9-47.

[36] Ballester M., Dubernard G, Lécuru F., Heitz D., Mathevet P., Marret H., et al. Detection rate and diagnostic accuracy of sentinel-node biopsy in early stage endometrial cancer: a prospective multicentre study (SENTI-ENDO). *Lancet Oncol. 2011*; 12:469–476. doi:10.1016/S1470-2045(11)70070-5.

[37] Holloway R. W., Gupta S., Stavitzski N. M., Zhu X., Takimoto E. L., Gubbi A., et al. Sentinel lymph node mapping with staging lymphadenectomy for patients with endometrial cancer increases the detection of metastasis. *Gynecol Oncol. 2016*;141:206–210. doi:10.1016/j.ygyno.2016.02.018.

[38] Kim C. H., Khoury-Collado F., Barber E. L., Soslow R. A., Makker V., Leitao M. M., et al. Sentinel lymph node mapping with pathologic ultrastaging: a valuable tool for assessing nodal metastasis in low-grade endometrial cancer with superficial myoinvasion. *Gynecol Oncol. 2013*;131:714–719. doi:10.1016/j.ygyno.2013.09.027.

[39] St Clair C. M., Eriksson A.G. Z., Ducie J. A., Jewell E. L., Alektiar K. M., Hensley M. L., et al. Low-Volume Lymph Node Metastasis Discovered During Sentinel Lymph Node Mapping for Endometrial Carcinoma. *Ann Surg Oncol. 2016*;23:1653–1659. doi:10.1245/s10434-015-5040-z.

[40] How J., Gauthier C., Abitbol J., Lau S., Salvador S., Gotlieb R., et al. Impact of sentinel lymph node mapping on recurrence patterns in endometrial cancer. *Gynecol Oncol. 2017*;144:503–509. doi:10.1016/j.ygyno.2017.01.013.

[41] Nagai T., Niikura H., Okamoto S., Nakabayashi K., Matoda M., Utsunomiya H., et al. A new diagnostic method for rapid detection of lymph node metastases using a one-step nucleic acid amplification (OSNA) assay in endometrial cancer. *Ann Surg Oncol. 2015*;22:980–986. doi:10.1245/s10434-014-4038-2.

[42] Fanfani F., Monterossi G., Ghizzoni V., Rossi E. D., Dinoi G., Inzani F., et al. One-Step Nucleic Acid Amplification (OSNA): A fast molecular test based on CK19 mRNA concentration for assessment of lymph-nodes metastases in early stage endometrial cancer. *PloS one. 2018*;13:e0195877. doi:10.1371/journal.pone.0195877.

[43] American College of Surgeons. *AJCC Cancer Staging Manual (Eighth Edition).* Springer. 2017.

[44] Han G., Lim D., Leitao M. M., Abu-Rustum N. R., Soslow R. A. Histological features associated with occult lymph node metastasis in FIGO clinical stage I, grade I endometrioid carcinoma. *Histopathology. 2014*;64:389–398. doi:10.1111/his.12254.

[45] Erkanli S., Bolat F., Seydaoglu G. Detection and importance of micrometastases in histologically negative lymph nodes in endometrial carcinoma. *Eur J Gynaecol Oncol. 2011*;32:619–625.

[46] Plante M., Stanleigh J., Renaud M. C., Sebastianelli A., Grondin K., Grégoire J. Isolated tumor cells identified by sentinel lymph node mapping in endometrial cancer: Does adjuvant treatment matter? *Gynecol Oncol. 2017*;146:240–246. doi: 10.1016/j.ygyno.2017.05.024.

In: The Sentinel Lymph Node
Editors: A. Londero, S. Bertozzi and C. Cedolini
ISBN: 978-1-53614-557-1


*Chapter 12*

# ULTRASOUND NODAL STAGING IN CERVICAL AND ENDOMETRIAL CANCER

***Anjeza Xholli*, Fabiana Cecchini, Ambrogio P. Londero and Angelo Cagnacci***
Clinic of Obstetrics and Gynecology, DAME,
University of Udine, University Hospital of Udine, Italy

**Abstract**

Imaging plays an important role in the diagnosis, staging and follow-up of patients with gynecological tumors. Although there is a variety of techniques that clinicians can use, ultrasound is a commonly available and affordable non-invasive imaging method associated with minimal discomfort perception among patients. Another diagnostic option is computed tomography, which can detect suspicious nodes in the case of an increase in size, but unlike ultrasound it cannot describe their morphological features. Magnetic resonance imaging and positron emission tomography are imaging technique based on the metabolic activity of neoplastic cells and are more accurate but at the same time more expensive, thus not suitable for routine preoperative staging. Unfortunately, even ultrasound has some limitations, such as the operator's ability and the patient's BMI. To overcome this last limit, a newly introduced ultrasonographic method, the intraoperative ultrasound, could be used, which is able to detect nodal metastases with a high sensitivity, sparing women with gynecological malignancy from unnecessary lymphadenectomy.

**Keywords:** endometrial cancer, cervix cancer, ultrasound imaging, nodal staging

## 1. Introduction

Ultrasound is a non-invasive, commonly available, and affordable imaging method associated with minimal risk and discomfort perception among patients. When performed by an experienced diagnostician, it is of great use in the primary diagnosis of gynecological

*Corresponding Author E-mail: anj160583@yahoo.it.

cancers, in the evaluation of tumor extension in the pelvic and abdominal cavity, in the evaluation of nodal basins involvement and in the post-treatment follow-up. Biopsy of advanced tumors and metastatic lesions is also allowed by ultrasound [1].

The accuracy of ultrasound is largely dependent on three variables: the operator, the equipment and the patient. To become an ultrasound expert in gynecological oncology it requires adequate practical expertise, which is developed through exposure to abnormal findings. It is of the utmost importance to use complementary imaging methods in questionable cases and to be present in the operating theater in order to maximize the knowledge of the characteristics and spread of tumors.

To examine oncological patients, a high-end ultrasound machine equipped with sensitive Doppler, endocavitary (micro-convex) and transabdominal (convex array probe for abdomen and linear probe for peripheral lymph node assessment) transducers are required. Although there have been significant improvements in scanning technology in recent years, in some cases there are still limitations due to certain characteristics of the patient. In particular, the evaluation of retroperitoneum in obese patients is very challenging, such as the assessment of the liver in the presence of abundant ascites or postoperative adhesions with intestinal loops causing acoustic shadowing.

Transvaginal ultrasound is the optimal approach for the examination of the uterus (including cervix, endometrium, endometrial-myometrial junction, myometrium, and perimetrium), the adnexa, the pelvic peritoneum, the bladder and the rectosigmoid colon. The transrectal insertion of the probe has an advantage in patients who are virgin, have a stenotic vagina or have undergone brachytherapy. It also eliminates the risk of bleeding from an exophytically growing tumor of the vagina or uterine cervix.

For transabdominal sonography, a convex array probe (3.5-7 MHz) is usually used, depending on the patient's body habitus. Ultrasound examination of the abdominal cavity must be performed systematically and the entire anatomy must be evaluated in both sagittal and transverse sections [2]. First of all, attention is paid to the visceral organs of the upper abdomen, their size and structure. Intraparenchymatous focal or diffuse lesions are evaluated, as well as capsular infiltration or visceral lymphadenopathy. Secondly, the parietal, visceral, mesenteric peritoneum and omentum are evaluated. Finally, the peripheral (superficial and deep inguinal) and retroperitoneal (also called parietal) lymph nodes are evaluated [3].

## 2. Cervical and Endometrial Cancer Sonographic Evaluation

### 2.1. Cervical Cancer

Ultrasound plays a role in the precise evaluation of tumor spread [4] either locally, through the infiltration of surrounding structures (paracolpium, pericervical fascia and parametria, urethra, urinary bladder, rectosigmoid), or in the form of peritoneal lesions in the pelvis and abdominal cavity (peritoneal carcinomatosis). In addition, the tumor may also spread through the lymphatic and vascular systems, as described by the TNM (primary Tumor, regional lymph Nodes and distant Metastasis) staging classification system [5].

The sonographic detection rate for cervical cancer is 93-94% [6, 7] and ultrasound is a highly accurate method in classifying early-stage tumors [6, 7, 8, 9]. When planning the individual patient treatment, it is important to focus on the following information needed by the clinicians from the ultrasound examiners:

- growth pattern of the tumor (exocervix/exophytic tumor growth, endocervix/infiltrative);
- tumor size, which is measured in three diameters;
- distance between the tumor and the internal cervical os. It is recommended in fertile individuals who may want to plan a later pregnancy. In order to maintain an adequate tumor-free margin and reduce the risk of future miscarriage, this distance should be $\geq$ 10 mm [10, 11, 12];
- extent of the stromal invasion. The proportion of stromal invasion can be defined as partial ($\leq 2/3$) or full thickness (¿2/3), or tumor-free. This is achieved by measuring the distance between the tumor and the pericervix, or pericervical fascia, at the point where the ventral (including vesicouterine and vesicovaginal), lateral and dorsal (including uterosacral and sacrovaginal) ligaments attach to the cervix on both sides.

The extent of the radical procedure (parametrectomy) can be planned on the basis of this data [13].

## 2.2. Endometrial Cancer

Ultrasound is widely accepted as an appropriate staging method for early-stage endometrial cancers [4]. Sonographic diagnosis should provide the clinician with information on the tumor location, size (three diameters), sonomorphology (e.g., echogenicity, homogeneity, endometrial-myometrial junction) and vascular pattern [14]. Moreover, it offers the possibility of evaluating the tumor infiltration into the myometrium and towards the cervix.

Ideally, the depth of the tumor invasion should be measured from the endometrial-myometrial interface to the deepest edge of the tumor extension into the myometrium and should be related to the width of the normal myometrium. However, sonographic measurement has its limitations. In fact, in some cases the normal myometrium is not accessible, as it is either consumed by the tumor or greatly thinned by pressure from an exophytically grown tumor. Another way of measuring the degree of the myometrial infiltration is to determine the relationship between the maximum tumor thickness (d1) and the antero-posterior diameter of the uterus (d2) in the sagittal plane. Invasion of less than half the myometrium is recorded when the ratio of d1 to d2 is $<50\%$ (Stage T1a), and invasion equal to or greater than half the myometrium is recorded when the ratio of d1 to d2 equals or exceeds 50% (Stage T1b) [15]. This approach seems less operator-dependent, although the extent of invasion may be overestimated in cases of large polypoid exophytic tumors with intact but thinned myometrium. Both techniques have an accuracy of over 80% in assessing the extent of myometrial infiltration [15, 16, 17]. Another option is to measure instead the shortest myometrial tumor-free distance to the serosa. This parameter is easy to assess and also appears to be a useful prognostic factor for recurrence, using a 10 mm cut-off (area under the receiver-operating characteristics curve is 0.76) [18].

Moreover, in the case of mainly polypoid growing tumors, the detection with Doppler of dominant feeding vessels enables a more detailed examination of the endometrial-myometrial junction at the insertion of the pedicle, in order to assess more accurately the depth of myometrial invasion. To exclude cervical stromal involvement, in cases where the endometrial tumor protrudes only into the cervical canal and has not infiltrated the cervical stroma, the sliding effect of tumor mass against the endocervical mucosa can be obtained and observed by applying light pressure with a transvaginal probe.

## 3. Lymph Node Assessment

The evaluation of the lymph nodes is a critical part of the clinical cancer staging and is important in determining prognosis and selecting optimal treatment. Magnetic resonance imaging (MRI) or computed tomography (CT) diagnoses of infiltrated lymph nodes are based mainly on their size, with the most widely accepted definition of lymph node involvement being as the node transverse diameter exceeding 10 mm [19].

Ultrasound differs from these two imaging techniques in its ability to accurately evaluate the morphology of lymph nodes, allowing the identification of changes in their inner structure, especially in infiltrated peripheral lymph nodes. With the use of power Doppler ultrasonography technique, the vascular pattern of the lymph nodes can also be evaluated.

The standard approach for visualizing the lymph nodes starts from the inguinal canal and proceeds towards the diaphragm (Figure 1A, B, C, and D). However, an initial transvaginal or transrectal examination will provide information about the location of the lymph nodes in the region of the external iliac vessels and the obturator fossa, as well as the branching of their feeding arteries from large vessels.

Once a lymph node is visualized in the setting of a patient with a pelvic malignancy, there are a number of potentially useful features to determine if it is involved with tumor or not. However, the sensitivity and specificity of these features are modest [20, 21, 22, 23].

## 4. Distribution and Classification of Lymph Nodes

Lymph nodes that may be involved in patients with gynecological cancers are divided into:

- peripheral lymph nodes (i.e., superficial and deep inguinal lymph nodes);
- non-peripheral lymph nodes, that include those showed in Figure 2 and Figure 3;
  - parietal and retroperitoneal lymph nodes (periaortic and iliac lymph nodes);
  - visceral lymph nodes (intraperitoneal lymph nodes), that receive lymph from the abdominal organs associated with the visceral branches of the aorta (along the course of the celiac trunk, including lymph nodes of the splenic and hepatic hilum and the superior and inferior mesenteric vessels) and from the pelvic organs [24, 25] (Figure 3).

The peripheral lymph nodes that may be examined in patients with gynecological cancer are:

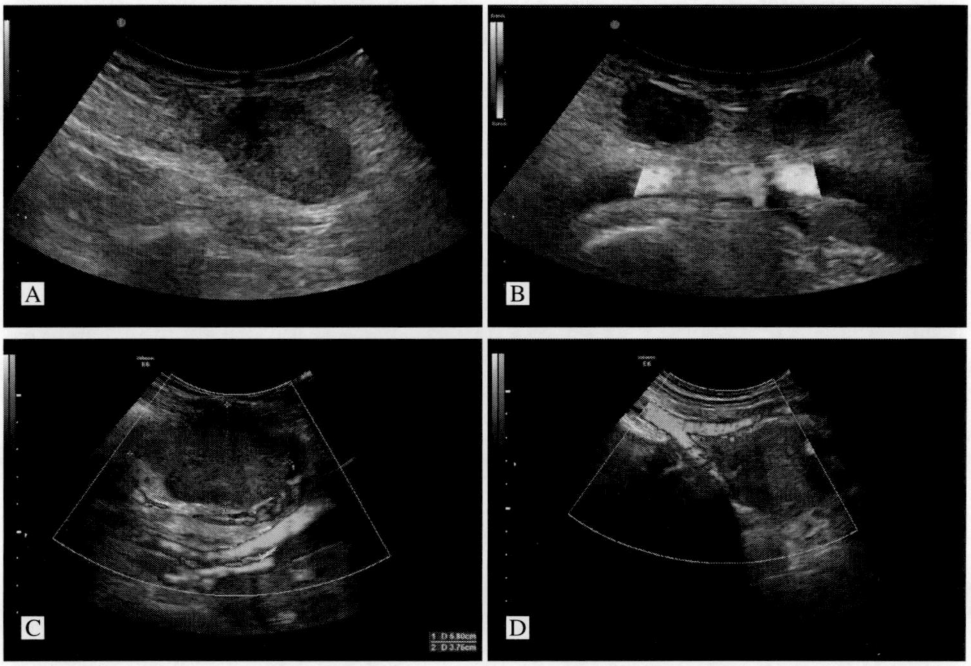


Figure 1. Panel A) Superficial inguinal metastatic lymph node. Panel B) Inguinal metastatic lymph nodes. Panel C) External iliac metastatic lymph node. Panel D) Interiliac (middle) node.

- Inguinal lymph nodes, in the case of vulvar, vaginal or ovarian cancer;
- Supraclavicular lymph nodes, in the case of disseminated or recurrent cancer.

Inguinal nodes are located inferior to the inguinal ligament level and to the external iliac node group. They can be grouped into superficial and deep inguinal nodes. Superficial inguinal lymph nodes are an organized chain of approximately 10 lymph nodes, located in the triangular area bounded by the inguinal ligament superiorly, the border of the sartorius muscle laterally and the adductor longus muscle medially. Deep inguinal lymph nodes are about 3-5 lymph nodes, located medial to femoral vein and beneath the cribriform fascia. The highest deep inguinal lymph node located inferior to the inguinal ligament is called "Cloquet's node".

After the evaluation of inguinal lymph nodes, the lymph nodes of the retroperitoneal compartment must be examined. The probe should be moved in an oblique section to evaluate the external iliac artery and the external iliac vein, which are located on the psoas major muscle. Beneath the external iliac vessels there is the obturator fossa, and at the pelvic margin there is the bifurcation of the internal and external iliac vessels.

Pelvic retroperitoneal lymph nodes are grouped as follows:

- External iliac lymph nodes (lateral, middle, medial and obturator lymph nodes). These nodes are in proximity of the external iliac artery and vein, caudal to the bifurcation of the common iliac vessels and cranial to the inguinal ligament. The relationship between the nodes and the vessels determines the nomenclature of their

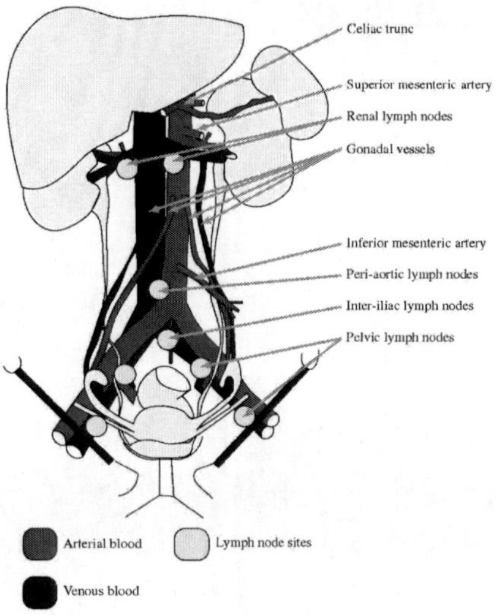


Figure 2. Schematic rappresentation of the anatomical distribution of parietal lymph nodes.

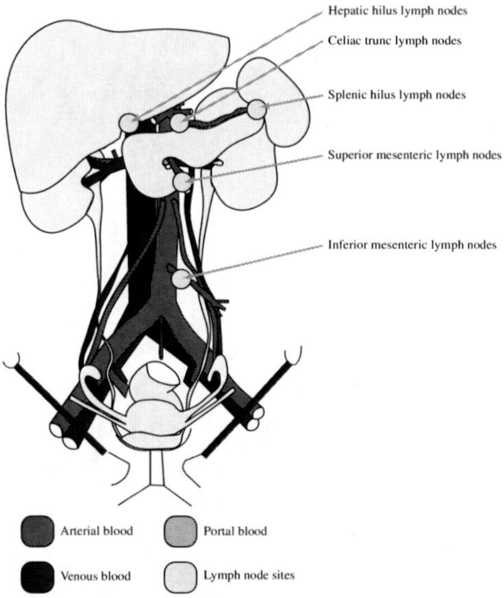


Figure 3. Schematic rappresentation of the anatomical distribution of visceral lymph nodes.

subgroups. In some cases, the medial external iliac lymph node group describes a node group postero-medial to the external iliac vessels. In the latter case, these nodes can be in proximity of the obturator internus muscle and are therefore called by some authors obturator nodes.

- Internal iliac lymph nodes (sacral, presacral and hypogastric nodes). These nodes are located adjacent to the internal iliac vessels and anterior to the origin of the proximal branches of the anterior division of the internal iliac arteries. They are generally subdivided according to the adjacent vessel. The lateral sacral nodes are close to the paired lateral sacral arteries. The presacral nodes are immediately anterior to the sacrum and posterior to the mesorectal fascia. The hypogastric nodes may describe the most cephalic of the internal iliac nodes, but also the entire internal iliac group.

- Common iliac lymph nodes (lateral, middle, medial). These nodes are located in proximity to the common iliac artery and vein and are therefore caudal to the aortic bifurcation and cranial to the bifurcation of the common iliac vessels.
- Periaortic and pericaval lymph nodes. To examine these nodes with ultrasound, it is necessary to obtain a sagittal plane in order to examine thetissue from the aorto-caval bifurcation to the diaphragm. Small movements of the probe from left to the right and vice versa should be used to evaluate the abdominal parietal lymph nodes (to the left of the aorta: lateral aortic nodes, pre- and post-aortic nodes, inter-aorto-caval intermediate lumbar nodes, pre- and post-caval nodes and lateral caval nodes). Based on the branching of the inferior mesenteric artery, the abdominal parietal lymph nodes can be further divided into lower level (infra-mesenteric, up to the branching of the inferior mesenteric artery) and upper level (supra-mesenteric, above the branching of the inferior mesenteric artery).

A disadvantage of ultrasound is that the retroperitoneal (parietal) lymph nodes are more difficult to visualize in obese patients or in cases of poor acoustic conditions, such as in women with postsurgical adhesions.

Visceral nodes include lateral vescical nodes, pre- and retro-vescical nodes, para-uterine nodes, para-vaginal nodes, para-rectal nodes. They can be visualized adequately by using a transvaginal probe. Abdominal infiltrated visceral lymph nodes in the branching area of the superior mesenteric artery and the celiac trunk may be visualized effectively on trans-abdominal ultrasound. Although ultrasound plays an important role in the initial staging of gynecological malignancies, the most accurate information on the lymph node status is obtained by systematic surgical staging.

# 5. Diagnostic Accuracy of Ultrasound Lymph Node Staging

## 5.1. Endometrial Cancer

Approximately 72% of endometrial cancers are diagnosed at FIGO stage I and about 10% have lymph node metastases. An ideal diagnostic test for nodal disease should be able to prevent both overtreatment (i.e., unnecessary lymphadenectomy) and undertreatment (i.e., withholding lymphadenectomy or adjuvant postoperative treatment to patients with lymph node metastases).

Lymph node involvement is an unfavorable prognostic factor, and the involvement of para-aortic lymph nodes is an independent predictor of poor outcome [26, 27]. However, given the favorable outcome for most cases, together with the potential complications of an extended procedure, the benefits of complete pelvic and para-aortic lymphadenectomy as part of the routine staging procedure remain controversial [27, 28, 29, 30, 31, 32, 33]. In particular, after lymphadenectomy 10.5% of patients develop lower limb lymphedema

[34, 35]. Other common complications are small bowel obstruction (4.4%), lymphocysts (7.6%) and deep venous thrombosis (2.6%), in addition to longer anesthesia time, hospital stay and higher estimated blood loss.

A major limitation of all radiologic techniques in the evaluation of lymph node metastases is the minimal size of the node suspected for metastases. Most authors consider enlarged a lymph node that exceeds 10 mm in size, although several reports suggest that metastatic lymph nodes can be 2 mm or less in diameter [36, 37, 38]. This also explains why lymph nodes may remain undiagnosed by sampling or selective lymphadenectomy: because they cannot be identified with the naked eye or by palpation, and this further reinforces the need for a complete lymphadenectomy.

In 2013, by reviewing the results of four radiologic modalities, Pelikan and colleagues found that CT has a low sensitivity (38.9%) and a high specificity (100%), and for this reason he defined CT as a poor diagnostic tool for evaluating lymph node status in patients with endometrial cancer [39], while positron emission tomography (PET) or positron emission tomography/computed tomography (PET/CT) had a reported sensitivity of 50% and a specificity of 100% [40, 41]. No study has been found that met his inclusion criteria for study evaluation, either with MRI or with ultrasound. Due to the lack of high-quality articles on preoperative tests for lymph node status in endometrial cancer, no proper comparison of these modalities has been performed.

Ryo is one of the authors who has most studied the utility of intraoperative ultrasound in detecting abnormal lymph nodes in gynecological malignancies [39]. He conducted a comparative study of three methods of detection of enlarged para-aortic lymph nodes in 163 women with ovarian and uterine corpus malignancy. CT, palpation during surgery and intraoperative ultrasound were the techniques used to assess metastatic lymph nodes. All of the women underwent para-aortic lymphadenectomy, and nodes were assessed for metastases. In this study, both specificity and positive predictive value were the highest for CT. If para-aortic lymphadenectomy was performed only in the presence of enlarged lymph nodes at CT, its high specificity would have allowed most women without metastases to avoid lymphadenectomy. However, lymph node metastases would have been missed in more than half of the women with involved lymph nodes. Therefore, CT was not a practical approach for the selection of women requiring para-aortic lymphadenectomy. Both sensitivity and negative predictive value were the highest for intraoperative ultrasound (Tables 1 and 2), which likely reduced the number of para-aortic lymphadenectomies performed by around 60%, while maintaining sensitivity for node metastases at around 90%. One of the advantages of intraoperative ultrasound is its high resolution, of less than 1 mm. However, when a new method is being tested, no data is initially available on which to base a decision concerning the criteria to be used. In this study, a lymph node was defined as abnormal simply when its diameter in the transverse plane was bigger than 5 mm, a value that was based on data from a CT imaging study [42, 43, 44]. In conclusion, intraoperative ultrasound can detect lymph node metastases with a high sensitivity, allowing to avoid unnecessary para-aortic lymphadenectomy in women with ovarian and uterine corpus malignancy [39].

Ryo and colleagues conducted another study in women with endometrial cancer to evaluate the accuracy of three methods in detecting abnormal para-aortic lymph node, using a combination of CT, intrauterine pathological findings (muscular invasion and grade of differentiation of the tumor) and intraoperative ultrasound. From these findings, the diag-

**Table 1. Sensitivity, specificity and positive and negative predictive values (PPV and NPV) of computed tomography, palpation during surgery, and intraoperative ultrasonography for the detection of para-aortic lymph node metastases [39]**

| Method | Sensitivity (%) | Specificity (%) | PPV (%) | NPV (%) |
|---|---|---|---|---|
| Computed Tomography | 42.9 | 96.1 | 75 | 86.0 |
| Palpation | 60.0 | 82.0 | 47.7 | 88.2 |
| Intraoperative ultrasonography | 91.4 | 69.5 | 45.1 | 96.7 |

**Table 2. P-values for the comparison of the accuracy of different methods for para-aortic lymph node metastases detection [39]**

| Modality pair | Sensitivity (Pv) | Specificity (Pv) | PPV (Pv) | NPV (Pv) |
|---|---|---|---|---|
| CT vs Palpation | 0.2318 | 0.0007 | 0.0773 | 0.7278 |
| IU vs Palpation | 0.0053 | 0.0286 | 0.9307 | 0.0458 |
| IU vs CT | ¡0.0001 | ¡0.0001 | 0.0344 | 0.0133 |

nostic accuracy of the association of CT and intraoperative ultrasound in evaluating para-aortic node metastases was calculated based on sensitivity, specificity, positive and negative predictive values. The diagnostic accuracy of intrauterine pathological findings was also calculated, although it was obtained retrospectively. It was assumed that para-aortic lymphadenectomy was performed only in the presence of enlarged lymph nodes detected by CT and intraoperative ultrasound. It was also assumed that only the women in the high-risk pathological findings group underwent para-aortic lymphadenectomy. Finally, the authors calculated the number of women who would have had missed para-aortic metastases and the number of women who could have avoided para-aortic lymphadenectomy [39].

The results of this study showed that no method had a superiority over all diagnostic indexes. To date, the only known accurate assessment procedure is a combination of lymphadenectomy and postoperative staging. Intraoperative ultrasound was the most effective technique in avoiding both unnecessary para-aortic lymphadenectomy and missed para-aortic node metastases (Table 3). Ultrasound scanning is operator-dependent, and most gynecologists are unfamiliar with intraoperative ultrasound. However, para-aortic areas are flat and the branching pattern of the vessels is simple, and images of enlarged lymph nodes are also easy to define. Although training is necessary before its actual clinical use, intraoperative ultrasound for para-aortic nodes is a procedure that can be easily mastered to a reliable level and is also safe and inexpensive [39].

In a systematic review, Selman and colleagues [45] showed that MRI and a successful SLNB were the most accurate tests for predicting the lymph node status in women with primary endometrial cancer. While other tests were low in accuracy. These results must be interpreted with caution as the quality of the studies available for review varied, with many of them of poor methodological quality, which may result in the introduction of bias.

**Table 3. Diagnostic accuracy of computed tomography (CT), intraoperative ultrasonoghraphy (IU), and intrauterine pathological finding (IPF) for para-aortic node metastases [39]**

| Method | Sensitivity (%) | Specificity (%) | PPV (%) | NPV (%) |
|---|---|---|---|---|
| CT | 38.9 | 100 | 100 | 86.9 |
| IU | 88.9 | 78.1 | 50.0 | 96.6 |
| IPF | 88.9 | 37.0 | 25.8 | 93.1 |

The three methods evaluated were CT, MRI and SLNB, and only one manuscript that had evaluated ultrasound was found [44].

Sawicki and colleagues [44] studied the effectiveness of transabdominal and transvaginal ultrasonography in the assessment of myometrial invasion, cervical involvement, pelvic lymph nodes, adnexal and omental metastases in endometrial cancer. Myometrial invasion evaluated with transvaginal ultrasound had an accuracy of 84.4%. The evaluation of tumor extension to the cervix was also accurate (sensitivity 86.4%, specificity 85.3%, positive predictive value 85.5%, and negative predictive value 95.1%). The efficiency in identifying adnexa was satisfactory (sensitivity 72.7%, specificity 97.5%, positive predictive value 80%, and negative predictive value 96.3%) and lymph node metastases were found with a sensitivity of 33.3% and a specificity of 100%. These results suggested that 2D transabdominal and transvaginal ultrasound evaluation of endometrial cancer are reliable methods for the preoperative assessment of selected prognostic factors, such as myometrial invasion, cervical involvement and adnexal metastases. However, in the assessment of lymph node metastases, they did not provide additional information [44].

Another multicenter prospective comparative study evaluated and compared the diagnostic performance of PET/CT, MRI and 2D ultrasound in the preoperative staging of endometrial cancer with special focus on myometrial infiltration, cervical infiltration and lymph nodes metastases. They concluded that none of the modalities can yet replace surgical staging. However, they all contributed to important knowledge and, furthermore, were able to upstage low-risk patients who would not have been recommended lymph node resection based on histology and grade alone. They did not evaluate the lymph node status by ultrasound and, when comparing the other two radiological methods they found that PET/CT had a higher sensitivity in detecting abnormal lymph nodes than MRI, but the difference was not significant ($p = 0.140$) [46].

A literature review summarized the reported staging performances of both conventional and novel preoperative imaging methods and provided an overview of other promising novel imaging methods for endometrial cancer care. Regarding 2D and 3D ultrasounds, they reported a high accuracy in assessing deep myometrial and cervical stroma invasion, but they found them unsuitable for a reliable assessment of pelvic and para-aortic lymph node metastases due to the small field of view and limited depth of penetration with high-frequency vaginal ultrasound probes [47].

In their meta-analysis, Gong and colleagues [48] evaluated the diagnostic performance of different imaging techniques and the associated diagnostic criteria for the preoperative detection of pelvic lymph node metastases in gynecological carcinomas. They demonstrated that diffusion-weighted imaging, MRI, PET, PET/CT were the top-priority imaging methods for the detection of metastatic pelvic lymph nodes in gynecological carcinoma. Diffusion-weighted imaging was recommended as the first choice for metastases exclusion and all other imaging techniques, including CT and MRI, were suitable for metastases confirmation. However, for early-stage lymph node malignancy, PET or PET/CT could represent a better choice. They showed that the pooled sensibility of the imaging techniques for detecting metastatic pelvic lymph nodes was 47% for CT, 50% for MRI, 84% for diffusion-weighted imaging, 56% for PET, 68% for PET/CT, and 71% for ultrasound. The pooled specificity ranged from 93% to 99% with limited variations, with the highest specificity achieved by ultrasound (99%) (Table 4).

**Table 4. P-value of the accuracy of the different methods [48]**

| Modality pair | Sensitivity (Pv) | Specificity (Pv) | PPV (Pv) | NPV (Pv) |
|---|---|---|---|---|
| CT vs IU | ¡ 0.01 | ¡ 0.001 | 0.032 | 0.090 |
| IU vs IPF | 0.596 | ¡ 0.001 | 0.040 | 0.843 |
| CT vs IPF | ¡ 0.01 | ¡ 0.001 | ¡ 0.001 | 0.572 |

They concluded that ultrasound, in particular transvaginal ultrasound, is safer, cost-effective and widely available. In clinical practice, laparoscopic, transvaginal and transabdominal ultrasound are frequently used for the detection of metastatic lymph nodes. Among all ultrasound types, laparoscopic ultrasound had the highest sensibility and specificity, followed by transvaginal ultrasound with an area under the curve of 87.6%. The results suggest that the detection of metastatic pelvic lymph nodes with transvaginal ultrasound might lead to misdiagnosis, but at the same time it may be a valuable technique for confirming metastatic lymph nodes.

Jisun and colleagues proposed a prediction model of lymph node metastases using preoperative grade tumor, transvaginal ultrasound and serum antigen 125 (CA 125) in patients with endometrial cancer. They studied patients at every stage of the disease. Deep myometrial invasion at preoperative transvaginal ultrasound (¿ 50%), high serum CA 125 level (¿ 35 IU/ml), preoperative grade 2 or 3 of tumors were significant preoperative factors predicting lymph node metastases. They calculated a simple model for the prediction of lymph node metastases based on preoperative tumor grade, transvaginal findings and CA 125 level using logistic regression analysis. The sensibility and specificity of this model were 94% and 57%, respectively [49].

## 5.2. Cervical Cancer

Lymph node metastases are the most important independent adverse prognostic factor for patients with cervical cancer [50]. Surgical lymphadenectomy is considered the gold standard procedure for the diagnosis of nodal metastases, but because it is an invasive and expensive procedure with a high-risk of complications, it is not routinely performed [51]. If metastatic pelvic nodes are found during surgery, adjuvant chemotherapy and radiation therapy are required, even if the tumor stage remains the same. Positive para-aortic or inguinal lymph nodes classify the tumor as stage IVB.

Even today, size (short axis ¿1 cm) is the main cross-sectional imaging criterion for discriminating normal lymph nodes from metastatic nodes. These results in moderate sensitivity and specificity values for both CT and MRI (43%-73%) in the detection of metastatic lymph nodes. Positron emission PET/CT has the highest diagnostic performance for the detection of nodal metastases in cervical cancer patients. However, its accuracy decreases for nodal size ¡ 5 mm.

Xhue and colleagues explored the diagnostic value of transvaginal ultrasound in lymph node metastases from cervical cancer patients. They found that transvaginal ultrasound specificity was 84.6% and sensitivity was 100%, thus concluding that transvaginal ultrasound has a high value in the clinical staging and treatment of the tumor [52].

Another Chinese group also studied the value of transvaginal color Doppler ultrasound in the diagnosis of obturator lymph node metastases from gynecological pelvic tumors. All patients underwent transvaginal ultrasonography before surgery to detect obturator lymph nodes. Subsequently, the findings were compared with surgery. The sensitivity and specificity of transvaginal ultrasonography were also assessed, 84.21% and 93.5%, respectively, and confirming that transvaginal ultrasound has clinical value in the diagnosis of obturator fossa lymph nodes metastases from gynecological pelvic tumors [53].

The same Chinese group conducted a study on the clinical application value of transvaginal ultrasound in the diagnosis of internal iliac lymph nodes metastases from pelvis cavity tumors. They performed a preoperative ultrasound of the pelvis with special attention to the internal iliac lymph nodes and the findings were confirmed by histological examination. In 42 patients analyzed, 39 cases of internal iliac lymph nodes were consistent with the pathology, the accuracy was 92.8% (39/42), 2 cases were misdiagnosed and in 1 case the diagnosis was missed. Therefore, transvaginal ultrasound can diagnose internal iliac lymph nodes metastases from gynecological pelvic tumors effectively and has a high value in clinical staging of gynecological cancer and treatment scheme [54].

# Conclusion

Imaging plays an important role in the diagnosis, staging and follow-up of patients with gynecological tumors. Although there are many different techniques available that the clinician can use, ultrasound is a non-invasive, commonly available and affordable imaging method associated with minimal discomfort perception among patients.

Unfortunately, ultrasound can be limited by the operator's ability and the patient's BMI. To overcome this last limit, a newly introduced ultrasonographic method could be used (i.e., the intraoperative ultrasound), which is able to detect node metastases with a high sensitivity, avoiding unnecessary lymphadenectomy in women with gynecological malignancy.

# References

[1] Fischerova D., Cibula D., Dundr P., Zikan M., Calda P., Freitag P., et al. Ultrasound-guided tru-cut biopsy in the management of advanced abdomino-pelvic tumors. *Int J*

*Gynecol Cancer. 2008*;18:833–837. doi:10.1111/j.1525-1438.2007.01015.x.

[2] Testa A. C., Van Holsbeke C., Mascilini F., Timmerman D. Dynamic and interactive gynecological ultrasound examination. *Ultrasound Obstet Gynecol. 2009*;34:225–229. doi:10.1002/uog.7309.

[3] Alcázar J. L., Castillo G., Jurado M., López-García G. Intratumoral blood flow in cervical cancer as assessed by transvaginal color doppler ultrasonography: Correlation with tumor characteristics. *Int J Gynecol Cancer. 2003*;13:510–514.

[4] Benedet J. L., Bender H., Jones H., Ngan H. Y., Pecorelli S. FIGO staging classifications and clinical practice guidelines in the management of gynecologic cancers. FIGO Committee on Gynecologic Oncology. *Int J Gynaecol Obstet. 2000*;70:209–262.

[5] International Union Against Cancer (UICC). *TNM Classification of Malignant Tumours (8th edition).* Wiley-Blackwell. 2016.

[6] Fischerova D., Cibula D., Stenhova H., Vondrichova H., Calda P., Zikan M., et al. Transrectal ultrasound and magnetic resonance imaging in staging of early cervical cancer. *Int J Gynecol Cancer. 2008*;18:766–772. doi:10.1111/j.1525-1438.2007.01072.x.

[7] Testa A. C., Ludovisi M., Manfredi R., Zannoni G., Gui B., Basso D., et al. Transvaginal ultrasonography and magnetic resonance imaging for assessment of presence, size and extent of invasive cervical cancer. *Ultrasound Obstet Gynecol. 2009*;34:335–344. doi:10.1002/uog.7325.

[8] Gaurilcikas A., Vaitkiene D., Cizauskas A., Inciura A., Svedas E., Maciuleviciene R., et al. Early-stage cervical cancer: agreement between ultrasound and histopathological findings with regard to tumor size and extent of local disease. *Ultrasound Obstet Gynecol. 2011*;38:707–715. doi:10.1002/uog.9037.

[9] Innocenti P., Pulli F., Savino L., Nicolucci A., Pandimiglio A., Menchi I., et al. Staging of cervical cancer: reliability of transrectal US. *Radiology. 1992*;185:201–205. doi:10.1148/radiology.185.1.1523308.

[10] Fischerova D., Cibula D., Zikan M., Pinkavova I., Dundr P., Calda P., OC23.01: Role of ultrasound in the referral of young patients with cervical cancer for fertility sparing surgery. *Ultrasound Obstet Gynecol. 2009*;34:43–43. doi:10.1002/uog.6589.

[11] Cibula D., Sláma J., Svárovský J., Fischerova D., Freitag P., Zikán M, et al. Abdominal radical trachelectomy in fertility-sparing treatment of early-stage cervical cancer. *Int J Gynecol Cancer. 2009*;19:1407–1411. doi:10.1111/IGC.0b013e3181b9549a.

[12] Rob L., Skapa P., Robova H. Fertility-sparing surgery in patients with cervical cancer. *Lancet Oncol. 2011*;12:192–200. doi:10.1016/S1470-2045(10)70084-X.

[13] Fischerova D., Cibula D., Calda P., Dundr P., Slama J, Pinkavova I. OC129: Role of ultrasound in guiding of surgery radicality in cervical cancer management. *Ultrasound Obstet Gynecol. 2008*;32:285–285. doi:10.1002/uog.5537.

[14] Leone F. P. G., Timmerman D., Bourne T., Valentin L., Epstein E., Goldstein S. R., et al. Terms, definitions and measurements to describe the sonographic features of the endometrium and intrauterine lesions: a consensus opinion from the International Endometrial Tumor Analysis (IETA) group. *Ultrasound Obstet Gynecol. 2010*;35:103–112. doi:10.1002/uog.7487.

[15] Karlsson B., Norström A., Granberg S., Wikland M. The use of endovaginal ultrasound to diagnose invasion of endometrial carcinoma. *Ultrasound Obstet Gynecol. 1992*;2:35–39. doi:10.1046/j.1469-0705.1992.02010035.x.

[16] Weber G., Merz E., Bahlmann F., Mitze M., Weikel W., Knapstein P. G. Assessment of myometrial infiltration and preoperative staging by transvaginal ultrasound in patients with endometrial carcinoma. *Ultrasound Obstet Gynecol. 1995*;6:362–367. doi:10.1046/j.1469-0705.1995.06050362.x.

[17] Savelli L., Ceccarini M., Ludovisi M., Fruscella E., De Iaco P. A., Salizzoni E., et al. Preoperative local staging of endometrial cancer: transvaginal sonography vs. magnetic resonance imaging. *Ultrasound Obstet Gynecol. 2008*;31:560–566. doi:10.1002/uog.5295.

[18] Lindauer J., Fowler J. M., Manolitsas T. P., Copeland L. J., Eaton L. A., Ramirez N. C., et al. Is there a prognostic difference between depth of myometrial invasion and the tumor-free distance from the uterine serosa in endometrial cancer? *Gynecol Oncol. 2003*;91:547–551.

[19] Nicolet V., Carignan L., Bourdon F., Prosmanne O. MR imaging of cervical carcinoma: a practical staging approach. *Radiographics. 2000*;20:1539–1549. doi:10.1148/radiographics.20.6.g00nv111539.

[20] Ahuja A. T., Ying M. Sonographic evaluation of cervical lymph nodes. *AJR Am J Roentgenol. 2005*;184:1691–1699. doi:10.2214/ajr.184.5.01841691.

[21] Hall T. B., Barton D. P. J., Trott P. A., Nasiri N., Shepherd J. H., Thomas J. M., et al. The role of ultrasound-guided cytology of groin lymph nodes in the management of squamous cell carcinoma of the vulva: 5-year experience in 44 patients. *Clin Radiol. 2003*;58:367–371.

[22] Poanta L., Serban O., Pascu I., Pop S., Cosgarea M., Fodor D. The place of CEUS in distinguishing benign from malignant cervical lymph nodes: a prospective study. *Medical ultrasonography. 2014*;16:7–14.

[23] Epstein E., Van Holsbeke C., Mascilini F., Masbäck A, Kannisto P., Ameye L., et al. Gray-scale and color Doppler ultrasound characteristics of endometrial cancer in relation to stage, grade and tumor size. *Ultrasound Obstet Gynecol. 2011*;38:586–593. doi:10.1002/uog.9038.

[24] Hernandez E., of Obstericians A. C., Gynecologists. ACOG Practice Bulletin number 65: management of endometrial cancer. *Obstet Gynecol. 2006*;107:952; author reply 952–952; author reply 953. doi:10.1097/01.AOG.0000209463.53764.e7.

[25] Fischerova D., Ultrasound scanning of the pelvis and abdomen for staging of gynecological tumors: a review. *Ultrasound Obstet Gynecol. 2011*;38:246–266. doi: 10.1002/uog.10054.

[26] Pelikan H. M. P., Trum J. W., Bakers F. C. H., Beets-Tan R. G. H., Smits L. J. M., Kruitwagen R. F. P. M. Diagnostic accuracy of preoperative tests for lymph node status in endometrial cancer: a systematic review. *Cancer Imaging. 2013*;13:314–322. doi:10.1102/1470-7330.2013.0032.

[27] Aalders J. G., Thomas G. Endometrial cancer–revisiting the importance of pelvic and para aortic lymph nodes. *Gynecol Oncol. 2007*;104:222–231. doi:10.1016/j.ygyno.2006.10.013.

[28] Amant F., Moerman P., Neven P., Timmerman D., Van Limbergen E., Vergote I. Endometrial cancer. *Lancet* (London, England). 2005;366:491–505. doi:10.1016/S0140-6736(05)67063-8.

[29] McMeekin D. S., Lashbrook D., Gold M., Johnson G., Walker J. L., Mannel R. Analysis of FIGO Stage IIIc endometrial cancer patients. *Gynecol Oncol. 2001*;81:273–278. doi:10.1006/gyno.2001.6157.

[30] Cragun J. M., Havrilesky L. J., Calingaert B., Synan I., Secord A. A., Soper J. T., et al. Retrospective analysis of selective lymphadenectomy in apparent early-stage endometrial cancer. *J Clin Oncol. 2005*;23:3668–3675. doi:10.1200/JCO.2005.04.144.

[31] Creasman W. T., Morrow C. P., Bundy B. N., Homesley H. D., Graham J. E., Heller P. B. Surgical pathologic spread patterns of endometrial cancer. A Gynecologic Oncology Group Study. *Cancer. 1987*;60:2035–2041.

[32] Chan J. K., Kapp D. S. Role of complete lymphadenectomy in endometrioid uterine cancer. *Lancet Oncol. 2007*;8:831–841. doi:10.1016/S1470-2045(07)70275-9.

[33] Orr J. W., Holimon J. L., Orr P. F. Stage I corpus cancer: is teletherapy necessary? *Am J Obstet Gynecol. 1997*;176:777–88; discussion 788–9.

[34] Abu-Rustum N. R., Alektiar K., Iasonos A., Lev G., Sonoda Y., Aghajanian C., et al. The incidence of symptomatic lower-extremity lymphedema following treatment of uterine corpus malignancies: a 12-year experience at Memorial Sloan-Kettering Cancer Center. *Gynecol Oncol. 2006*;103:714–718. doi:10.1016/j.ygyno.2006.03.055.

[35] Kodama J., Seki N., Ojima Y., Nakamura K., Hongo A., Hiramatsu Y. Risk factors for early and late postoperative complications of patients with endometrial cancer. *Eur J Obstet Gynecol Reprod Biol. 2006*;124:222–226. doi:10.1016/j.ejogrb.2005.06.027.

[36] Ayhan A., Celik H., Dursun P. Lymphatic mapping and sentinel node biopsy in gynecological cancers: a critical review of the literature. *World J Surg Oncol. 2008*;6:53. doi:10.1186/1477-7819-6-53.

[37] Boran N., Akdag D., Halici F., Tulunay G., Turan T., Bozok S., et al. A retrospective analysis of the diameter of metastatic lymph nodes in apparently early stage endometrial cancer. *Tumori. 2008*;94:681–685.

[38] Girardi F., Petru E., Heydarfadai M., Haas J., Winter R. Pelvic lymphadenectomy in the surgical treatment of endometrial cancer. *Gynecol Oncol. 1993*;49:177–180. doi:10.1006/gyno.1993.1103.

[39] Ryo E., Yasugi T., Mizutani K., Kita T., Takeshita S., Ayabe T. Diagnostic usefulness of intraoperative ultrasonography in avoiding unnecessary para-aortic lymphadenectomy in women with endometrial carcinoma. *Int J Gynecol Cancer. 2011*;21:859–863. doi:10.1097/IGC.0b013e31821a35ef.

[40] Horowitz N. S., Dehdashti F., Herzog T. J., Rader J. S., Powell M. A., Gibb R. K., et al. Prospective evaluation of FDG-PET for detecting pelvic and para-aortic lymph node metastasis in uterine corpus cancer. *Gynecol Oncol. 2004*;95:546–551. doi: 10.1016/j.ygyno.2004.08.009.

[41] Nayot D., Kwon J. S., Carey M. S., Driedger A. Does preoperative positron emission tomography with computed tomography predict nodal status in endometrial cancer? A pilot study. *Curr Oncol. 2008*;15:123–125.

[42] Dorfman R. E., Alpern M. B., Gross B. H., Sandler M. A. Upper abdominal lymph nodes: criteria for normal size determined with CT. *Radiology. 1991*;180:319–322. doi:10.1148/radiology.180.2.2068292.

[43] Tempany C. M., Zou K. H., Silverman S. G., Brown D. L., Kurtz A. B., McNeil B. J. Staging of advanced ovarian cancer: comparison of imaging modalities–report from the Radiological Diagnostic Oncology Group. *Radiology. 2000*;215:761–767. doi:10.1148/radiology.215.3.r00jn25761.

[44] Sawicki W., Spiewankiewicz B., Stelmachów J., Cendrowski K. The value of ultrasonography in preoperative assessment of selected prognostic factors in endometrial cancer. *Eur J Gynaecol Oncol. 2003*;24:293–298.

[45] Selman T. J., Mann C. H., Zamora J., Khan K. S. A systematic review of tests for lymph node status in primary endometrial cancer. *BMC Womens Health. 2008*;8:8. doi:10.1186/1472-6874-8-8.

[46] Antonsen S. L., Jensen L. N., Loft A., Berthelsen A. K., Costa J., Tabor A., et al. MRI, PET/CT and ultrasound in the preoperative staging of endometrial cancer - a multicenter prospective comparative study. *Gynecol Oncol. 2013*;128:300–308. doi: 10.1016/j.ygyno.2012.11.025.

[47] Haldorsen I. S., Salvesen H. B. What Is the Best Preoperative Imaging for Endometrial Cancer? *Curr Oncol Rep. 2016*;18:25. doi:10.1007/s11912-016-0506-0.

[48] Gong Y., Wang Q., Dong L., Jia Y., Hua C., Mi F., et al. Different imaging techniques for the detection of pelvic lymph nodes metastasis from gynecological malignancies: a systematic review and meta-analysis. *Oncotarget. 2017*;8:14107–14125. doi:10.18632/oncotarget.12959.

[49] Lee J., Kong T. W., Paek J., Chang S. J., Ryu H. S. Predicting Model of Lymph Node Metastasis Using Preoperative Tumor Grade, Transvaginal Ultrasound, and Serum CA-125 Level in Patients With Endometrial Cancer. *Int J Gynecol Cancer. 2016*; 26:1630–1635. doi:10.1097/IGC.0000000000000820.

[50] Bourgioti C., Chatoupis K., Moulopoulos L. A. Current imaging strategies for the evaluation of uterine cervical cancer. *World journal of radiology. 2016*;8:342–354. doi:10.4329/wjr.v8.i4.342.

[51] Plante M., Renaud M. C., Tétu B., Harel F., Roy M. Laparoscopic sentinel node mapping in early-stage cervical cancer. *Gynecol Oncol. 2003*;91:494–503.

[52] Xue X., Zhao Z., Tian X. The diagnostic value of transvaginal ultrasound in lymph node metastasis of cervical cancer patients. *Chinese Journal of Clinical Oncology and Rehabilitation. 2013*;2:034.

[53] Li Y., Zhao Z., Yang J., Liang Y. The Value of Transvaginal Color Doppler Ultrasonography in the Diagnosis of Obturator Lymph Nodes Metastases of Gynecological Pelvic Tumors. *Chinese Journal of Medical Imaging. 2011*;12:014.

[54] Li Y., Zhao Z. Value of transvaginal ultrasound in diagnosis of internal iliac lymph nodes metastasis of cavitas pelvis tumor. *Journal of Clinical Ultrasound in Medicine. 2011*;12:025.

In: The Sentinel Lymph Node
Editors: A. Londero, S. Bertozzi and C. Cedolini ISBN: 978-1-53614-557-1


*Chapter 13*

# Complications of Lymphadenectomy and Sentinel Lymph Node Biopsy in Patients with Gynecological Cancer

*Nicoletta Biglia*, Valentina E. Bounous, Elisabetta Robba and Guido Menato*
Academic Division of Obstetric and Gynacology,
Mauriziano Umberto I Hospital, University of Turin, Italy

**Abstract**

Inguino-femoral and pelvic lymphadenectomy are an essential part of surgery for gynecological malignancies, as lymph node status and the presence of distant metastatic lesions are the most relevant factors to define the prognosis and the subsequent adjuvant therapy in these conditions. Acute complications related to inguino-femoral lymphadenectomy include vascular and neurological injuries, urinary and gastrointestinal tracts damage. In most cases, these complications are caused by an inadequate visualization of the pelvic anatomy and the principal structures, which must be always achieved during both laparotomic and laparoscopic gynecological interventions. Unlike vascular injuries, nervous and urinary tract lesions may not be intraoperatively recognized, causing a variety of postoperative complications. As regards para-aortic lymphadenectomy, the most frequent intraoperative complications are injuries to poorly visualized ureters and bleeding from the inferior vena cava or its perforators. Postoperative complications include wound infections and dehiscence, hernias, lymphedema and pelvic lymphocyst formation. Lymphedema is by far the most common late complication. Systemic complications such as thromboembolic events can also occur, due to patient comorbidities, prolonged immobilization and hospital stay.

**Keywords:** gynecological cancer, surgical complications, postoperative complications, lymphadenectomy, sentinel lymph node biopsy

*Corresponding Author E-mail: nicoletta.biglia@unito.it.

# 1. Introduction

The lymph node status and the presence of distant metastatic lesions are the most relevant factors to define the prognosis and the subsequent adjuvant therapy in gynecological cancer. However, complete pelvic and para-aortic lymphadenectomy can cause severe and disabling surgical and postoperative complications, often under-recognized [1, 2, 3, 4].

Since the therapeutic benefit of lymphadenectomy is controversial [5, 6], the associated risks must be evaluated with caution. The introduction of the sentinel lymph node biopsy (SLNB) for endometrial, cervical and vulvar cancer is a promising alternative to standard lymphadenectomy, as it has the same diagnostic capability to detect metastases while minimizing morbidity [7, 8, 9, 10].

Complications related to lymphadenectomy include vascular and neurological injuries, damage to the urinary and gastrointestinal tract, wound infections and dehiscence, hernias, deep venous thrombosis, pulmonary embolism, lymphedema and pelvic lymphocyst formation [1, 2, 3, 4, 11, 12]. As regards para-aortic lymphadenectomy, the most frequent intraoperative complications are injuries to poorly visualized ureters and bleeding from the inferior vena cava or its perforators, while lymphedema is the most common late complication [12]. As to inguinal lymphadenectomy, delayed wound healing and chronic lymphedema are the most frequent complications. Thromboembolic events can occur as well, due to the long hospital stay [12]. In the next sections we will discuss the most common complications.

# 2. Vascular Injury

Severe and hemodynamically significant bleeding with subsequent blood transfusions is one of the most important complications of any surgical operation. Major bleeding causes the loss of overall anatomical view, increases the operation time and indirectly contributes to the damage of other structures. The outcome of uncontrolled bleeding is a life-threatening hypovolemic shock [12].

The lymphatics that drain the uterus and the cervix are surrounded by major vascular structures, including the external and internal iliac artery and vein. Many studies have reported the incidence of vascular injuries amounting to 0.01% of open or laparoscopic gynecological procedures [13]. The most frequent sites of vascular injuries for pelvic and lombo-aortic lymphadenectomy are the inferior epigastric vessels, the terminal aorta, the vena cava and the obturator vessels. In the literature, an association of arterial and venous lesions is reported in 10% of all cases [14, 15, 16].

Surgeons must recognize immediately the damage and carry out a provisional, rapid and efficient hemostasis. Failure in vascular repair can complicate the immediate postoperative period with acute ischemia and venous thrombosis, eventually leading to intermittent claudicatio or lower limb edema respectively in the case of arterial or venous involvement. If the diagnosis of vascular injury is delayed, the mortality can increase up to 33% [17].

In laparoscopic surgery, vascular injury is the second most common cause of mortality [18]. Vascular injuries may involve abdominal wall vessels or retroperitoneal vessels. Preventive and therapeutic ligature of the internal iliac artery or coagulation of the uterine artery at its origin may be considered (Figure 1). To minimize the potential effects of iatrogenic vascular injuries, the gynecologist should operate with the vascular surgeon on hand.

In the case of a major injury to the main vessels, immediate manual compression is the first thing to do, pending the vascular surgeon's arrival (Figure 2).

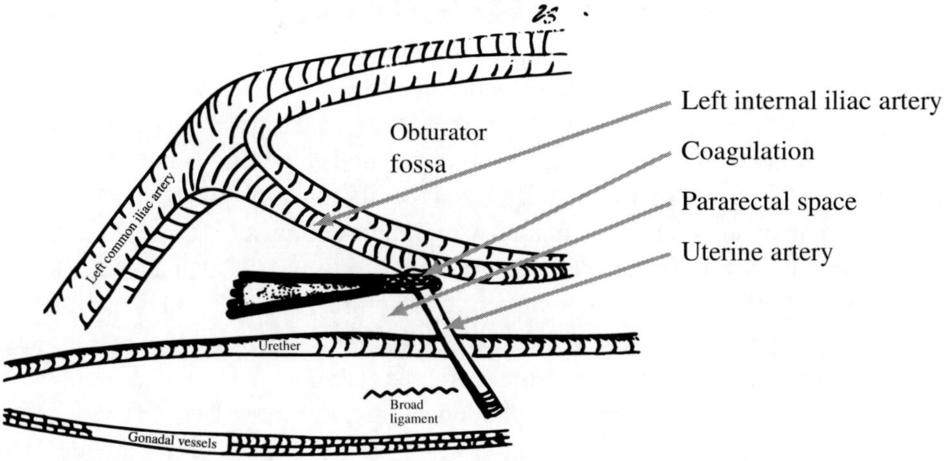


Figure 1. Preventive coagulation of the uterine artery at its origin (drawing by Valentina E. Bounous).

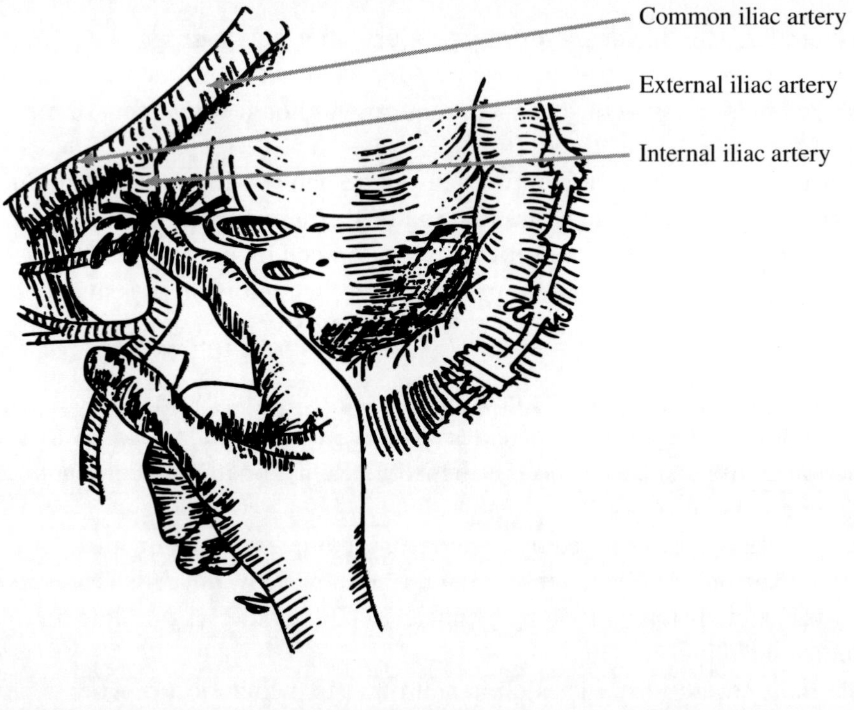


Figure 2. Immediate manual compression is the first thing to do in the case of major injury to the main vessels (drawing by Valentina E. Bounous).

Usually, arterial lesions may be repaired by arteriorrhaphy, using interrupted monofilament sutures to avoid stenosis. When arteriorrhaphy is not feasible, the use of patch angioplasty is indicated. In the case of large arterial damage or when arterial resection is requested (cases of intimal flap), the implantation of autologous or synthetic graft is necessary to achieve arterial continuity [15]. Whenever manual hemostasis is prolonged, arterial thrombectomy using a Fogarty probe is recommended [18].

Blunt tearing of the perforators, often due to excessive traction, causes most of the venous hemorrhages on the adipose tissue. When venous bleeding occurs, the management depends on the origin site of the blood. Bipolar coagulation may be considered if perforators are involved. The gynecologist can manage small hemorrhages from the inferior vena cava with a cotton ball, while in the case of massive bleeding, the damage to the vein wall may be sutured with a smooth, nonwoven, 5-0 suture [12]. Venous ligation should be always avoided to prevent significant venous insufficiency. Venorrhaphy may be suggested, although it carries the risk of subsequent thrombosis [18].

In the case of inguino-femoral lymphadenectomy, the most frequent vascular injuries occur to the long saphenous vein and the femoral artery or vein. For damage to the long saphenous vein, coagulation or ligatures proximal and distal to the injury may be considered, while the injury of the femoral vessel is repaired with a monofilament suture up to size 4-0 [12].

## 3. Nerve Injuries

In the literature, the incidence of nerve injury after pelvic surgery is reported at around 1.1-1.9%. A good prognosis is generally reported, with only a minority of the patients suffering from long-term consequences requiring prolonged treatment or reparative surgery [19, 20, 21].

The mechanism of intraoperative neurologic damage involves a combination of compression, stretch, entrapment or transection of the nerve fibres, and thermal injury. Compression and stretch injuries are ordinarily determined by the inapposite placement of self-retaining retractors such as Balfour or Bookwalter retractors, in patients in prolonged lithotomic position. Transection damage is widely related to incorrectly sited surgical incisions [22].

Three types of postoperative neuropathy can occur in gynecological surgery. Neuropraxia represents the outcome of external nerve compression leading to a disruption of conduction across a small portion of the axon. Remyelination occurs in weeks or months resulting in nerve recovery.

Axonotmesis is determined by severe nerve compression or traction. The injury is limited to the axon only, while the reserve of the support Schwann cells is preserved. Although the recovery time is longer than for neuropraxia, renovation is possible because these support cells remain intact.

The most severe form of lesion is neurotmesis, which occurs when a complete nerve transection or ligation takes place, with a severe disruption of both the axon and the Schwann cells. Regeneration is impossible and prognosis is poor without restorative surgery [23].

### 3.1. Femoral Nerve

The femoral nerve is responsible for both sensory and motor functions. This nerve represents the largest branch of the lumbar plexus, originating from the dorsal divisions of the ventral branches of the second, third and fourth lumbar nerves. Then, the nerve descends through the fibers of the psoas muscle, emerging from the lateral border of the muscle approximately 4 cm above the inguinal ligament, beneath the fascia of the iliac muscle. The femoral nerve passes into the thigh laterally to the femoral vessels, and at about 1-4 cm distally to the inguinal ligament it separates into an anterior and a posterior division.

The anterior division comprises one muscular branch for the sartorius and two sensorial branches: the intermediate and medial cutaneous nerves of the thigh. The posterior division provides the quadriceps femoris and articularis genus and then gives origin to the saphenous nerve, the sensorial nerve of the medial side of the leg and the foot. Moreover, this nerve innervates the knee and the hip joints. Because the femoral nerve receives blood from the ilio-lumbar artery of the pelvis and from the circumflex arteries, injuries can occur in both the intra-pelvic and extra-pelvic regions [24].

Gynecological surgery is the most common cause of iatrogenic femoral nerve injury, especially when an extensive pelvic surgery, such as lymphadenectomy, is carried out. Although femoral nerve injury is considered a rare complication, its incidence ranges from 0.1% to 11% in pelvic surgery [25].

Femoral neuropathy is usually caused by compression of the nerve against the pelvic side wall, as it emerges from the lateral border of the psoas muscle. This damage occurs when the pelvic blades apply excessive traction and a rotation on the plane of the ring is exerted to elevate the rectus muscle and expose the circumflex iliac vein and the deep pelvis. A study reported an incidence of 8% of femoral nerve injury when self-retaining retractors were used during gynecological surgery, compared to an incidence of less than 1% when not used [22, 26].

Injuries can occur bilaterally, but damage on the left side is more frequently reported [27]. Femoral nerve injury causes weakness in hip flexion and adduction and knee extension. There is a loss of the knee jerk reflex and anterior and medial thigh paresthesia, as well as of the medial aspect of the calf [28]. The typical presentation of femoral neuropathy is patients falling out of bed when attempting ambulation in the postoperative period. Permanent deficiency usually consists in paresthesia and numbness [20].

Diagnosis is allowed by physical and neurological examination, but electromyography must confirm the suspicion. Promptly recognized injuries enable an effective physiotherapy program, which was able to fully restore muscular function within about 2 months in 75% of patients.

Nevertheless, prevention is always better than treatment, so surgeons must be careful when performing radical gynecological surgery with the use of the Bookwalter retractor. Operators should use the shortest retractor and maximal traction must be maintained only for as long as is necessary to expose the deep pelvis. The rotation on the ring plane must be cautiously practised, avoiding the direct contact of the blades with the psoas up to the circumflex iliac vein [22].

### 3.2. Lateral Cutaneous Nerve

The lateral cutaneous nerve of the thigh is a sensorial nerve of the lumbar plexus. It arises from the dorsal divisions of the second and the third lumbar nerve, which emerge from the lateral border of the psoas muscle. This nerve obliquely crosses the iliac muscle, towards the anterior superior iliac spine. Then, it passes below the inguinal ligament, through the lacuna muscolorum and on to over the sartorius muscle in the thigh, where it divides into an anterior and a posterior branch.

The anterior branch, about 10 cm below the inguinal ligament, becomes superficial, and divides into branches that provide the skin of the anterior and lateral parts of the thigh and knee. The terminal filaments of the nerve communicate with the anterior cutaneous branches of the femoral nerve and with the intra-patellar branch of the saphenous nerve, establishing the peri-patellar plexus jointly with them. The posterior branch perforates the fascia lata, and divides into filaments that pass across the lateral and posterior surfaces of the thigh, providing skin from the greater trochanter to the middle of the thigh [24].

The mechanism of lateral cutaneous nerve neuropathy is similar to that of the femoral nerve. In particular, entrapment caused by the compression of the nerve adjacent to the anterior superior iliac spine and inguinal ligament leads to anterior and posterolateral thigh paresthesia and pain, usually referred to as meralgia paresthetica and also known as Bernhardt-Roth syndrome [28].

### 3.3. Genito-Femoral Nerve

The genito-femoral nerve arises from the primary ventral divisions of the first and the second lumbar spinal nerve roots and then crosses the anterior surface of the psoas muscle, immediately lateral to the external iliac vessels. The genital branch enters the deep inguinal ring, while the femoral branch passes deep into the inguinal ligament, within the femoral sheath. In women, the genito-femoral nerve accompanies the round ligament of the uterus, where it terminates as the nerve that supplies the skin overlying the labia majora and the mons pubis [24].

In women, the genital ramus terminates in sensory branches that supply the external genital organs; in men, the branch constitutes part of the spermatic cord and performs a motor function for the cremasteric reflex. The femoral branch serves exclusively for sensory perception in both genders.

Genito-femoral nerve injuries may occur during pelvic side wall surgery and external iliac lymph node dissection. The consequence of this neuropathy is paresthesia of the mons pubis, the labia majora and the femoral triangle [28]. In the case of inguino-femoral lymphadenectomy, paresthesia of the medial thigh may occur due to injuries to the genital branch of the genito-femoral nerve, but without motor disorders or major consequences for the quality of life [12].

### 3.4. Obturator Nerve

The obturator nerve is a mixed sensory and motor nerve that originates from the anterior divisions of the ventral branches of the second, third and fourth lumbar spinal nerves within the psoas muscle. It derives from the unification of the branches and descends through the psoas muscle to emerge from its medial border at the pelvic brim. Then, it passes over the pelvic brim into the lesser pelvis, in front of the sacroiliac joint and behind the common iliac vessels to enter the thigh through the obturator foramen. At this level, the nerve divides into an anterior and a posterior branch.

The anterior branch provides the adductor longus, the gracilis and the adductor brevis muscles. It also emits sensory fibers, that supply the skin and fascia of the medial part of the thigh. The posterior division innervates the obturator externus muscle. Then, the nerve passes between the adductor brevis and magnus muscles, and divides into a motor branch that supplies the adductor magnus, and a sensory branch direct to the knee joint that provides the articular capsule, the cruciate ligaments, and the synovial membrane of the knee joint [24].

The obturator nerve is an important landmark during pelvic lymph node dissection and its injuries are frequent in gynecological surgery. The incidence does not seem to differ between open and laparoscopic approach [29]. Obturator neuropathy causes sensory alteration in the medial thigh, including paresthesia, numbness, sensory loss and pain. Deep pain may be reported in the region of origin of the adductor at the pubic bone and may extend to the medial thigh up to the knee. In the case of severe injury, weakness or even loss of adduction and internal rotation can occur. The hip is rotated externally and abducted abnormally, resulting in a circumducting, wide base gait. Ipsilateral loss of the hip adductor tendon reflex may be possible, but it is only suggestive and not pathognomonic of the obturator neuropathy [30].

In the case of complete nerve damage, surgeons must provide an immediate repair of the obturator nerve. In the case of iatrogenic nerve transection, microsurgical epineural end-to-end tension free coaptation is currently considered the most efficient method to restore the anatomy and the function of the nerve. Nevertheless, in many cases of loss of neural substance, the collagen and elastin present in the nerve cause a retraction of the divided ends, preventing the chance of tension-free primary anastomosis [31].

Nerve grafting is a reconstructive procedure widely reported in the literature for the correction of different instances of nerve injury. Many variations in the technique are described, concerning the materials, the choice of donor site, the number of grafts used and the specific features of the injury to be treated [32, 33].

The sural nerve is the most common source of donor nerve graft. In fact, this nerve can provide large tract of grafts without significant morbidity. The calibre of the obturator nerve is usually much larger than the sural nerve, and therefore the number of grafts must be sufficient to occupy the entire area of the transacted nerve and to allow the bulk of regenerating axons reaching the distal stump of the nerve. Less frequently, other nerves may be used, such as the saphenous nerve, the superficial branch of the radial nerve, the medial cutaneous nerve of the forearm and the greater auricular nerve. All these nerves are sensory, so their removal only results in sensory alteration without motor deficiency [34].

The prognosis of obturator nerve transection depends on the nature and severity of the injury. However, patients who have undergone reparative neurological surgery followed by physiotherapy usually develop complete symptom resolution with complete motor recovery within one year of injury [35].

# 4. Urinary Tract Injuries

The female genital and urinary tract are anatomically closely related, so potential urological injury must always be considered in the case of pelvic and abdominal surgical procedures. It has been reported that 75% of urinary tract injuries are caused by gynecological surgery [36]. Urological injuries occur in up to 1% of all gynecological procedures. Actual incidence is difficult to estimate because the majority of studies report only those patients who have become symptomatic, requiring an intervention [37]. The risk of damage increases when the normal anatomy is altered or incorrectly identified due to intraoperative complications such as severe bleeding or pelvic adhesions.

## 4.1. Bladder Injuries

Although the bladder is the most frequently injured organ during gynecological surgery, bladder injury is not a frequent complication of lymphadenectomy. Reduced exposure and/or visibility due to large pelvic masses, pelvic hemorrhage, obesity, malignant disease, anatomical distortions in the case of adhesions, previous pelvic surgery and radiation therapy are the main risk factors for bladder injuries [38].

Prompt recognition allows for immediate repair, so constant attention from surgeons is crucial. During surgical procedures, signs of bladder injuries include the presence of clear fluid in the operative field, visible laceration and gas distension of the urinary drainage bag in laparoscopic techniques [38].

The most frequent site of injury is the roof of the bladder at the site of the peritoneal reflection on the anterior abdominal wall [39]. Injuries that are sufficiently distant from the ureteral ostia can be easily managed with sutures. When injuries are adjacent to or involve the ureters, there is a risk of ureter stenosis and the urologist participation is essential [40].

The closure technique depends on the thickness of the bladder wall. When only the muscularis layer is damaged, interrupted sutures with PDS, Vicryl, 3-0 or 2-0 are suggested and a second layer can be performed with the interposition of the peritoneum. When the bladder lumen is opened, mucosa and muscularis must be closed together with a 3-0 atraumatic, continuous, absorbable suture and then the peritoneum is closed as well.

## 4.2. Ureteral Injuries

More than 80% of ureteral injuries occur during pelvic surgery, however ureteral injuries are relatively infrequent during pelvic lymph node dissection, occurring in less than 1% of cases in large series [11]. One of the most common areas of ureteral injury during lymphadenectomy is adjacent to the pelvic brim, in close relation to the peritoneal fold of the gonadal vessels at the level of the infundibulo-pelvic ligament [39, 12]. The type of lymph node dissection (open or laparoscopic) does not seem to influence the incidence of this rare injury [11].

Urinary tract injuries are usually divided into two categories: acute, if identified at the time of the surgery, and chronic, if they occur subsequently. Only about 50% of ureteral injuries are recognized during surgery. By this fact alone, it is clear that the best protection against injury to the ureter is its exact visualization. To avoid urological injuries, surgeons must have an accurate knowledge of the pelvic anatomy and a meticulous surgical technique

[41]. The ureters must always be isolated and, if necessary, marked with a rubber loop. Direct visualization of the ureter, especially in complicated procedures, seems safer than palpation [42].

In the case of laparoscopic surgery, heat damage is frequent and often under-recognized, as it determines necrosis and leakage only in the postoperative period. If surgeons have any doubts on ureteral injuries during laparoscopic surgery, 5-10 ml of indigo carmine may be injected intravenously to check for dye leakage through the ureter [43].

Obstructive uropathy may follow accidental stapling of the ureter or thermal injury resulting in a stricture, leading to hydroureter and hydronephrosis. A super-imposed infection may cause pyonephrosis.

Unrecognized ureteral injury causes prolonged postoperative morbidity, leading to fistula formation, sepsis, or renal function loss. Early detection and treatment can prevent the deterioration of renal function, leading to a good prognosis, as injuries not corrected during initial hospitalization can lead to serious disruption in the patient's quality of life and to potential legal action [42, 44].

Prophylactic ureteral stenting during gynecological surgery is a controversial issue. Some studies have reported that prophylactic ureteral stenting did not prevent surgical damage to the ureter, but the ureteral stents can predispose to injury by reducing their pliability. However, in the case of gynecological surgery with severe pelvic adhesion, methylene blue injection or intraoperative cystoscopy is recommended [45].

## 5. Gastrointestinal Tract Injuries

Small and large bowel injuries can occur during adhesiolysis previous to lymphadenectomy both by direct trauma or traction to separate the tissues. The defects are closed transversely to the long axis of the bowel with atraumatic absorbable material (4-0, 3-0), to avoid intestinal stenosis [12].

## 6. Wound Infections

Wound infections can occur after lymphadenectomy, especially in patients with predisposing factors such as obesity, diabetes mellitus, tobacco smoking or concomitant use of immunosuppressive drugs. Long operating time, incomplete intraoperative asepsis and postoperative hematoma or seroma formation increase the risk of wound infection as well. The main symptoms of wound infection are hyperpyrexia associated with pain and erythema in the wound area.

Antibiotics may be sufficient for initial infections, while in the case of abscess or infected hematoma, surgical opening and cleaning of the wound is necessary. Wound dehiscence is due to suture rupture, favored by wound infection and increased intra-abdominal pressure, as in the case of vomiting or persistent cough. Other factors that interfere with wound healing are hypoproteinemia, diabetes mellitus, anemia and the concomitant use of steroid drugs.

Complete wound dehiscence with exposed bowel must be immediately repaired under antibiotic coverage. After inguino-femoral lymphadenectomy, wound infection and dehiscence are frequent complications, reported in about 20-40% of patients [19].

## 7. Hernias

Because a vertical midline incision is required for pelvic and para-aortic lymphadenectomy, hernias are a common late complication, reported in up to 1% of cases after laparotomy, and up to 10% after postoperative wound infections. In particular, acquired umbilical hernia is frequent after this type of surgery.

The incisional hernia is due to incomplete healing of the fascial layers, favored by infections, obesity, increased intra-abdominal pressure, suture breakdown or corticosteroid therapy [12].

## 8. Thromboembolic Events

Deep venous thrombosis and/or pulmonary embolism have been reported in approximately 0-8% of pelvic node dissections [46]. The risk of thromboembolic events is quite high as a result of the underlying malignant disease, surgery of the lower limbs and pelvic veins, elderly, obesity, comorbidities, long operating times in the lithotomy position and post-operative immobilization (especially after vulvectomy). Consequently, thromboembolic prophylaxis with low-molecular-weight heparin derivatives, antithrombosis compression stockings and early mobilization is essential [11].

## 9. Lymphedema and Pelvic Lymphocysts

Lymphadenectomy is frequently associated with lower limb lymphedema, which is a chronic condition due to an impaired ability to absorb the fluid excess given by the disruption of the pelvic lymphatic system, which generally develops in the first year after surgery [47, 48]. Lymphatic system insufficiency, impaired lymph transport and decreased membrane permeability cause fluids, cells and proteins to escape into the extracellular spaces, with consequent swelling [49]. Persistent edema can cause fibrosis, due to long-term proliferation of parenchymal and stromal elements and excessive extracellular matrix deposition, while protein pooling provides a medium for cellulitis and lymphangitis [47, 50]. The most used system to describe lymphedema of the limbs is the International Society of Lymphology 4-stage classification [51] (Table 1).

Lymphedema can be asymptomatic or associated with pain, erythema or heaviness, often requiring lifelong treatment and psychosocial support [52]. Lymphedema limits physical activity [53, 54] and normal daily activities such as walking, standing or housework. Financial difficulties are also reported [54, 55], due to costs of rehabilitation [56], changes of clothing to hide the appearance of swollen legs or compression garments [57], or the inability to continue working [55, 57].

The most accurate diagnostic method for lymphedema is physical examination performed by an experienced lymphedema specialist [58]. Objective evaluation of lymphedema is performed by a comparative circumferential measurement, in which one limb is compared with the opposite at four specific points. A circumferential difference of 2-2.5

**Table 1. International Society of Lymphology 4-stage classification of lymphedema [51]**

| Stage | Characteristics |
|---|---|
| 0 | Latent or sub-clinical condition where swelling is not yet evident despite impaired lymph transport, subtle changes in tissue fluid/composition, and changes in subjective symptoms |
| I | Early accumulation of fluid relatively high in protein content which subsides with limb elevation |
| II | Limb elevation alone rarely reduces tissue swelling and pitting is evident |
| III | Lymphostatic elephantiasis where pitting can be absent and skin changes such as acanthosis, further deposition of fat and fibrosis, and warty overgrowths have developed |

cm between the two legs seems consensual for making a diagnosis of lymphedema [59]. In the case of lymphedema located in the feet, a specific diagnostic test consists in pinching the skin between the toes; lymphedema is diagnosed if the pinched skin does not fold up (Stemmer's sign) [50].

The latest technologies including 3D magnetic resonance imaging (MRI) [60], lymphoscintigraphy, computed tomography (CT), ultrasound [61] and bioelectrical impedance analysis, are reserved for patients with bilateral lymphedema without final diagnosis or in cases where lymphatic obstruction is suspected for malignancy. Ultrasound is useful for excluding other etiologies such as deep venous thrombosis or venous insufficiency and can also help identify tissue changes and masses that could be the cause of lymphatic compression. CT and MRI can investigate soft tissue edema with high sensitivity and specificity, but they are expensive [50].

With regard to subjective evaluation, general scales focus poorly on lymphedema. A specific scale for the evaluation of lymphedema in gynecological cancer patients is the Gynecologic Cancer Lymphedema Questionnaire [62], which is a 20-item self-reporting questionnaire that analyzes the physical functioning, numbness, swelling, infections, heaviness and pain during the previous month.

Lymphadenectomy is associated with a variable rate of lymphedema depending on many concomitant risk factors regarding the anatomy of regional lymphatics, the presence of alternative lymphatic drainage pathways, surgical aggressiveness, the number of nodes removed, the removal of specific nodes, the use of adjuvant radiotherapy, and the individual characteristics of the patient (BMI, comorbidities and age) [49].

Since there is no consensus on a uniform evaluation of lymphedema, the reported incidence is broadly different, ranging from 0% to 70% through the literature [63, 64]. This enormous difference may depend on the cancer histotype (endometrial, cervical, ovarian or vulvar) and on the stage, type of treatment, surgical radicality, differences in measurement techniques and assessment. In particular, the highest lymphedema rates are reported after inguino-femoral lymphadenectomy for vulvar cancer.

Lymphadenectomy is associated also with other sequelae involving the lymphatic system, such as lymphocele, lymphocysts, and seromas formation, reported in around 20-30% of patients and mostly an incidental finding during postoperative imaging [65]. In order to reduce the incidence and severity of lymphedema, risk-reducing strategies must be considered. SLNB is the most effective strategy to reduce the risk of lymphedema, but it is not yet the standard procedure in gynecologic oncology.

## 9.1. Endometrial Cancer

The incidence of lymphedema after treatment for endometrial cancer varies between 1.2% and 47%, depending on the method of assessment [66, 67]. For endometrial cancer, the proven risk factors for the lymphedema development are obesity (BMI ¿35 kg/$m^2$) [67, 68, 69], the number of lymph nodes removed, the lymphadenectomy extent and the removal of the circumflex iliac lymph nodes [70].

Furthermore, postoperative radiotherapy is a debated risk factor for lymphedema development, since radiotherapy-induced fibrosis may concur in the alteration of the lymphatic flow, especially in patients with a lymphatic vessel alteration due to the presence of metastatic disease [71, 72].

For endometrial cancer, SLNB can be a feasible option that has the advantage of a limited disruption of the lymphatic channels.

## 9.2. Cervical Cancer

The incidence of lymphedema in patients treated for cervical cancer ranges from 0% to 55.9% [63, 72]. In women with early-stage cervical cancer (tumor size ¡2 cm) who wish to preserve fertility after undergoing radical trachelectomy with lymphadenectomy, an incidence of 11-24.1% [73, 74] has been reported.

The postoperative radiotherapy [75, 48, 51, 72, 76, 77, 78], the number of lymph nodes removed [72, 79] and supra-femoral node dissection [77] are the most cited factors related to the development of lymphedema.

SLNB is a promising option for early-stage cervical cancer, but it is not yet accepted as a standard of treatment. Many studies have established its feasibility, with high detection rates and low false-negative rates, in particular when the sentinel node is detected bilaterally. In contrast, large tumors (¿2 cm) and lymphovascular space invasion are associated with a higher false-negative rate [7, 80].

## 9.3. Ovarian Cancer

The reported incidence of lymphedema among ovarian cancer patients ranges from 4.7% to 40.8% [75, 81]. The most frequently reported risk factors for lymphedema are a high number of lymph nodes removed [72], cellulitis [70] and the removal of circumflex iliac lymph nodes [70, 82].

Lymphocele is a frequent condition after lymphadenectomy for ovarian cancer. In fact, ovarian cancer represents an independent risk factor for lymphocele formation (OR=3.137), as well as for symptomatic lymphocele (OR=2.310) [65].

### 9.4. Vulvar Cancer

Permanent lower body lymphedema is reported in about 30-70% of cases after inguino-femoral lymphadenectomy for vulvar cancer [64]. After inguino-femoral lymphadenectomy for vulvar cancer, lymphocele is observed in up to 40% of cases. Draining the wound may reduce lymphocele formation.

According to some authors, the preservation of the saphenous vein during inguinal lymphadenectomy is associated with a lower risk of lymphedema [83], but this approach is not widely accepted. Protecting the lower extremity from infection or trauma is very important for the prevention of lymphedema [84]. However, SLNB appears to be the most effective strategy to reduce lymphedema in selected women with squamous early-stage (¡4 cm) unifocal vulvar cancer not suspect for nodal involvement at imaging [7].

Educating healthcare professionals and women is key to identifying early signals and helping patients access appropriate care. In fact, patients should be referred to a specialist as soon as possible in order to begin a treatment and avoid further complications. Collaborating with a lymphedema therapist and working in a multidisciplinary team is necessary for managing patients with lymphedema.

There is no consensus on the best treatment for lymphedema. As it is a chronic disease, lymphedema management is permanent and generally conservative, reserving operative methods for failed medical therapies [85]. For conservative treatment, combined physical therapy consists in a two-step program carried out by a team of professionals including specially trained lymphologists, nurses and physiotherapists. The first step includes skin care to keep the skin intact, a light manual massage to avoid damage to the lymphatic vessels, an exercise that, by increasing muscle mass, stimulates the lymph flow, and protein absorption and compression with a multi-layered bandage. The second step consists in compression with elastic garments and manual lymph drainage [50].

Pharmacological therapy with diuretics and benzopyrones may also be considered. However, diuretics must be used with caution in patients with malignancy, as they can cause electrolyte imbalance. Other conservative alternatives with uncertain benefits include intermittent pneumatic compression, thermal therapy, limb elevation, mesotherapy and immunological therapy [51, 86].

When conservative therapy is unsuccessful, surgical treatment is taken into account. Surgery for lymphedema includes both the physiologic and ablative approaches. Physiologic techniques consist in microsurgery techniques (lymphatic collector implantation, vein and lymph segments transplantation and lymphatic-venous or lymph nodal-venous shunts), which aim to improve the rate of the lymph flow into the venous circulation. This approach can only be considered for early-stage lymphedema without severe tissue damage and has a low complication rate, but the success rate varies widely among studies [51, 87]. Ablative procedures (liposuction and direct excision) should be reserved for patients with advanced lymphedema, fat deposition and tissue fibrosis [51, 88].

## Acknowledgments

The authors would like to thank Prof. Piero Sismondi for revising the manuscript.

## References

[1] Agar N., Philippe A. C., Bourdel N., Rabischong B., Canis M., Le Bouedec G., et al. [Morbidity of pelvic lymphadenectomy and para-aortic lymphadenectomy in endometrial cancer]. *Bull Cancer (Paris). 2015*;102:428–435. doi:10.1016/j.bulcan.2015.04.001.

[2] Frost J. A., Webster K. E., Bryant A., Morrison J. Lymphadenectomy for the management of endometrial cancer. *Cochrane Database Syst Rev. 2015*;CD007585. doi: 10.1002/14651858.CD007585.pub3.

[3] Todo Y., Kato H., Kaneuchi M., Watari H., Takeda M., Sakuragi N. Survival effect of para-aortic lymphadenectomy in endometrial cancer (SEPAL study): a retrospective cohort analysis. *Lancet. 2010*;375:1165–1172. doi:10.1016/S0140-6736(09)62002-X.

[4] Benedetti Panici P., Basile S., Maneschi F., Alberto Lissoni A., Signorelli M., Scambia G, et al. Systematic pelvic lymphadenectomy vs. no lymphadenectomy in early-stage endometrial carcinoma: randomized clinical trial. *J Natl Cancer Inst. 2008*;100:1707–1716. doi:10.1093/jnci/djn397.

[5] ASTEC study group, Kitchener H., Swart A. M. C., Qian Q., Amos C., Parmar M. K. B. Efficacy of systematic pelvic lymphadenectomy in endometrial cancer (MRC ASTEC trial): a randomised study. *Lancet. 2009*;373:125–136. doi: 10.1016/S0140-6736(08)61766-3.

[6] Maggioni A., Benedetti Panici P., Dell'Anna T., Landoni F., Lissoni A., Pellegrino A., et al. Randomised study of systematic lymphadenectomy in patients with epithelial ovarian cancer macroscopically confined to the pelvis. *Br J Cancer. 2006*;95:699–704. doi:10.1038/sj.bjc.6603323.

[7] Cibula D., Oonk M. H. M., Abu-Rustum N. R. Sentinel lymph node biopsy in the management of gynecologic cancer. *Curr Opin Obstet Gynecol. 2015*;27:66–72. doi: 10.1097/GCO.0000000000000133.

[8] Sullivan S. A., Rossi E. C., Sentinel Lymph Node Biopsy in Endometrial Cancer: a New Standard of Care? *Curr Treat Options Oncol. 2017*;18:62. doi: 10.1007/s11864-017-0503-z.

[9] Rossi E. C., Kowalski L. D., Scalici J., Cantrell L., Schuler K., Hanna R. K., et al. A comparison of sentinel lymph node biopsy to lymphadenectomy for endometrial cancer staging (FIRES trial): a multicentre, prospective, cohort study. *Lancet Oncol. 2017*;18:384–392. doi:10.1016/S1470-2045(17)30068-2.

[10] Bodurtha Smith A. J., Fader A. N., Tanner E. J. Sentinel lymph node assessment in endometrial cancer: a systematic review and meta-analysis. *Am J Obstet Gynecol. 2017*;216:459–476.e10. doi:10.1016/j.ajog.2016.11.1033.

[11] Loeb S., Partin A. W., Schaeffer E. M. Complications of pelvic lymphadenectomy: do the risks outweigh the benefits? *Rev Urol. 2010*;12:20–24.

[12] Wallwiener D., Becker S., Beckmann M. W., Brucker S. Y., Friese K., Isaacson K. B., et al. Atlas of Gynecologic Surgery (Fourth Edition). *Thieme. 2014.*

[13] Chapron C., Querleu D., Mage G., Madelenat P., Dubuisson J. B., Audebert A., et al. [Complications of gynecologic laparoscopy. Multicentric study of 7,604 laparoscopies]. *J Gynecol Obstet Biol Reprod (Paris). 1992*;21:207–213.

[14] Chapron C. M., Pierre F., Lacroix S., Querleu D., Lansac J., Dubuisson J. B. Major vascular injuries during gynecologic laparoscopy. *J Am Coll Surg. 1997*;185:461–465.

[15] Baadsgaard S. E., Bille S., Egeblad K. Major vascular injury during gynecologic laparoscopy. Report of a case and review of published cases. *Acta Obstet Gynecol Scand. 1989*;68:283–285.

[16] Geers J., Holden C. Major vascular injury as a complication of laparoscopic surgery: a report of three cases and review of the literature. *Am Surg. 1996*;62:377–379.

[17] Nordestgaard A. G., Bodily K. C., Osborne R. W., Buttorff J. D. Major vascular injuries during laparoscopic procedures. *Am J Surg. 1995*;169:543–545.

[18] Barbosa Barros M., Lozano F. S., Queral L. Vascular injuries during gynecological laparoscopy–the vascular surgeon's advice. *Sao Paulo Med J. 2005*;123:38–41. doi: /S1516-31802005000100009.

[19] Hoffman M. S., Roberts W. S., Cavanagh D. Neuropathies associated with radical pelvic surgery for gynecologic cancer. *Gynecol Oncol. 1988*;31:462–466.

[20] Cardosi R. J., Cox C. S., Hoffman M. S. Postoperative neuropathies after major pelvic surgery. *Obstet Gynecol. 2002*;100:240–244.

[21] Bohrer J. C., Walters M. D., Park A., Polston D., Barber M. D. Pelvic nerve injury following gynecologic surgery: a prospective cohort study. *Am J Obstet Gynecol. 2009*;201:531.e1–531.e7. doi:10.1016/j.ajog.2009.07.023.

[22] Maneschi F., Nale R., Tozzi R., Biccirè D., Perrone S., Sarno M. Femoral nerve injury complicating surgery for gynecologic cancer. *Int J Gynecol Cancer. 2014*;24:1112–1117. doi:10.1097/IGC.0000000000000141.

[23] Bradshaw A. D., Advincula A. P. Postoperative neuropathy in gynecologic surgery. *Obstet Gynecol Clin North Am. 2010*;37:451–459. doi:10.1016/j.ogc.2010.05.008.

[24] Standring S. *Gray's Anatomy: The Anatomical Basis of Clinical Practice*, 41e. Elsevier. 2015.

[25] Chan J. K., Manetta A. Prevention of femoral nerve injuries in gynecologic surgery. *Am J Obstet Gynecol. 2002*;186:1–7.

[26] Irvin W., Andersen W., Taylor P., Rice L. Minimizing the risk of neurologic injury in gynecologic surgery. *Obstet Gynecol. 2004*;103:374–382. doi:10.1097/01.AOG.0000110542.53489.c6.

[27] Huang W. S., Lin P. Y., Yeh C. H., Chin C. C., Hsieh C. C., Wang J. Y. Iatrogenic femoral neuropathy following pelvic surgery: a rare and often overlooked complication–four case reports and literature review. *Chang Gung Med J. 2007*; 30:374–379.

[28] Kuponiyi O., Alleemudder D. I., Latunde-Dada A., Eedarapalli P. Nerve injuries associated with gynaecological surgery. *The Obstetrician & Gynaecologist. 2014*; 16:29–36. doi:10.1111/tog.12064.

[29] Dias A. R., Silva E Silva A., Carvalho J. P., Baracat E. C., Favero G. Correction of iatrogenic injury of the obturator nerve during pelvic laparoscopic lymphadenectomy by the use of sural nerve grafts. *Gynecologic oncology reports. 2014*;10:16–18. doi: 10.1016/j.gore.2014.08.001.

[30] Hallgren A., Björkman A., Chemnitz A., Dahlin L. B. Subjective outcome related to donor site morbidity after sural nerve graft harvesting: a survey in 41 patients. *BMC Surg. 2013*;13:39. doi:10.1186/1471-2482-13-39.

[31] Tipton J. S. Obturator neuropathy. *Curr Rev Musculoskelet Med. 2008*;1:234–237. doi:10.1007/s12178-008-9030-7.

[32] Vasilev S. A. Obturator nerve injury: a review of management options. *Gynecol Oncol. 1994*;53:152–155. doi:10.1006/gyno.1994.1108.

[33] Ricciardi E., Jakimovska M., Maniglio P., Schimberni M., Frega A., Kobal B., et al. Laparoscopic injury of the obturator nerve during fertility-sparing procedure for cervical cancer. *World J Surg Oncol. 2012*;10:177. doi:10.1186/1477-7819-10-177.

[34] Spiliopoulos K., Williams Z. Femoral branch to obturator nerve transfer for restoration of thigh adduction following iatrogenic injury. *J Neurosurg. 2011*;114:1529–1533. doi:10.3171/2011.1.JNS101239.

[35] Martins R. S., Bastos D., Siqueira M. G., Heise C. O., Teixeira M. J. Traumatic injuries of peripheral nerves:a review with emphasis on surgical indication. *Arq Neuropsiquiatr. 2013*;71:811–814. doi:10.1590/0004-282X20130127.

[36] Thompson J. *TeLinde's operative gynecology (8th ed.)*, chapter "Operative injuries to the ureter: prevention, recognition, and management.", 1135–74. Philadelphia: Lippincott Williams & Wilkins. 1997.

[37] Gilmour D. T., Dwyer P. L., Carey M. P. Lower urinary tract injury during gynecologic surgery and its detection by intraoperative cystoscopy. *Obstet Gynecol. 1999*;94:883–889.

[38] Gomez R. G., Ceballos L., Coburn M., Corriere J. N., Dixon C. M., Lobel B., et al. Consensus statement on bladder injuries. *BJU Int. 2004*;94:27–32. doi:10.1111/j.1464-410X.2004.04896.x.

[39] Liapis A., Bakas P., Giannopoulos V., Creatsas G. Ureteral injuries during gynecological surgery. *Int Urogynecol J Pelvic Floor Dysfunct. 2001*;12:391–3; discussion 394.

[40] Ibeanu O. A., Chesson R. R., Echols K. T., Nieves M., Busangu F., Nolan T. E. Urinary tract injury during hysterectomy based on universal cystoscopy. *Obstet Gynecol. 2009*; 113:6–10. doi:10.1097/AOG.0b013e31818f6219.

[41] Neuman M., Eidelman A., Langer R., Golan A., Bukovsky I., Caspi E. Iatrogenic injuries to the ureter during gynecologic and obstetric operations. *Surg Gynecol Obstet. 1991*;173:268–272.

[42] Aronson M. P., Bose T. M. Urinary tract injury in pelvic surgery. *Clin Obstet Gynecol. 2002*;45:428–438.

[43] Li T. C., Saravelos H., Richmond M., Cooke I. D. Complications of laparoscopic pelvic surgery: recognition, management and prevention. *Hum Reprod Update. 1997*; 3:505–515.

[44] Lee J. S., Choe J. H., Lee H. S., Seo J. T. Urologic complications following obstetric and gynecologic surgery. *Korean journal of urology. 2012*;53:795–799. doi:10.4111/kju.2012.53.11.795.

[45] Ozdemir E., Ozturk U., Celen S., Sucak A., Gunel M., Guney G., et al. Urinary complications of gynecologic surgery: iatrogenic urinary tract system injuries in obstetrics and gynecology operations. *Clin Exp Obstet Gynecol. 2011*;38:217–220.

[46] Raboy A., Adler H., Albert P. Extraperitoneal endoscopic pelvic lymph node dissection: a review of 125 patients. *J Urol. 1997*;158:2202–4; discussion 2204–5.

[47] Hareyama H., Hada K., Goto K., Watanabe S., Hakoyama M., Oku K., et al. Prevalence, classification, and risk factors for postoperative lower extremity lymphedema in women with gynecologic malignancies: a retrospective study. *Int J Gynecol Cancer. 2015*;25:751–757. doi:10.1097/IGC.0000000000000405.

[48] Ryan M., Stainton M. C., Slaytor E. K., Jaconelli C., Watts S., Mackenzie P. Aetiology and prevalence of lower limb lymphoedema following treatment for gynaecological cancer. *Aust N Z J Obstet Gynaecol. 2003*;43:148–151.

[49] Biglia N., Zanfagnin V., Daniele A., Robba E., Bounous V. E. Lower Body Lymphedema in Patients with Gynecologic Cancer. *Anticancer Res. 2017*;37:4005–4015. doi:10.21873/anticanres.11785.

[50] Lockwood-Rayermann S. Lymphedema in gynecologic cancer survivors: an area for exploration? *Cancer Nurs. 2007*;30:E11–E18. doi:10.1097/01.NCC.0000281734.48479.33.

[51] International Society of Lymphology. The diagnosis and treatment of peripheral lymphedema: 2013 Consensus Document of the International Society of Lymphology. *Lymphology. 2013*;46:1–11.

[52] Achouri A., Huchon C., Bats A. S., Bensaid C., Nos C., Lécuru F. Complications of lymphadenectomy for gynecologic cancer. *Eur J Surg Oncol. 2013*;39:81–86. doi: 10.1016/j.ejso.2012.10.011.

[53] Dunberger G., Lindquist H., Waldenström A. C., Nyberg T., Steineck G., Avall Lundqvist E. Lower limb lymphedema in gynecological cancer survivors–effect on daily life functioning. *Support Care Cancer. 2013*;21:3063–3070. doi:10.1007/s00520-013-1879-3.

[54] de Melo Ferreira A. P., de Figueiredo E. M., Lima R. A., Cândido E. B., de Castro Monteiro M. V., de Figueiredo Franco T. M. R., et al. Quality of life in women with vulvar cancer submitted to surgical treatment: a comparative study. *Eur J Obstet Gynecol Reprod Biol. 2012*;165:91–95. doi:10.1016/j.ejogrb.2012.06.027.

[55] Kim S. I., Lim M. C., Lee J. S., Lee Y., Park K., Joo J., et al. Impact of lower limb lymphedema on quality of life in gynecologic cancer survivors after pelvic lymph node dissection. *Eur J Obstet Gynecol Reprod Biol. 2015*;192:31–36. doi:10.1016/j.ejogrb.2015.06.011.

[56] Finnane A., Hayes S. C., Obermair A., Janda M. Quality of life of women with lower-limb lymphedema following gynecological cancer. *Expert Rev Pharmacoecon Outcomes Res. 2011*;11:287–297. doi:10.1586/erp.11.30.

[57] Ryan M., Stainton M. C., Jaconelli C., Watts S., MacKenzie P., Mansberg T. The experience of lower limb lymphedema for women after treatment for gynecologic cancer. *Oncol Nurs Forum. 2003*;30:417–423. doi:10.1188/03.ONF.417-423.

[58] Kim J. H., Choi J. H., Ki E. Y., Lee S. J., Yoon J. H., Lee K. H., et al. Incidence and risk factors of lower-extremity lymphedema after radical surgery with or without adjuvant radiotherapy in patients with FIGO stage I to stage IIA cervical cancer. *Int J Gynecol Cancer. 2012*;22:686–691. doi:10.1097/IGC.0b013e3182466950.

[59] Brown J. A clinically useful method for evaluating lymphedema. *Clin J Oncol Nurs. 2004*;8:35–38. doi:10.1188/04.CJON.35-38.

[60] Liu N., Wang C., Sun M. Noncontrast three-dimensional magnetic resonance imaging vs lymphoscintigraphy in the evaluation of lymph circulation disorders: A comparative study. *J Vasc Surg. 2005*;41:69–75. doi:10.1016/j.jvs.2004.11.013.

[61] Suehiro K., Morikage N., Murakami M., Yamashita O., Samura M., Hamano K. Significance of ultrasound examination of skin and subcutaneous tissue in secondary lower extremity lymphedema. *Annals of vascular diseases. 2013*;6:180–188. doi: 10.3400/avd.oa.12.00102.

[62] Carter J., Raviv L., Appollo K., Baser R. E., Iasonos A., Barakat R. R. A pilot study using the Gynecologic Cancer Lymphedema Questionnaire (GCLQ) as a clinical care tool to identify lower extremity lymphedema in gynecologic cancer survivors. *Gynecol Oncol. 2010*;117:317–323. doi:10.1016/j.ygyno.2010.01.022.

[63] Abu-Rustum N. R., Gemignani M. L., Moore K., Sonoda Y., Venkatraman E., Brown C., et al. Total laparoscopic radical hysterectomy with pelvic lymphadenectomy using the argon-beam coagulator: pilot data and comparison to laparotomy. *Gynecol Oncol. 2003*;91:402–409.

[64] Van der Zee A. G. J., Oonk M. H., De Hullu J. A., Ansink A. C., Vergote I., Verheijen R. H., et al. Sentinel node dissection is safe in the treatment of early-stage vulvar cancer. *J Clin Oncol. 2008*;26:884–889. doi:10.1200/JCO.2007.14.0566.

[65] Zikan M., Fischerova D., Pinkavova I., Slama J., Weinberger V., Dusek L., et al. A prospective study examining the incidence of asymptomatic and symptomatic lymphoceles following lymphadenectomy in patients with gynecological cancer. *Gynecol Oncol. 2015*;137:291–298. doi:10.1016/j.ygyno.2015.02.016.

[66] Abu-Rustum N. R., Alektiar K., Iasonos A., Lev G., Sonoda Y., Aghajanian C., et al. The incidence of symptomatic lower-extremity lymphedema following treatment of uterine corpus malignancies: a 12-year experience at Memorial Sloan-Kettering Cancer Center. *Gynecol Oncol. 2006*;103:714–718. doi:10.1016/j.ygyno.2006.03.055.

[67] Yost K. J., Cheville A. L., Al-Hilli M. M., Mariani A., Barrette B. A., McGree M. E., et al. Lymphedema after surgery for endometrial cancer: prevalence, risk factors, and quality of life. *Obstet Gynecol. 2014*;124:307–315. doi:10.1097/AOG.0000000000000372.

[68] Mendivil A. A., Rettenmaier M. A., Abaid L. N., Brown J. V., Micha J. P., Lopez K. L., et al. Lower-extremity lymphedema following management for endometrial and cervical cancer. *Surg Oncol. 2016*;25:200–204. doi:10.1016/j.suronc.2016.05.015.

[69] Nicholas Z., Hu N., Ying J., Soisson P., Dodson M., Gaffney D. K. Impact of comorbid conditions on survival in endometrial cancer. *Am J Clin Oncol. 2014*;37:131–134. doi: 10.1097/COC.0b013e318277d5f4.

[70] Hareyama H., Ito K., Hada K., Uchida A., Hayakashi Y., Hirayama E., et al. Reduction/prevention of lower extremity lymphedema after pelvic and para-aortic lymphadenectomy for patients with gynecologic malignancies. *Ann Surg Oncol. 2012*; 19:268–273. doi:10.1245/s10434-011-1863-4.

[71] Tada H., Teramukai S., Fukushima M., Sasaki H. Risk factors for lower limb lymphedema after lymph node dissection in patients with ovarian and uterine carcinoma. *BMC Cancer. 2009*;9:47. doi:10.1186/1471-2407-9-47.

[72] Biglia N., Librino A., Ottino M. C., Panuccio E., Daniele A., Chahin A. Lower limb lymphedema and neurological complications after lymphadenectomy for gynecological cancer. *Int J Gynecol Cancer. 2015*;25:521–525. doi:10.1097/IGC.0000000000000341.

[73] Froding L. P., Ottosen C., Mosgaard B. J., Jensen P. T. Quality of life, urogynecological morbidity, and lymphedema after radical vaginal trachelectomy for early-stage cervical cancer. *Int J Gynecol Cancer. 2015*;25:699–706. doi:10.1097/IGC.0000000000000395.

[74] Lanowska M., Mangler M., Spek A., Grittner U., Hasenbein K., Chiantera V., et al. Radical vaginal trachelectomy (RVT) combined with laparoscopic lymphadenectomy: prospective study of 225 patients with early-stage cervical cancer. *Int J Gynecol Cancer. 2011*;21:1458–1464. doi:10.1097/IGC.0b013e3182216aa7.

[75] Beesley V., Janda M., Eakin E., Obermair A., Battistutta D. Lymphedema after gynecological cancer treatment: prevalence, correlates, and supportive care needs. *Cancer. 2007*;109:2607–2614. doi:10.1002/cncr.22684.

[76] Nakamura K., Kitahara Y., Satoh T., Takei Y., Takano M., Nagao S., et al. Analysis of the effect of adjuvant radiotherapy on outcomes and complications after radical hysterectomy in FIGO stage IB1 cervical cancer patients with intermediate risk factors (GOTIC Study). *World J Surg Oncol. 2016*;14:173. doi:10.1186/s12957-016-0931-4.

[77] Ohba Y., Todo Y., Kobayashi N., Kaneuchi M., Watari H., Takeda M., et al. Risk factors for lower-limb lymphedema after surgery for cervical cancer. *Int J Clin Oncol. 2011*;16:238–243. doi:10.1007/s10147-010-0171-5.

[78] Hosaka M., Watari H., Takeda M., Moriwaki M., Hara Y., Todo Y., et al. Treatment of cervical cancer with adjuvant chemotherapy versus adjuvant radiotherapy after radical hysterectomy and systematic lymphadenectomy. *J Obstet Gynaecol Res. 2008*; 34:552–556. doi:10.1111/j.1447-0756.2008.00739.x.

[79] Füller J., Guderian D., Köhler C., Schneider A., Wendt T. G. Lymph edema of the lower extremities after lymphadenectomy and radiotherapy for cervical cancer. *Strahlenther Onkol. 2008*;184:206–211. doi:10.1007/s00066-008-1728-3.

[80] Lécuru F., Mathevet P., Querleu D., Leblanc E., Morice P., Daraï E., et al. Bilateral negative sentinel nodes accurately predict absence of lymph node metastasis in early cervical cancer: results of the SENTICOL study. *J Clin Oncol. 2011*;29:1686–1691. doi:10.1200/JCO.2010.32.0432.

[81] Lim M. C., Lee J. S., Nam B. H., Seo S. S., Kang S., Park S. Y. Lower extremity edema in patients with early ovarian cancer. *Journal of ovarian research. 2014*;7:28. doi:10.1186/1757-2215-7-28. Original DateCompleted: 20140317.

[82] Abu-Rustum N. R., Barakat R. R. Observations on the role of circumflex iliac node resection and the etiology of lower extremity lymphedema following pelvic lymphadenectomy for gynecologic malignancy. *Gynecol Oncol. 2007*;106:4–5. doi: 10.1016/j.ygyno.2007.03.026.

[83] Zhang S. H., Sood A. K., Sorosky J. I., Anderson B., Buller R. E. Preservation of the saphenous vein during inguinal lymphadenectomy decreases morbidity in patients with carcinoma of the vulva. *Cancer. 2000*;89:1520–1525.

[84] Gaarenstroom K. N., Kenter G. G., Trimbos J. B., Agous I., Amant F., Peters A. A. W., et al. Postoperative complications after vulvectomy and inguinofemoral lymphadenectomy using separate groin incisions. *Int J Gynecol Cancer. 2003*;13:522–527.

[85] Douglass J., Graves P., Gordon S. Self-Care for Management of Secondary Lymphedema: A Systematic Review. *PLoS Negl Trop Dis. 2016*;10:e0004740. doi: 10.1371/journal.pntd.0004740.

[86] Korpan M. I., Crevenna R., Fialka-Moser V. Lymphedema: a therapeutic approach in the treatment and rehabilitation of cancer patients. *Am J Phys Med Rehabil. 2011*; 90:S69–S75. doi:10.1097/PHM.0b013e31820be160.

[87] Basta M. N., Gao L. L., Wu L. C. Operative treatment of peripheral lymphedema: a systematic meta-analysis of the efficacy and safety of lymphovenous microsurgery and tissue transplantation. *Plast Reconstr Surg. 2014*;133:905–913. doi:10.1097/PRS.0000000000000010.

[88] Brorson H., Ohlin K., Olsson G., Svensson B., Svensson H. Controlled compression and liposuction treatment for lower extremity lymphedema. *Lymphology. 2008*;41:52–63.

In: The Sentinel Lymph Node
Editors: A. Londero, S. Bertozzi and C. Cedolini
ISBN: 978-1-53614-557-1


*Chapter 14*

# SENTINEL LYMPH NODE BIOPSY IN ANAL CARCINOMA

*Giovanni Terrosu*[1]*, *Carla Cedolini*[2], *Edoardo Scarpa*[1], *Ambrogio P. Londero*[3] and *Serena Bertozzi*[2]

[1]Clinic of Surgery, University Hospital of Udine, Italy
[2]Breast Unit, University Hospital of Udine, Italy
[3]Clinic of Obstetrics and Gynecology, University Hospital of Udine, Udine, Italy

**Abstract**

Anal carcinoma is a rare disease usually treated with combined radio- and chemotherapy. Given the low incidence of metachronous lymph node metastases and the significant side effects of complete inguinal node dissection or irradiation, it is of crucial importance to identify the lymph node metastases. However, both clinical examination and imaging studies are not accurate enough to detect inguinal lymph node metastases. According to the current literature, in order to detect occult inguinal metastatic disease and to spare node-negative patients from unnecessary surgical or radiation treatment, sentinel lymph node biopsy is a safe and effective procedure, with low morbidity rates, minor self-limiting complications and could be considered the procedure of choice for the assessment of the status of inguinal lymph node. The combination of radiotracer and blue dye techniques can maximize the inguinal detection rate. Nevertheless, no consensus has yet been reached on the treatment of inguinal basins, particularly in node-negative patients, due to the small sample size and suboptimal quality of the studies included, and current data does not yet support the routine use of this technique. Large scale multicenter studies with long-term consistent follow-up are needed to better estimate the outcome of node-negative patients who have undergone sentinel lymph node biopsy and inguinal node-sparing irradiation and to validate this technique conclusively.

**Keywords:** anal cancer, sentinel lymph node biopsy, inguinal metastatic disease, inguinal lymph node

*Corresponding Author E-mail: giovanni.terrosu@uniud.it.

# 1. Introduction

Anal carcinoma represents approximately 2.6% of all digestive tract cancers [1], with an incidence rate of 1.8 per 100,000 new cases per year in the United States [2]. Although still considered an uncommon type of cancer, its prevalence in the United States has increased from 1.5 to 1.9-fold since 1973, and constitutes a substantial burden in specific risk subgroups [3, 4, 5, 6].

Taking into account factors predisposing to anal carcinoma, tobacco smoking represents an important and widespread risk factor, as is the case for several other cancers. Also, some viral infections are strongly correlated with the occurrence of anal cancer, such as Human Papilloma Virus (HPV) infection and Human Immunodeficiency Virus (HIV) seropositivity. As a consequence, also cervical dysplasia or cancer, and low CD4 count represent a predisposing factor for anal cancer, as well as any type of immunosuppressing condition, such as immunodeficiency following solid organ transplantation [7, 2, 8, 9].

The most common histotype of anal cancer is the squamous cell carcinoma [10]. Over the natural course of this disease, approximately 12% of patients develop distant metastases, most commonly in the liver and lung, while lymph node metastases occur in about 10-25% of cases [11, 12, 13]. Superficial inguinal lymph nodes are involved in 15-25% of carcinomas of size T2 or smaller and up to 50% of carcinomas classified as T3 or T4 [10, 14, 15] according to the latest TNM classification system developed by the American Joint Committee on Cancer [16]. The presence of inguinal lymph node metastases in anal cancer has been shown to reduce overall survival to 30-58% [17].

Tumor site, size and nodal status are considered the most important prognostic factors [18, 19, 20, 21]. According to the multivariate analysis of certain prospective studies, such as the European Organization for Research and Treatment of Cancer trial (EORTC 22861), Radiation Therapy Oncology Group trial (RTOG 98-11), and more recently the United Kingdom Coordinating Committee on Cancer Research Anal Cancer Trial (ACT I), inguinal lymph node involvement is reported to be a major independent prognostic factor for local recurrence, disease-free survival and overall survival [22, 18, 19, 23, 24, 15, 17, 20]. In particular, survival rates drop from 70% in the case of negative nodes to 30-58% in the case of nodal involvement [15, 17].

As expected, prognosis is worsened by 50% in tumors larger than 5 cm associated with nodal involvement [10]. Synchronous inguinal metastases are strongly related to the size of the tumor and occur in 10-25% of patients, while metachronous metastases are found in 5-25% of node-negative patients at diagnosis [25]. Despite the high prevalence of patients undergoing radio- and chemotherapy, approximately 7% of patients suffer from tumor recurrence in the inguinal lymphatic basin [26]. Conversely, the presence of a concomitant involvement of the perirectal lymph nodes is more frequent, but does not significantly affect the prognosis, as the perirectal lymph nodes are always routinely included in the primary pelvic radiotherapy fields [13, 27].

In the next sections we will describe the surgical treatment of anal cancer, the evaluation method of lymph nodes and the clinical implications of nodal involvement in the treatment and prognosis of the disease.

## 2. Rationale of Sentinel Lymph Node Biopsy

Initially, the traditional surgical treatment for anal cancer was the abdomino-perineal resection with permanent colostomy. This type of intervention had a survival rate of 40% to 70% at 5 years [10]. Subsequently, a combined radio- and chemotherapy treatment has progressively replaced surgical resection since Nigro and colleagues introduced their protocol in 1974, which prospected a treatment for anal carcinoma without surgical intervention and the concurrent morbidity of a permanent colostomy [28]. This non-surgical combined treatment has increased survival rates to 70-90% in selected patients [29, 30], with a reported 5-year overall survival rate of 58% to 92% [31, 15], and is currently considered the standard of care [32, 33, 10].

Although the standard treatment for the primary site of anal cancer is established, the ideal approach to inguinal lymph nodes remains debated. As with other types of cancers, the approach to lymph nodes must be justified by some important considerations about the expected prevalence of nodal metastases and their clinical significance in terms of prognostic impact on overall and disease-free survival.

Currently, most authors agree that clinically suspicious synchronous inguinal nodes should be histologically examined. In the case of lymph node metastatic localizations of the disease, the treatment of choice is irradiation of the inguinal region [34]. However, this type of presentation involves only 10% to 20% of patients [27, 25]. In addition, elective inguinal dissection for clinically suspected nodal involvement has revealed lymph node metastases in only about 55% of cases at definitive histological examination [21, 34].

About 80% to 90% of patients have no clinical signs of inguinal metastases at the time of diagnosis of anal cancer, although a clinically negative groin does not imply absolute absence of metastatic disease [31, 21]. For this reason, when comparing the consequences of a false-negative diagnosis with a false-positive one, inguinal lymph node management in clinically negative inguinal nodes is much debated and varies across the different centers [21, 14, 12, 25].

However, there is a delicate balance between undertreatment and overtreatment, which has already been discussed in the previous chapters. In fact, it is probably more acceptable to excise a negative node than to misdiagnose a metastatic node. In particular, the underestimation of nodal involvement can increase the incidence of locoregional recurrences with a clear consequent impact on the patient's quality of life and potentially on the overall survival, while overtreatment is surely correlated with a greater prevalence of complications, such as lower limb lymphedema in the case of complete inguinal lymph node dissection. As a consequence, the clinician must make accurate decisions based on these risks.

Routine inguinal lymph node dissection can cause severe complications and, due to the absence of a significant survival benefit and high morbidity, it is currently not recommended for anal cancer [20]. On the other hand, bilateral prophylactic groin irradiation can lead to adequate locoregional control of the disease in the majority of patients. In several series, this approach has proved to be effective in avoiding the development of late nodal metastases as compared with data obtained from patients treated with elective inguinal lymph node surgery [35, 24]. In particular, several series concerning patients affected by anal cancer and treated with inguinal node irradiation have reported a reduction in the incidence of metachronous inguinal metastases from 15-25% to 2.5-4% [35, 14, 36].

However, systematic inguinal irradiation is not immune from complications either. In fact, this approach requires large volumes of radiotherapy, which are related to a relevant toxicity in around 15% of patients [25, 37]. The irradiation fields involving the inguinal lymph node chain may cause short-term complications such as inguinal fibrosis, external genitalia edema, erythema, skin burns and epidermolysis with cutaneous superinfection. In addition, some long-term complications may also arise in patients undergoing inguinal irradiation, such as necrosis of the femoral head, hip fracture and stenosis of the iliac artery [13, 38, 39, 37, 25, 35]. Despite its rarity, death related to radiation toxicity is reported in 2% to 2.7% of patients [25, 22, 40, 41]. Furthermore, by looking at the follow-up of patients after inguinal irradiation, Jung and colleagues have shown that the annual risk of radiation side effects does not decrease over time and may pose a lifelong risk of late complications [38, 9].

Again, taking into consideration only patients without any pathological inguinal lymph node involvement, there is even more controversy about the inguinal lymph node treatment, since both surgery and irradiation have demonstrated significant morbidity [24, 35]. Therefore, in opposition to this type of management, some authors have evaluated the possibility of excluding the inguinal basins from the standard radiotherapy fields, reserving lymph node irradiation only to those patients who eventually develop groin metastases during a close follow-up [42].

Papillon and colleagues [43] and Gerard and colleagues [25] examined a wide range of respectively 223 and 270 clinically node-negative patients who had not undergone inguinal irradiation, and observed inguinal metachronous recurrence in respectively 7.4% and 7.8% of cases. In a retrospective study of 181 patients with clinically uninvolved inguinal lymph nodes, Ortholan and colleagues showed a 5-year cumulative rate of inguinal recurrence of 12% in T1-T2 tumors, and of 30% in T3-T4 tumors [24]. These results suggest that almost 90% of patients who have undergone prophylactic inguinal irradiation can definitely be overtreated [12, 43, 25].

However, despite the lower recurrence rate, even early-stage node-negative patients are at risk of recurrence, and a conservative approach does not prevent from the development of a restrained percentage of inguinal metastases, which could otherwise be prevented via radiotherapy [27, 13, 44]. Inguinal recurrences in patients with early-stage anal cancer may also lead to a potential decrease in survival in some cases. In fact, during the follow-up of patients treated for anal cancer, some studies report an inguinal recurrence of up to 20%, which can be very difficult to successfully eradicate [20, 27].

Certainly, taking into account both the risk of recurrence in the absence of any type of lymph node treatment and the morbidity related to complete inguinal lymph node dissection or irradiation, new therapeutic strategies have been developed for clinically node-negative anal cancer patients, in order not to subject their inguinal nodes to undertreatment nor to overtreatment. In particular, as has happened for many other cancers, sentinel lymph node biopsy (SLNB) technique has been pursued with the aim of reducing surgical morbidity by offering an adequate staging of the disease.

## 3. Nodal Status Assessment

Currently, the main issue in the treatment of anal carcinoma is the identification of a reliable nodal staging system and strategies to achieve a better long-term survival while reducing radiation side effects [21]. Early detection of metastatic subclinical lymph nodes could improve the outcome, allowing a distinction to be made between patients who would actually benefit from inguinal irradiation and those who would be unnecessarily exposed to the risks of this treatment [27, 13, 44, 21, 42].

Since combined chemo- and radiotherapy, unlike surgery, does not produce a specimen for histopathological examination, it is difficult to determine the real incidence of inguinal node involvement [13, 27, 21]. Wade and colleagues showed that 44% of all lymph node metastases have a diameter of less than 5 mm and are therefore difficult to detect with conventional imaging [45]. On the other hand, Pintor and colleagues shown that 50% of the larger nodes appear to be inflammatory [46]. To confirm this data, a series of De Nardi and colleagues demonstrated that smaller lymph nodes (4-7 mm) are more likely to harbor metastases than larger ones [47], which means that the size is not always a reliable parameter for assessing nodal involvement. With a sensitivity of 36-87% and a specificity of 56-89%, ultrasound remains an operator-dependent technique with little reliability, even when associated with fine needle aspiration cytology (FNAC) [14, 13].

Even more advanced imaging techniques, such as magnetic resonance imaging (MRI), are not accurate enough in identifying metastatic lymph nodes [27, 13]. Positron emission tomography / computer tomography (PET/CT) has recently been shown to detect inguinal metastases in up to 20% of patients with clinically and radiologically uninvolved nodes resulting from conventional imaging, proving a better detection rate for abnormal inguinal lymph nodes than standard clinical staging with computed tomography (CT) scan and physical examination [48, 49]. Recently, De Nardi and colleagues have reported a sensitivity of 33% and a specificity of 84% for PET/CT [21]. Other recent studies have evaluated the role of PET/CT in anal squamous cell carcinoma, either alone or in combination with traditional CT scan, showing that contrast-enhanced PET/CT, both alone or in combination with standard CT, is superior to CT scan alone in the recognition of inguinal lymph node metastases. In particular, PET/CT combined with traditional CT provided an upstaging in up to 17% of cases and a modification of radiotherapy fields in up to 23% of cases compared with PET/CT or CT scan alone [50, 51].

In accordance with these studies, Mistrangelo and colleagues compared the detection of inguinal metastases of PET/CT combined with traditional CT and SLNB in a series of 27 patients, demonstrating that the latter was superior in terms of inguinal lymph nodes staging, mainly due to a low specificity and a positive predictive value of PET/CT and CT scan [52]. PET/CT and CT imaging detected inguinal lymph nodes in 7 patients, while histological examination of SLNB confirmed metastases in 3 of these 7 patients. Although it has a sensitivity of 100% and a negative predictive value of 100%, PET/CT in combination with CT showed a specificity of 83% and a positive predictive value of 43%. Both these values were lower than those of SLNB, which showed no false-positive results and no metachronous metastases during the follow-up period [52].

In this scenario, the sentinel node evaluation seems to be a promising minimally invasive method for the accurate assessment of nodal status [20, 27, 14]. Two reports published by Spratt and colleagues in 2000 and by Keshtgar and colleagues in 2001 suggested that prophylactic surgical dissection may be curative in the case of positive SLNB [53, 54]. Since then, several other studies demonstrated the feasibility and effectiveness of SLNB in anal cancer, confirming its usefulness for a more selective approach to patients [47, 55, 56, 57, 58, 17, 59, 60, 61, 62, 26].

The technique has been proven safe and highly effective for the sampling of inguinal lymph nodes and has been increasingly applied to anal canal cancer, improving the accuracy of inguinal staging and the indication for radiotherapy, while preventing prophylactic inguinal radiotherapy and related morbidity in patients with negative nodes [17, 59, 58, 56, 62, 60, 55, 20, 21].

# 4. Technical Aspects of Sentinel Lymph Node Biopsy

As with other primary cancers, radiotracer and vital dye injection are the most commonly used techniques for detecting the sentinel lymph node in anal cancer. The first technique consists in a preoperative local submucosal injection of a radioisotope, commonly a technetium-99-labelled nanocolloid, directly around the site of the anal lesion in the four cardinal points with the aid of an anoscope. Subsequently, a lymphoscintigraphy is usually performed to identify the lymphatic drainage and the first node where the tracer is captured. The node is then located intraoperatively by a gamma probe and sent for histological and immunohistochemical examination [14].

The second option for the detection of the sentinel lymph node is the injection of blue dye around the tumor site during surgery, which allows visual identification of the sentinel lymph node. These two techniques can be used individually or in combination.

Surgical excision of the node can be performed under local anesthesia, followed by histopathological analysis using either intraoperative frozen section analysis or postoperative paraffin-embedded formalin-fixed block sectioning and histological examination [14, 21].

The effectiveness of the two sentinel node detection techniques has been analyzed in several studies [47, 55, 56, 57, 58, 17, 59, 60, 61, 62, 26, 63, 13, 52] involving patients with T1-T4 anal tumors with clinical or imaging negative inguinal nodes. The detection rate of inguinal sentinel lymph nodes was generally high, ranging from 47% to 100% in studies using radiotracer alone [58, 13, 55, 17], and from 67% to 100% in studies using both radiotracer and blue dye methods combined [26, 56, 60, 57, 59, 62, 63, 47, 52, 56]. In their review study, Tehranian and colleagues [20] reported a pooled inguinal detection rate of 86.2%. However, this review was affected by a large heterogeneity of data between the studies evaluated. In particular, the detection rate was 90.1% (78.7-95.8) for studies using both blue dye and radiotracer and 72.4% (46.3-88.9) for studies using radiotracer alone. Most authors suggest that combined tracer method rather than radiotracer alone is more effective at locating the sentinel lymph node [21, 20, 14]. In any case, some studies that used radioisotope alone had inguinal detection rates of 100% or nearly [13, 55], suggesting therefore that the superiority of neither method can be definitely concluded.

In their 2010 series, Hirche and colleagues used indocyanine green fluorescent dye technique and near-infrared imaging, comparing the results with the conventional combined blue dye and radiotracer technique [64]. They reported an inguinal detection rate of 83%

with the first method versus 75% with the second, since in one patient infrared imaging showed the sentinel node despite the failure of its detection with the conventional method. These results seem promising, but need to be further validated in larger randomized trials.

In terms of the time of injection, most authors argue that the injection of the radiotracer should be given the day before the surgery [56, 60, 58, 27, 55, 26, 64, 15, 65]. The rationale is to give the lymphatic system enough time for the radiotracer to move into the inguinal nodes [13]. However, other groups [57, 63, 13] reported comparable results by performing the injection on the same day of intervention, which is in accordance with the reports on the sentinel lymph node mapping in breast cancer [20].

Lymphoscintigraphic imaging was performed in all studies and is currently considered an indispensable part of the sentinel node mapping. As reported by Gretschel and colleagues and De Nardi and colleagues, not all patients have an inguinal drainage of the radiotracer, and preoperative imaging would help select only those patients with an inguinal sentinel node visible at the lymphoscintigraphy [55, 15].

The rate of metastatic nodes among sentinel lymph nodes varied between 0% and 33%. Again, the series were very heterogeneous and included all T stages, from T1 to T4, although the majority of patients were clinically node-negative [21, 44]. The overall rate of inguinal metastases reported in the literature is 26,2%, and considering T stages separately is 22.2% in the case of T1 cancers, 17.3% in the case of T2, 38.5% in the case of T3, and 28.6% in the case of T4 [66].

Taking into account the sensitivity of the technique, in a review of Tehranian and colleagues from 16 studies, which included a total of 323 patients, the sensitivity value of SLNB ranged from 79% to 97%, with a calculated pooled sensitivity of 90% [20]. However, the accuracy of SLNB in predicting inguinal node involvement in anal cancer remains controversial and results should be interpreted with caution, due to the limited number of studies and the fact that a negative SLNB has usually not been followed by systematic lymph node dissections to assess the actual status of inguinal lymph nodes [34, 20, 14].

At present, false-negative rates can only be identified by follow-up of patients undergoing SLNB without subsequent radiation therapy due to sentinel node negativity. In this perspective, Bobin and colleagues followed up for a period of 18 months a group of patients with anal canal carcinoma and negative SLNB, treated without radiotherapy to the inguinal basins [60]. None of the patients developed late inguinal metastases. This type of follow-up was also performed by other authors, with a metachronous inguinal lymph node metastases rate ranging from 0% to 18.75% [55, 13, 26, 52, 64, 66].

In a series published in 2009 and updated in 2013, Mistrangelo and colleagues did not observe any inguinal recurrence during the follow-up of 28 and 50 node-negative patients, respectively [13, 66]. The sensitivity, specificity, negative and positive predictive value reported in the 2013 series were 100%, 83%, 100% and 43%, respectively. In the same series, Mistrangelo and colleagues reviewed 14 clinical trials with a total of 163 patients, obtaining a false-negative rate of 3.7%, which was considered acceptable [66]. In addition, the authors concluded that the SLNB procedure is easy and perfectly feasible in patients with anal carcinoma, presenting a high detection rate of up to 98.4% [66].

According to Gretschel and colleagues [55], the sentinel lymph node assessment was able to modify the treatment plan recommended by the national guidelines in about 50% of patients. In the group of patients who underwent SLNB without subsequent inguinal irradiation, inguinal recurrences were found in two out of 20 patients. In detail, one patient had a disseminated T4 tumor, and the other was affected by a T1 tumor previously treated with local excision. Similarly, in a prospective study of 50 patients, De Jong and colleagues [26] reported that SLNB provided treatment variation in at least 11 of the 21 patients. Inguinal recurrences within 12-24 months were observed in only two out of 14 node-negative patients who underwent node-sparing irradiation.

Inguinal sentinel node laterality depends on the location of the primary tumor. In fact, the anal canal has an extremely rich lymphatic system that drains into three different lymphatic basins: inguinal, lateral pelvic and mesorectal [21, 20]. The incidence of inguinal drainage increases for anal carcinomas further from the dentate line and closer to the anal verge [20]. Many authors reported mesorectal rather than inguinal drainage in patients with high tumor location in the anal canal, above the dentate line [57, 55, 15]. In these cases, lymphoscintigraphy plays a key role in avoiding unnecessary inguinal surgery [20].

Also the unilateral or bilateral inguinal drainage is strongly dependent on the location of the tumor. Damin and colleagues observed that tumors located on a single side of the anal canal without a midline extension had only an ipsilateral inguinal drainage, while tumors involving the midline of the anal canal drained to bilateral inguinal nodes in 94% of cases [27]. As a result, Mistrangelo and colleagues underline that an unilateral inguinal lymph node drainage in the case of a midline location should always give rise to reasonable suspicion of potential inguinal lymph node involvement in the contralateral inguinal basin [13].

The complication rate of the SLNB procedure is reported in the literature between 4.5% to 23.8% and includes wound infection, hematoma, seroma, lymphatic fistula, lymphedema, lymphocele and lymphorrea [15, 64, 26, 55, 27, 58].

Palpable inguinal lymph nodes are considered by some authors as an absolute contraindication for SLNB in anal cancer. According to these authors, metastatic or even reactive nodes may be associated with false-negative results, as they may alter the lymphatic drainage pattern via alternative pathways to secondary non-sentinel nodes, thereby rendering the SLNB unreliable [27, 55, 67]. Nonetheless, Mistrangelo and colleagues mentioned that palpable lymph nodes are generally superficial, whereas inguinal sentinel lymph nodes are usually located in deeper layers. They documented no metachronous metastases in 8 patients with palpable inguinal nodes who underwent SLNB. However, diagnostic biopsy is recommended instead of intraoperative SLNB in the case of massive or multiple palpable inguinal nodes [66, 13].

Gretschel and colleagues also suggest that SLNB in anal cancer can be used to adequately select patients for inguinal irradiation, especially in T1 and T2 tumors, while currently not recommended for larger T3 or T4 tumors due to their high incidence of inguinal lymph node involvement, which may lead to false-negative sentinel node results [55]. Other authors do not corroborate this recommendation. According to Mistrangelo and colleagues, since two out of three patients with T3-T4 anal cancers do not have inguinal node involvement, they could benefit from SLNB and node-sparing radiotherapy [66, 12]. To date, no study has reported any association between tumor size and false-negative results [65, 20], and cases of inguinal recurrences in sentinel node-negative T1 or T2 patients have also occurred [55, 26].

Previous inguinal surgery is not a well-established contraindication for SLNB. However, previous surgical manipulation of an anal tumor can theoretically change the lymphatic drainage pattern and may be associated with false-negative results [20, 27, 55, 67]. Gretschel and colleagues reported two detection failures and one false-negative result in patients with previous surgical manipulation for anal cancer [55]. On the other hand, Mistrangelo and colleagues included 5 patients with previous surgical manipulation of the anal mass without any reported problem in the subsequent sentinel node mapping [66]. More extensive studies are needed to clarify the effect of these conditions on the false-negative rate in SLNB for anal cancer.

## Conclusion

Despite the low incidence of anal canal carcinoma, considerable progress has been made over the past 30 years in understanding its etiology, biological behavior and therapy. The current therapeutic approach is primarily combined radio- and chemotherapy. The identification of lymph nodes metastases, especially in the inguinal area, is one of the main issues to be addressed. The low incidence of metachronous metastases and the significant side effects of complete inguinal node dissection and radiotherapy do not justify any of these prophylactic treatments [21].

At present, there is no imaging test capable of detecting metastases in small subcentimetric lymph nodes, which according to a study by Wade and colleagues carry about 44% of lymph node metastases in anal carcinoma [45]. In many cases, clinical examination and imaging studies, such as CT, MRI and endoscopic ultrasound, are not always able to adequately detect the presence of inguinal lymph node metastases.

As a consequence, consensus on the treatment of the inguinal region is still lacking, particularly in node-negative patients. The current inguinal treatment is mostly empirical and based on the single-institution routine. Some centers follow protocols of prophylactic inguinal irradiation, while others reserve inguinal irradiation for patients with histologically confirmed inguinal metastases [13]. In addition, there remains the need for a more selective approach to individualize treatment regimens for patients with anal squamous cell carcinoma.

An accurate nodal staging method to accurately identify the extent of the disease could lead to an individualized therapy. In this context, SLNB is a minimally invasive procedure that can improve inguinal lymph node staging and may be useful in selecting patients who would benefit from inguinal radiation, help detect occult inguinal metastatic disease and spare node-negative patients from unnecessary and unjustified radiation treatment and associated morbidity [21, 20, 14].

The combined radiotracer and blue dye techniques method can maximize the inguinal detection rate. The tumor location is highly associated with the detection of inguinal sentinel nodes. According to the current literature, SLNB is an easy and feasible procedure, with low morbidity rates, minor self-limiting complications and could be considered the procedure of choice for assessing inguinal lymph node status. The feasibility and effectiveness of SLNB have been addressed in several reports, together with its clinical utility in changing the therapeutic plan [47, 55, 56, 57, 58, 17, 59, 60, 61, 62, 26, 63, 13, 52].

Nevertheless, despite the high pooled sensitivity, it is not possible to draw definitive conclusions on the false-negative rate of SLNB in anal cancer due to the small sample size and sub-optimal quality of the studies included. Moreover, the current data does not yet support the routine use of this technique. Large-scale multicenter studies with consistent long-term follow-up are needed to better estimate the outcome in node-negative patients undergoing inguinal node-sparing irradiation and to validate this technique permanently.

## References

[1] Siegel R. L., Miller K. D., Jemal A. Cancer Statistics, 2017. *CA Cancer J Clin. 2017*; 67:7–30. doi:10.3322/caac.21387.

[2] SEER Cancer Stat Facts: Anal Cancer National Cancer Institute Bethesda, MD. *Anal Cancer - Cancer Stat Facts.* https://seer.cancer.gov/statfacts/html/anus.html. acessed 2018-05-07.

[3] Jemal A., Simard E. P., Dorell C., Noone A. M., Markowitz L. E., Kohler B., et al. Annual Report to the Nation on the Status of Cancer, 1975-2009, featuring the burden and trends in human papillomavirus(HPV)-associated cancers and HPV vaccination coverage levels. *J Natl Cancer Inst. 2013*;105:175–201. doi:10.1093/jnci/djs491.

[4] Johnson L. G., Madeleine M. M., Newcomer L. M., Schwartz S. M., Daling J. R. Anal cancer incidence and survival: the surveillance, epidemiology, and end results experience, 1973-2000. *Cancer. 2004*;101:281–288. doi:10.1002/cncr.20364.

[5] Nelson R. A., Levine A. M., Bernstein L., Smith D. D., Lai L. L. Changing patterns of anal canal carcinoma in the United States. *J Clin Oncol. 2013*;31:1569–1575. doi: 10.1200/JCO.2012.45.2524.

[6] Shiels M. S., Kreimer A. R., Coghill A. E., Darragh T. M., Devesa S. S. Anal Cancer Incidence in the United States, 1977-2011: Distinct Patterns by Histology and Behavior. *Cancer Epidemiol Biomarkers Prev. 2015*;24:1548–1556. doi:10.1158/1055-9965.EPI-15-0044.

[7] Daling J. R., Madeleine M. M., Johnson L. G., Schwartz S. M., Shera K. A., Wurscher M. A., et al. Human papillomavirus, smoking, and sexual practices in the etiology of anal cancer. *Cancer. 2004*;101:270–280. doi:10.1002/cncr.20365.

[8] Benson A. B., Venook A. P., Cederquist L., Chan E., Chen Y. J., Cooper H. S., et al. *Anal Carcinoma (Version 2.2017).* techreport, NCCN Clinical Practice Guidelines in Oncology (NCCN Guidelines). 2017.

[9] Glynne-Jones R., Nilsson P. J., Aschele C., Goh V., Peiffert D., Cervantes A., et al. Anal cancer: ESMO-ESSO-ESTRO clinical practice guidelines for diagnosis, treatment and follow-up. *Eur J Surg Oncol. 2014*;40:1165–1176. doi: 10.1016/j.ejso.2014.07.030.

[10] Ryan D. P., Compton C. C., Mayer R. J. Carcinoma of the anal canal. *N Engl J Med. 2000*;342:792–800. doi:10.1056/NEJM200003163421107.

[11] Sato H., Koh P. K., Bartolo D. C. C. Management of anal canal cancer. *Dis Colon Rectum. 2005*;48:1301–1315. doi:10.1007/s10350-004-0934-z.

[12] Mistrangelo M., Bellò M, Mobiglia A., Beltramo G., Cassoni P., Milanesi E., et al. Feasibility of the sentinel node biopsy in anal cancer. *Q J Nucl Med Mol Imaging. 2009*;53:3–8.

[13] Mistrangelo M., Morino M. Sentinel lymph node biopsy in anal cancer: a review. *Gastroenterol Clin Biol. 2009*;33:446–450. doi:10.1016/j.gcb.2009.01.009.

[14] Noorani A., Rabey N., Durrani A., Walsh S. R., Davies R. J. Systematic review of sentinel lymph node biopsy in anal squamous cell carcinoma. *Int J Surg. 2013*; 11:762–766. doi:10.1016/j.ijsu.2013.07.005.

[15] De Nardi P., Carvello M., Staudacher C. New approach to anal cancer: individualized therapy based on sentinel lymph node biopsy. *World J Gastroenterol. 2012*;18:6349–6356. doi:10.3748/wjg.v18.i44.6349.

[16] American Joint Committee on Cancer. *AJCC Cancer Staging Manual (7th Edition).* Springer. 2011.

[17] Ulmer C., Bembenek A., Gretschel S., Markwardt J., Koswig S., Schneider U., et al. Refined staging by sentinel lymph node biopsy to individualize therapy in anal cancer. *Ann Surg Oncol. 2004*;11:259S–262S.

[18] Ajani J. A., Winter K. A., Gunderson L. L., Pedersen J., Benson A. B., Thomas C. R., et al. Fluorouracil, mitomycin, and radiotherapy vs fluorouracil, cisplatin, and radiotherapy for carcinoma of the anal canal: a randomized controlled trial. *JAMA. 2008*;299:1914–1921. doi:10.1001/jama.299.16.1914.

[19] Glynne-Jones R., Sebag-Montefiore D., Adams R., Gollins S., Harrison M., Meadows H. M., et al. Prognostic factors for recurrence and survival in anal cancer: generating hypotheses from the mature outcomes of the first United Kingdom Coordinating Committee on Cancer Research Anal Cancer Trial (ACT I). *Cancer. 2013*;119:748–755. doi:10.1002/cncr.27825.

[20] Tehranian S., Treglia G., Krag D. N., Dabbagh Kakhki V. R., Zakavi S. R., Sadeghi R., et al. Sentinel node mapping in anal canal cancer: systematic review and meta-analysis. *J Gastrointestin Liver Dis. 2013*;22:321–328.

[21] De Nardi P., Carvello M. How reliable is current imaging in restaging rectal cancer after neoadjuvant therapy? *World J Gastroenterol. 2013*;19:5964–5972. doi: 10.3748/wjg.v19.i36.5964.

[22] Bartelink H., Roelofsen F., Eschwege F., Rougier P., Bosset J. F., Gonzalez D. G., et al. Concomitant radiotherapy and chemotherapy is superior to radiotherapy alone in the treatment of locally advanced anal cancer: results of a phase III randomized trial of the European Organization for Research and Treatment of Cancer Radiotherapy and Gastrointestinal Cooperative Groups. *J Clin Oncol. 1997*;15:2040–2049. doi: 10.1200/JCO.1997.15.5.2040.

[23] Magalhães M. N., Barbosa L. E. R. Anal canal squamous carcinoma. *Journal of Coloproctology. 2017*;37:72–79. doi:10.1016/j.jcol.2016.08.003.

[24] Ortholan C., Resbeut M., Hannoun-Levi J. M., Teissier E., Gerard J. P., Ronchin P., et al. Anal canal cancer: management of inguinal nodes and benefit of prophylactic inguinal irradiation (CORS-03 Study). *Int J Radiat Oncol Biol Phys. 2012*;82:1988–1995. doi:10.1016/j.ijrobp.2011.02.010.

[25] Gerard J. P., Chapet O., Samiei F., Morignat E., Isaac S., Paulin C., et al. Management of inguinal lymph node metastases in patients with carcinoma of the anal canal: experience in a series of 270 patients treated in Lyon and review of the literature. *Cancer. 2001*;92:77–84.

[26] de Jong J. S., Beukema J. C., van Dam G. M., Slart R., Lemstra C., Wiggers T. Limited value of staging squamous cell carcinoma of the anal margin and canal using the sentinel lymph node procedure: a prospective study with long-term follow-up. *Ann Surg Oncol. 2010*;17:2656–2662. doi:10.1245/s10434-010-1063-7.

[27] Damin D. C., Rosito M. A., Schwartsmann G. Sentinel lymph node in carcinoma of the anal canal: a review. *Eur J Surg Oncol. 2006*;32:247–252. doi: 10.1016/j.ejso.2005.08.006.

[28] Nigro N. D., Vaitkevicius V. K., Considine B. Combined therapy for cancer of the anal canal: a preliminary report. *Dis Colon Rectum. 1974*;17:354–356.

[29] Tomaszewski J. M., Link E., Leong T., Heriot A., Vazquez M., Chander S., et al. Twenty-five-year experience with radical chemoradiation for anal cancer. *Int J Radiat Oncol Biol Phys. 2012*;83:552–558. doi:10.1016/j.ijrobp.2011.07.007.

[30] Bilimoria K. Y., Bentrem D. J., Ko C. Y., Stewart A. K., Winchester D. P., Talamonti M. S., et al. Squamous cell carcinoma of the anal canal: utilization and outcomes of recommended treatment in the United States. *Ann Surg Oncol. 2008*;15:1948–1958. doi:10.1245/s10434-008-9905-2.

[31] Fuchshuber P. R., Rodriguez-Bigas M., Weber T., Petrelli N. J. Anal canal and perianal epidermoid cancers. *J Am Coll Surg. 1997*;185:494–505.

[32] Czito B. G., Willett C. G. Current management of anal canal cancer. *Curr Oncol Rep. 2009*;11:186–192.

[33] Zilli T., Schick U., Ozsahin M., Gervaz P., Roth A. D., Allal A. S. Node-negative T1-T2 anal cancer: radiotherapy alone or concomitant chemoradiotherapy? *Radiother Oncol. 2012*;102:62–67. doi:10.1016/j.radonc.2011.09.015.

[34] Schulze T., Bembenek A., Schlag P. M. Sentinel lymph node biopsy progress in surgical treatment of cancer. *Langenbecks Arch Surg. 2004*;389:532–550. doi: 10.1007/s00423-004-0484-9.

[35] Myerson R. J., Kong F., Birnbaum E. H., Fleshman J. W., Kodner I. J., Picus J., et al. Radiation therapy for epidermoid carcinoma of the anal canal, clinical and treatment factors associated with outcome. *Radiother Oncol. 2001*;61:15–22.

[36] Mitchell S. E., Mendenhall W. M., Zlotecki R. A., Carroll R. R. Squamous cell carcinoma of the anal canal. *Int J Radiat Oncol Biol Phys. 2001*;49:1007–1013.

[37] Wagner J. P., Mahe M. A., Romestaing P., Rocher F. P., Berger C., Trillet-Lenoir V., et al. Radiation therapy in the conservative treatment of carcinoma of the anal canal. *Int J Radiat Oncol Biol Phys. 1994*;29:17–23.

[38] Jung H., Beck-Bornholdt H. P., Svoboda V., Alberti W., Herrmann T. Quantification of late complications after radiation therapy. *Radiother Oncol. 2001*;61:233–246.

[39] Lim F., Glynne-Jones R., Chemotherapy/chemoradiation in anal cancer: a systematic review. *Cancer Treat Rev. 2011*;37:520–532. doi:10.1016/j.ctrv.2011.02.003.

[40] UKCCCR Anal Cancer Trial Working Party. Epidermoid anal cancer: results from the UKCCCR randomised trial of radiotherapy alone versus radiotherapy, 5-fluorouracil, and mitomycin. UKCCCR Anal Cancer Trial Working Party. UK Co-ordinating Committee on Cancer Research. *Lancet* (London, England). 1996;348:1049–1054.

[41] Flam M., John M., Pajak T. F., Petrelli N., Myerson R., Doggett S., et al. Role of mitomycin in combination with fluorouracil and radiotherapy, and of salvage chemoradiation in the definitive nonsurgical treatment of epidermoid carcinoma of the anal canal: results of a phase III randomized intergroup study. *J Clin Oncol. 1996*;14:2527–2539. doi:10.1200/JCO.1996.14.9.2527.

[42] Matthews J. H. L., Burmeister B. H., Borg M., Capp A. L., Joseph D., Thompson K. M., et al. T1-2 anal carcinoma requires elective inguinal radiation treatment–the results of Trans Tasman Radiation Oncology Group study TROG 99.02. *Radiother Oncol. 2011*;98:93–98. doi:10.1016/j.radonc.2010.10.005.

[43] Papillon J., Montbarbon J. F. Epidermoid carcinoma of the anal canal. A series of 276 cases. *Dis Colon Rectum. 1987*;30:324–333.

[44] Shridhar R., Shibata D., Chan E., Thomas C. R. Anal cancer: current standards in care and recent changes in practice. *CA Cancer J Clin. 2015*;65:139–162. doi: 10.3322/caac.21259.

[45] Wade D. S., Herrera L., Castillo N. B., Petrelli N. J. Metastases to the lymph nodes in epidermoid carcinoma of the anal canal studied by a clearing technique. *Surg Gynecol Obstet. 1989*;169:238–242.

[46] Pintor M. P., Northover J. M., Nicholls R. J. Squamous cell carcinoma of the anus at one hospital from 1948 to 1984. *Br J Surg. 1989*;76:806–810.

[47] De Nardi P., Carvello M., Canevari C., Passoni P., Staudacher C. Sentinel node biopsy in squamous-cell carcinoma of the anal canal. *Ann Surg Oncol. 2011*;18:365–370. doi:10.1245/s10434-010-1275-x.

[48] Trautmann T. G., Zuger J. H. Positron Emission Tomography for pretreatment staging and posttreatment evaluation in cancer of the anal canal. *Mol Imaging Biol. 2005*; 7:309–313. doi:10.1007/s11307-005-0003-6.

[49] Cotter S. E., Grigsby P. W., Siegel B. A., Dehdashti F., Malyapa R. S., Fleshman J. W., et al. FDG-PET/CT in the evaluation of anal carcinoma. *Int J Radiat Oncol Biol Phys. 2006*;65:720–725. doi:10.1016/j.ijrobp.2006.01.009.

[50] Bannas P., Weber C., Adam G., Frenzel T., Derlin T., Mester J., et al. Contrast-enhanced [(18)F]fluorodeoxyglucose-positron emission tomography/computed tomography for staging and radiotherapy planning in patients with anal cancer. *Int J Radiat Oncol Biol Phys. 2011*;81:445–451. doi:10.1016/j.ijrobp.2010.05.050.

[51] Nguyen B. D., Ram P. C., Roarke M. C. F-18 FDG PET/CT imaging of anal canal squamous cell carcinoma. *Clin Nucl Med. 2007*;32:234–236. doi: 10.1097/01.rlu.0000255224.20271.3a.

[52] Mistrangelo M., Pelosi E., Bellò M., Castellano I., Cassoni P., Ricardi U., et al. Comparison of positron emission tomography scanning and sentinel node biopsy in the detection of inguinal node metastases in patients with anal cancer. *Int J Radiat Oncol Biol Phys. 2010*;77:73–78. doi:10.1016/j.ijrobp.2009.04.020.

[53] Spratt J. S. Cancer of the anus. *J Surg Oncol. 2000*;74:173–174. doi:10.1002/1096-9098(200006)74:2¡173::AID-JSO19¿3.0.CO;2-1.

[54] Keshtgar M. R., Amin A., Taylor I., Ell P. J. The sentinel node in anal carcinoma. *Eur J Surg Oncol. 2001*;27:113–114. doi:10.1053/ejso.2000.1019.

[55] Gretschel S., Warnick P., Bembenek A., Dresel S., Koswig S., String A., et al. Lymphatic mapping and sentinel lymph node biopsy in epidermoid carcinoma of the anal canal. *Eur J Surg Oncol. 2008*;34:890–894. doi:10.1016/j.ejso.2007.11.013.

[56] Péley G., Farkas E., Sinkovics I., Kovács T., Keresztes S., Orosz Z., et al. Inguinal sentinel lymph node biopsy for staging anal cancer. *Scand J Surg. 2002*;91:336–338. doi:10.1177/145749690209100405.

[57] Perera D., Pathma-Nathan N., Rabbitt P., Hewett P., Rieger N. Sentinel node biopsy for squamous-cell carcinoma of the anus and anal margin. *Dis Colon Rectum. 2003*; 46:1027–9; discussion 1030–1. doi:10.1097/01.DCR.0000081212.29821.FB.

[58] Ulmer C., Bembenek A., Gretschel S., Markwardt J., Koswig S., Slisow W., et al. Sentinel node biopsy in anal cancer - a promising strategy to individualize therapy. *Onkologie. 2003*;26:456–460. doi:10.1159/000072979.

[59] Damin D. C., Rosito M. A., Gus P., Spiro B. L., Amaral B. B., Meurer L., et al. Sentinel lymph node procedure in patients with epidermoid carcinoma of the anal canal: early experience. *Dis Colon Rectum. 2003*;46:1032–1037. doi: 10.1097/01.DCR.0000075208.76925.15.

[60] Bobin J. Y., Gérard J. P., Chapet O., Romestaing P., Isaac S. [Lymphatic mapping and inguinal sentinel lymph node biopsy in anal canal cancers to avoid prophylactic inguinal irradiation]. *Cancer Radiother. 2003*;7 Suppl 1:85s–90s.

[61] Mistrangelo M., Mobiglia A., Mussa B., Bellò M., Pelosi E., Goss M., et al. The sentinel node in anal carcinoma. *Tumori. 2002*;88:S51–S52.

[62] Rabbitt P., Pathma-Nathan N., Collinson T., Hewett P., Rieger N. Sentinel lymph node biopsy for squamous cell carcinoma of the anal canal. *ANZ J Surg. 2002*;72:651–654.

[63] Castro L. S., Mali Junior J., Rezende Neto J. F., Pedras D. d. S. V., Stoduto G., Pacheco J. S., et al. Inguinal sentinel node biopsy in epidermoid carcinoma of the anal canal: a pilot study. *Applied Cancer Research (Impresso). 2005*;25:71–74.

[64] Hirche C., Dresel S., Krempien R., Hünerbein M. Sentinel node biopsy by indocyanine green retention fluorescence detection for inguinal lymph node staging of anal cancer: preliminary experience. *Ann Surg Oncol. 2010*;17:2357–2362. doi: 10.1245/s10434-010-1010-7.

[65] Mistrangelo M., Pelosi E., Bellò M., Ricardi U., Milanesi E., Cassoni P., et al. Role of positron emission tomography-computed tomography in the management of anal cancer. *International journal of radiation oncology, biology, physics. 2012*;84:66–72. doi:10.1016/j.ijrobp.2011.10.048.

[66] Mistrangelo D. M., Bellò M., Cassoni P., Milanesi E., Racca P., Munoz F., et al. Value of staging squamous cell carcinoma of the anal margin and canal using the sentinel lymph node procedure: an update of the series and a review of the literature. *Br J Cancer. 2013*;108:527–532. doi:10.1038/bjc.2012.600.

[67] Damin D. C., Tolfo G. C., Rosito M. A., Spiro B. L., Kliemann L. M. Sentinel lymph node in patients with rectal cancer invading the anal canal. *Tech Coloproctol. 2010*; 14:133–139. doi:10.1007/s10151-010-0582-3.

In: The Sentinel Lymph Node
Editors: A. Londero, S. Bertozzi and C. Cedolini ISBN: 978-1-53614-557-1


*Chapter 15*

# SENTINEL LYMPH NODE BIOPSY IN COLORECTAL CANCER

*Giovanni Terrosu*[1,*], *Edoardo Scarpa*[1] *Serena Bertozzi*[2] *and Ambrogio P. Londero*[3]
[1]Clinic of Surgery, University Hospital of Udine, Italy
[2]Breast Unit, University Hospital of Udine, Italy
[3]Clinic of Obstetrics and Gynecology,
University Hospital of Udine, Udine, Italy

**Abstract**

One of the most important prognostic factors in colorectal cancer is locoregional lymph status. However, the role of the sentinel lymph node biopsy remains controversial due to its highly variable sensitivity rate and negative predictive value among studies. Sentinel node detection does not imply any alteration in the surgical procedure, but can achieve an improvement in staging accuracy, especially in the subgroup of patients with high-risk stage II colorectal cancer, probably due to occult lymph node metastases undetected by conventional hematoxylin-eosin staining. Sentinel node detection techniques include the use of blue vital dye, radiotracer or indocyanine green and may be performed in vivo before colic resection or ex vivo after specimen resection. Experience with sentinel lymph node biopsy in rectal cancer is still limited. Results show a lower sensitivity rate than for colon cancer, possibly due to a diversity of lymphatic drainage and to neoadjuvant irradiation leading to native lymphatic vessel disrupture. In conclusion, to date data on sentinel lymph node biopsy in colorectal cancer suggests that the sensitivity of this method remains too low to support a clinical guideline. Further studies are needed in order to assess the feasibility of sentinel lymph node biopsy in specific colorectal cancers subgroups.

**Keywords:** colorectal cancer, rectal cancer, colon cancer, sentinel lymph node biopsy, micrometastases

*Corresponding Author E-mail: giovanni.terrosu@uniud.it.

# 1. Introduction

With an estimated incidence of 17.2 cases per 100,000 people per year, colorectal cancer is the fourth most common cancer in the world, accounting for 9.7% of all cancers, and the fourth leading cause of cancer-related mortality [1]. Many staging systems have been proposed for colorectal cancer, although the American Joint Committee on Cancer (AJCC) classification based on tumor size, nodal status and possible metastases presence (TNM) remains the most widely applied [2].

According to AJCC recommendations, primary treatment for stage I colorectal cancer (T1-2 tumors without nodal involvement) is surgical resection of the primary tumor with en-bloc resection of the mesentery bearing the regional nodes. Similarly, the therapeutic management for stage III colorectal cancer (any T tumor with nodal involvement) is clearly outlined, as all patients undergo surgical treatment and adjuvant chemotherapy, which usually includes 5-fluorouracil [3].

On the other hand, conflicting data emerges on the role of adjuvant therapy in stage II colorectal cancer (T3-4 tumors without nodal involvement). Most recent studies suggest that there is little or no benefit to treating patients with low-risk colorectal cancer with adjuvant treatment, while there are chemotherapy-related adverse effects, regardless of the regimen used [4, 5, 6]. Nevertheless, patients with high-risk features such as T4, poorly differentiated tumors, bowel perforation or inadequate lymph node harvest show a recurrence rate similar to stage IIIA colorectal cancer (T1-2 with nodal involvement) and are therefore routinely considered for adjuvant chemotherapy [7, 8, 3, 9, 10].

However, the indication for adjuvant therapy still depends primarily on the lymph node status. Regional lymphadenectomy allows local disease control, cancer staging, adjuvant treatment planning and affects overall survival [11, 12, 13]. Therefore, optimal lymph node staging provides more precise indications for adjuvant therapy and may consequently have a paramount clinical and prognostic impact [14, 15]. In fact, appropriate staging and treatment reduces the recurrence rate by 40% and the mortality rate by 33% [13].

Survival rates depend mainly on the TNM stage at diagnosis, going from a 5-year overall survival of 92% in early-stage localized tumors to 11% in distant metastatic disease [16]. In particular, the most critical factor for the prognosis in colorectal cancer is the status of regional lymph nodes [17, 18, 11]. The 5-year survival rate in patients with metastatic regional lymph nodes (TNM Stage III) is 21-32%, thus lower than in patients with disease-free lymph nodes (TNM Stages I and II) [19, 20, 16].

However, when considering the substages, we can see that survival rates for stage IIB (T4 tumor without nodal involvement) are very similar or even worse than for stage IIIB (T1 to 4 tumor with nodal involvement). In particular, the US Surveillance, Epidemiology and End Results (SEER) study outlines a 5-year survival rate of 72.2% for stages IIB-IIC, compared to 83.4% for stages IIIA, probably due to adjuvant therapy, which is included as a standard of care for stage III colorectal cancer [16]. In particular, up to 20-30% of patients with early-stage node-negative colorectal cancer will experience regional or metastatic disease recurrence following potentially curative resection, probably because some node-positive patients are not offered an adequate postoperative treatment [10, 15, 19, 1, 21].

Inadequate nodal staging may result from incomplete surgical resection, insufficient pathological regional nodal retrieval, sampling error, aberrant lymphatic drainage or overlooked small-volume nodal disease. With regard to nodal retrieval, the current standard of care recommended by the AJCC calls for at least 12 nodes collected per specimen for an accurate nodal staging [22, 23, 4, 24]. In fact, lymph node staging accuracy increases with the number of lymph nodes examined. Nonetheless, in their multicenter review, Mitchell and colleagues have reported a high variability in the number of nodes found in the surgical specimen, with more than 50% of specimens containing less than 12 nodes, with a significant variation for Dukes B stages (T2 to T4N0) [25].

With regard to the sampling method, in the current practice only one 4-m-thick hematoxylin-eosin-stained section per 5 mm of each lymph node is assessed for metastases [26]. This means that only a limited area of the lymph node is analyzed, while a large area potentially bearing tumor cells remains unexamined. Serial sectioning, additional immunohistochemistry to detect cytokeratin-positive cells or molecular reverse transcriptase polymerase chain reaction (RT-PCR) may increase the accuracy of lymphatic spread detection.

Using molecular detection techniques, such as immunohistochemistry or RT-PCR, various studies have shown occult tumor cells in regional lymph nodes in 25% to 50% of patients with node-negative colorectal cancer at routine histopathological analysis, concluding that patients who meet the 12-node minimum benchmark, and are negative at cumulative pathological and molecular methods, are likely to be treated with surgery alone [27, 28, 29]. Moreover, nodal staging in colorectal cancer may also include isolated tumor cells (ITCs, deposits smaller than 0.2 mm) and micrometastases (deposits between 0.2 and 2 mm) in the lymph nodes, which are easily missed by routine histopathological examination [2, 30].

In a prospective study conducted on 26 patients affected by stage II colorectal cancer, Liefers and colleagues used RT-PCR, reporting the detection of lymph node micrometastases in 54% of cases, with a 5-year adjusted survival rate and a 5-year recurrence rate of 50% and 58%, respectively, in the group with lymph node micrometastases [21]. In a prospective multicenter trial, Bilchik and colleagues reported a 31.5% nodal upstaging out of 92 node-negative patients at conventional staining, with a micrometastases prevalence of 23.9%. The recurrence rate was 13% in the overall population and 6.5% in patients with micrometastases. The cancer-related mortality was 5.4%, and 3.2% when considering only patients with micrometastases. Therefore, they concluded that the detection of micrometastases may be clinically relevant in colorectal cancer, leading to improved patient selection for adjuvant systemic chemotherapy [28].

In a subsequent prospective study using immunohistochemistry ultrastaging, Bilchik and colleagues showed a nodal upstaging of 20% in node-negative patients at conventional staining, with a statistically significant 22% recurrence rate in patients with micrometastases [27].

A meta-analysis revealed a statistically significant difference in 3-year overall survival by analyzing with RT-PCR negative nodes by traditional staining, reporting a survival rate among patients with or without molecularly detected micrometastases of 78% and 98%, respectively [31]. Another recent meta-analysis found that the presence of micrometastases increases the likelihood of disease recurrence in patients with stage I-II colorectal cancer, while the presence of ITCs has no predictive value [32]. A report by Messerini and colleagues also shows that node-negative patients with or without ITCs show similar survival rates (77.7% and 78.3%, respectively), while patients with micrometastases have a lower survival rate of about 64% [33].

In contrast, a reduced relative survival was associated with the presence of occult tumor cells in patients with stage II colorectal cancer in a study conducted by Buckholm and colleagues, suggesting a clinical significance of ITCs [34].In addition, a recent meta-analysis of 4087 patients from 39 relevant studies concluded that the detection of either micrometastases and ITCs is associated with a poorer overall survival rate and that their regional disease recurrence was 23% versus 7%, respectively [35].

This data suggests that not only macrometastases, but also micrometastases and ITCs should be taken into account in the staging process of the disease. However, until the prognostic significance of ITCs is assessed, the AJCC recommends additional treatment to be considered only in patients with micrometastases.

Finally, all regional lymph nodes should ideally be examined with immunohistochemistry and RT-PCR because of their higher accuracy than traditional staining alone, but such a technique would be too expensive and time-consuming and therefore is not feasible in daily practice [30, 26, 13]. Thereafter, at present, immunohistochemical evaluation is adopted only in the case of a negative lymph node by traditional histological examination.

## 2. Rationale of Sentinel Lymph Node Biopsy

The concept of sentinel lymph node biopsy (SLNB) in colon cancer staging was introduced in 1999 by Joosten and colleagues in order to reduce false node-negative rates, given the importance of nodal involvement in determining further therapy and survival rates of these patients [36]. The sentinel lymph node is the closest node to the tumor in the lymphatic drainage pathways and therefore bears the highest risk of neoplastic involvement.

Using lymphatic mapping it is possible to identify 2 to 4 lymph nodes, which can be thoroughly examined, also by multi-sectioning and immunohistochemistry, thus optimizing the possibility of detecting metastases [15]. Evaluation of the sentinel node can lead to more precise staging, possibly identifying a subgroup of node-positive patient, who might have been understaged by conventional techniques and who may benefit from adjuvant therapy [37]. In addition, lymphatic mapping can help identify the pattern and status of lymph node basins, promoting adequate nodal yield and recognition of aberrant lymphatic drainages that can alter radical lymphadenectomy extent [38].

Unlike its application in other settings, SLNB is only an adjunctive procedure to conventional primary resection and regional lymphadenectomy. Its main advantage in colorectal cancer is the identification of nodes with the highest risk of metastases, particularly of micrometastases and ITCs [39]. However, the role of micrometastatic nodal disease in patients' survival and therapeutic decision making has not yet been determined.

Many studies have compared the performance of SLNB using hematoxylin-eosin staining or immunohistochemical analysis. Despite some promising results, there is no uniformity in histological processing or in the definition of nodal metastases [39, 40, 17, 41]. Therefore, the SLNB procedure in colorectal cancer is not standardized. However, since the sentinel node has the highest probability of lymphatic tumor spread, its routine histopathological examination promises to be a simple and effective technique to properly upstage patients who have otherwise been classified as N0 by traditional lymph node examination in high-risk stage II colorectal cancer [42].

Upstaging is a subject of great debate, given the clinical importance of occult tumor cells and micrometastases [26]. Asides from improving staging by selective additional staining, sentinel node mapping has been shown to increase the yield of the collected lymph nodes, increasing the percentage of N1 patients and consequently improving their prognosis compared to the N0 patient group [43, 44].

# 3. Technical Aspects of Sentinel Lymph Node Biopsy

Two approaches have been proposed for the identification of the sentinel lymph node in colorectal cancer. The in vivo method involves the injection of lymphatic blue dye into the subserosa around the tumor site, prior to the mobilization and resection of the tumor-bearing colon. After 5-10 minutes, the first blue-colored lymph node is removed and sent separately to the pathologist [19]. The ex vivo method is generally performed approximately 30 minutes after resection on a table apart from the operating field. It involves the injection of lymphatic dye into the subserosa and around the circumference of the tumor site along with area massage to push the tracer into the lymphatic vessels. Again, the first stained lymph node is defined as the sentinel lymph node [45].

Results from various studies have shown that in vivo mapping has the same accuracy as ex vivo, but the latter can disrupt native lymphatics flow, leading to false sentinel nodes. It is also deficient in detecting aberrant lymphatic drainage, a feature that can help improve nodal collection during surgery [46]. Aberrant drainage of lymphatics outside the field of an oncologic mesenteric resection has been reported in some studies [47, 48, 49]. So far, the frequency seems to vary between 0% and 10% [46]. Ex vivo mapping, on the other hand, allows the injection of dye into the submucosa, presumably the site where the tumor cells have access to the lymphatic system, and avoids the intraoperative manipulation of the tumor necessary in the in vivo technique, thus reducing the theoretical tumor cell shedding. In addition, it has the advantage of not adding operative time and not exposing patients to dye, which has a reported incidence of allergic reaction in 1-1.5% of patients [46, 42].

Nodal mapping can be performed with various substances: isosulfan blue dye, patent blue dye, methylene blue dye, radioactive tracers, and recently, near-infrared fluorescence after injection of indocyanine green [37, 50, 51, 52]. The vast majority of studies have used intraoperative blue dye injection, for both in vivo and ex vivo techniques.

Although it is an essential tool for SLNB in breast cancer and malignant melanoma, the preoperative use of radiocolloids in cancers of the gastrointestinal tract poses some issues, such as the need for an additional colonoscopy to inject the tracer. [42]. Radiocolloid particles, which size is relatively large, travel through the lymphatic channels at a slow rate. In addition, radiocolloids are incorporated in the first echelon lymph node by phagocytosis and remain trapped for a longer period than blue dye, making it more likely that the lymph node detected with this method is a proper sentinel node [53].

However, radioactive tracers involve the problem of overlapping radioactivity from the injection site to the primary tumor and the first paracolic lymph nodes. Conversely, because of its fairly rapid migration to the sentinel node through the lymphatic channels, the blue dye method is a preferable intraoperative technique that allows dye injection and sentinel node detection within several minutes. Potential disadvantages are the risk of secondary nodes receiving dye and confusing sentinel lymph node detection in the case of a prolonged preparation, rupture of the afferent lymphatic channels and dye diffusion to the abdominal situs in case of traumatic preparation [19, 54]. In addition, due to the small size of the particles, the blue dye travels through the lymphatic channels relatively quickly and passes on to the second echelon lymph node rapidly. For this reason, up to four or more lymph nodes can be regarded as sentinels and up to four or more colored lymph node must be analyzed [53].

Fluorescence navigation with indocyanine green requires a special camera, intraoperative dye injection around the tumor and its real-time visualization in the lymph nodal compartments after a few minutes. Fluorescence detection in colorectal cancer patients allows both ultrastaging and aberrant lymphatic detection, as it has been shown to conjoin the advantages of both dye and radiocolloid methods [55]. The main disadvantage of this procedure is the high cost of the required materials.

Published studies on SLNB in colorectal cancer show considerable heterogeneity in detection techniques, practical definition of the sentinel node, time interval chosen between dye injection and sentinel node detection, histopathological techniques applied and composition of patient groups. As a result, detection rate, sensitivity and upstaging rate vary considerably [42]. Most studies used blue dye tracer (either patent, isosulfan or methylene blue) [56, 57, 58, 59, 60, 61, 62, 63, 64, 65, 66, 67, 68, 69, 70, 71, 72, 43, 73, 74, 75, 39, 76, 24, 77, 46, 78, 79, 80, 81, 82, 83, 84, 40, 85, 86, 87, 88, 89, 48, 90, 36], while other studies used both blue dye and technetium-99 radiotracer [91, 92, 93, 94, 95, 96, 97, 73] or radiotracer only [98, 99, 100], and a few studies evaluated indocyanine green [101, 52, 102, 103, 104, 105, 55, 106, 101].

The reported success rate of lymphatic mapping ranged from 58% to 100%, with the majority of studies showing a detection rate above 90%, with a number of identified sentinel nodes ranging from 1.3 to 5.9 and an overall lymph node collection ranging from 5.3 to 33.9. According to the systematic review by van der Zaag and colleagues, the identification rate was significantly higher in studies including more than 100 patients, with a mean rate of 94.5%, and in studies involving ex vivo rather than in vivo procedures with a mean rate of 93.7% versus 89.2% [11]. On the other hand, the in vivo procedure allowed the identification of aberrant lymphatic drainage outside of the planned resection area in 1.6% to 15% of cases, thus improving staging accuracy compared to conventional colectomy with lymphadenectomy [58, 93, 96, 70, 68, 72, 73, 71, 91, 69, 46, 92, 40, 48, 87, 89, 36].

In the above mentioned review, there is a statistically significant difference between the reported detection rates of 93.1% and 83.1% in studies analyzing colon and rectal tumors, respectively [11]. A study by Vilcea and colleagues showed an identification rate of 86.3% for patients with colon cancer and of 68.9% for patients with rectal cancer. In particular, methylene blue dye injection was performed peritumorally and subserosally in vivo in colon cancers and ex vivo in rectal cancers [56]. Other factors that seem to influence the accuracy of the technique are female gender, tumor stage, previous abdominal surgery, intraoperative visualization of the blue lymphatic vessels, nodal status, body mass index (BMI) and volume of the injected dye [107, 13].

The sensitivity of SLNB ranged from 33.3% to 100% across studies, with a calculated overall sensitivity of 69.6% in the study by Van der Zaag and colleagues on 3944 performed procedures. An increased mean sensitivity of 80.2% was found when immunohistochemical findings were included in the accuracy parameters [11]. There seems to be a strong correlation between sensitivity and the number of identified sentinel nodes, with a good predictive value for lymph node involvement when four or more sentinel nodes are identified, while no correlation has been reported between sensitivity and the detection method or tracer used [11].

Two of the largest prospective multicenter trials up-to-date involved 315 and 500 patients, rescpectively [68, 76]. Bembenek and colleagues enrolled 315 patients with colon cancers alone, reporting a detection rate of 85% with a sensitivity of 54%, which were associated with the patient's BMI and with the number of metastatic lymph nodes [68]. Saha and colleagues reported more encouraging results, as they studied 408 colon cancers and 92 rectal cancers using the blue dye method with in vivo injection, with a sensitivity of 96%, a negative predictive value of 90% and a 2-year recurrence rate of 7% as compared to the conventional surgery group, which had a 2-years recurrence rate of up to 25% [76].

Among studies with separate results for colon and rectal cancer, a significantly higher sensitivity of 77.6% was found in the former, compared to 65.7% for the latter [56, 57, 59, 74, 75, 76, 79, 90]. When it was possible to calculate separately the test performance measures for early (T1 or T2) and advanced (T3 or T4) cancers, a significantly higher sensitivity was observed in the early-stage group than in the advanced carcinomas group (93.4% vs. 58.8%), although a smaller number of patients were included in this subgroup [59, 66, 73, 76, 98, 100].

No statistical differences have been found with regard to the ex vivo versus the in vivo technique, or the blue dye versus the radiocolloid injection. The false-negative results reported in sentinel node mapping vary from 0% to 60% for the in vivo technique and from 0% to 44% for the ex vivo one [46]. In rectal cancer, the sentinel lymph node is usually identified through the ex vivo technique, because the mobilization of the middle and inferior rectum is necessary, thus lymphatic drainage is strongly influenced [15]. A study conducted by Vilcea and colleagues reported better detection and sensitivity rates for colon cancers (86.4% and 66.7%, respectively) compared to rectal cancers (61.9% and 50%, respectively) [56].

Cahill and colleagues evaluated 225 patients with early-stage disease and 666 patients with advanced disease, achieving false-negative rates of 8% and 17%, respectively, with a negative predictive value of more than 95% for the former [108]. Opposing conclusions emerge from a systematic review conducted in 2011, which reported a non-significant sensitivity difference of 86% versus 82% for colon and rectal cancers, respectively, together with a non-significant difference in stratification by cancer stage when comparing T1 to T4 tumor nor in the type of tracer involved [26]. Another study comparing blue dye and radiocolloid techniques found a fewer sentinel nodes detected using radiotracers (1.38 vs 2.48 per patient), although metastases were more frequently found in nodes detected both by blue dye and radiocolloid, suggesting a more effective mapping with a combined injection technique [109].

The sensitivity rate in studies using indocyanine green ranged from 55% to 100%, with a negative predictive value from 0% to 100% [101, 110, 52, 111, 112, 102, 103, 104, 105, 55, 106]. Combined submucosal and subserosal injection has been shown to achieve the highest sensitivity, while subserosal injection reached the lowest sensitivity [18]. Two trials investigated the role of indocyanine green near-infrared fluorescence in the sentinel node mapping of rectal cancer, reporting contrasting results. Handgraaf and colleagues documented 21 positive sentinel nodes, using the indocyanine green, all free from malignancy, while the only micrometastatic lymph node was negative for indocyanine green, thus yielding a sensitivity rate of 0% [103]. On the other hand, Noura and collegues yielded a sensitivity rate of 100% in 25 patients with distal rectal cancer [105].

Likewise other dyes, according to the study conducted by Van der Zaag and colleagues [11], indocyanine green seems to attain higher sensitivity and accuracy in early-stage rather than advanced carcinomas [18]. According to Bembenek and colleagues, the most important factor to influence sensitivity rate was the BMI [42]. They reported a false-negative rate of 56% for patients with a BMI of more than 24, compared to 12% for patients with a BMI of less than 24, suggesting that visualization of the blue sentinel node in obese patients is a major problem [42].

The upstaging rate varied from 0% to 50%, with a mean weighted rate from 15% to 19% [26, 11]. This means that from 15% to 19% of patients with negative sentinel nodes evaluated with conventional histopathological staining presented micrometastases or ITCs after further detailed investigation. Most studies performed immunohistochemical staining only after a negative traditional hematoxylin-eosin staining [56, 57, 58, 60, 59, 65, 61, 64, 63, 66, 95, 67, 93, 96, 70, 68, 43, 72, 73, 74, 91, 69, 75, 77, 97, 24, 76, 46, 79, 78, 84, 83, 98, 48, 87, 36, 68, 86, 82, 88, 99, 62, 39, 85, 80], while only few studies used RT-PCR [62, 94]. Since not all studies have subclassified a finding of occult tumor cells into micrometastases or ITCs, 7.7% of the proper upstaging rate of stage I to II patients becoming stage III is difficult to interpret and not fully representative of the population [58, 64, 95, 70, 68, 73, 69, 77].

In a recent multicenter study involving 174 stage I to III patients, an upstaging of over 15% was shown for stages I and II [113]. A prospective multicenter trial conducted by Bilchik and collegues employed both immunohistochemistry and quantitative RT-PCR on hematoxylin-eosin negative sentinel nodes [28]. They reported a significantly higher sensitivity of 75% versus 36% for colon cancer than for rectal cancer, respectively, and 4 out of 92 patients node-negative at routine histopathological evaluation have developed a systemic recurrence. All of these four patients were found to have positive sentinel nodes after RT-PCR ultrastaging, while none of the 26 patients who resulted negative at the ultrastaging had a recurrence [28].

It has been hypothesized that in larger tumors with serosal and mesocolon infiltration, obstruction of the lymphatic vessels may lead to failure to detect the sentinel node or false-negative results [42]. Apart from the extraluminal extent, Cahill and colleagues suggest that SLNB may be more effective in early-stage rather than advanced cancers, since in the latter the obstruction of efferent lymph vessels or nodes by widespread tumor growth would force lymph drainage to take another route, leading to the detection of a second or third echelon lymph node rather than a proper sentinel node [114]. The results from uni- and multivariate analyses for factors influencing detection and sensitivity rates in a German multicenter study conducted by Bembenek and colleagues, suggest that extensive lymphatic tumor growth often leads to a complete blockage of lymph flow, and as a result, to a failure in the detection of the sentinel node and to a false-negative result [68].

In rectal cancer, the identification of the sentinel lymph node appears to be more difficult, and radiotherapy has been shown to induce fibrosis and alter lymphatic flow, leading to a false sentinel node identification [64]. However, in study conducted on 58 patients with rectal cancer, where 88% of the patients received neoadjuvant therapy, the sentinel lymph node detection rate was 85%, with an average sentinel lymph node harvest of 2.2 nodes per patient. In addition, 26% of patients had sentinel lymph node metastases at routine hematoxylin-eosin staining. The sensitivity of sentinel lymph node mapping was 53%, while the negative predictive value 79%. The authors concluded that for rectal cancer ex vivo sentinel node mapping is a technically feasible procedure after proctectomy, even after radiotherapy, although it does not improve staging [60].

# Conclusion

One of the most important prognostic factors in colorectal cancer is the locoregional lymph node status. Since the sentinel node is the first node that drains a tumor, it is most likely to become positive for metastases. However, the role of SLNB in colorectal cancer remains far from widely accepted. In fact, this minimally invasive technique is safe, with a reliable detection rate and accuracy, but its highly variable sensitivity rate and negative predictive value among studies still prevent it from being included in the surgical guidelines.

The detection of the sentinel node does not imply any alteration in the surgical procedure, but can achieve an improvement in the staging accuracy, especially in the high-risk subgroup of stage II colorectal cancer patients, probably due to occult nodal metastases undetected by conventional staining. In fact, these patients have poorer 5-year overall and disease-free survival than stage IIIA patients. The upstaging of high-risk stage II tumors into stage III tumors, based on the positive sentinel nodal status, can include them in the adjuvant therapy protocols, thus improving their survival rate by 33% and 5-year disease-free period by 40%. Therefore, precise identification and analysis of the sentinel node will improve the tumor staging and consequently establish a more appropriate postoperative treatment.

Lymphatic mapping allows a greater number of small lymph nodes to be detected and examined, in addition to the identification of aberrant lymphatic drainage, which can take place in up to 10% of patients. Nevertheless, the blue dye injection method, considered the best currently and most used, together with pathological examination in order to achieve better staging, remains a topic of discussion. Alternative detection techniques using radiocolloids alone or in combination with blue dye, or fluorescent dyes may also play a role in the future, but still need further evaluation.

When lymph node are analyzed by conventional methods, up to 15 - 20% of metastases may be missed, excluding patients from adjuvant chemotherapy. Immunohistochemical staining and RT-PCR permit a more precise nodal staging and the identification of micrometastases and ITCs. However, the prognostic value of this microscopic nodal disease is still unclear. Liefers and colleagues [21] showed that micrometastases corresponded to a significant reduction in 5-year survival of 50% compared to 91% for stage II colorectal cancer. Bukholm and colleagues [34] reported a reduced survival associated with the presence of ITCs in stage II colorectal cancer. Large randomized trials are still needed to demonstrate the clinical significance of micrometastases and ITCs and whether adjuvant chemotherapy can improve survival in this group of patients.

Among the pathological techniques used for the identification of lymph nodes, RT-PCR seems to provide the most accurate upstaging, albeit being the most expensive. The immunohistochemical evaluation of the sentinel nodes is more sensitive than the traditional hematoxylin-eosin staining but the molecular procedure is more specific and more accurate than immunohistochemistry in finding ITCs. In order to assess their feasibility on a large scale, an accurate analysis of sentinel and non-sentinel nodes should be carried out using RT-PCR technique.

On the other hand, high false-negative rates do not allow to date to avoid complete lymph node resection in node-negative cases. A sensitivity of 33% to 100% for the prediction of lymph node metastases was found, with a high variability across the studies, due to clinical heterogeneity in patient selection, technical details, and pathological analysis. The rationale for SLNB to be integrated into clinical protocols should be the evidence that the sentinel node is highly representative for a minimal residual disease. This hypothesis cannot be confirmed considering the relatively high false-negative rates for the identification of lymph node metastases [42].

Despite the overall disappointing sensitivity rate, subgroups with higher sensitivity rates could be identified. Sensitivity can be influenced by several factors, such as the tumor size and localization, volume of injected dye, the number of identified sentinel nodes and the patient's BMI, and seems to be higher especially in early-stage colorectal cancer, which in most studies represent the minority of the population. Lymphatic channels blockage by tumor masses and insufficient dye visualization in obese patients are the main disadvantages of the SLNB procedure. A careful patient selection (preferably early-stage T1 to T2 cancers) and technical improvements must be made before a final conclusion can be drawn on these issues.

In addition, sentinel node mapping requires a learning curve of up to 20-30 cases [62]. The increase in the detection rate observed in studies involving more than 100 patients indicates the existence of such learning-curve effect. Evidence suggests that when the mapping of the sentinel node has been done by a skilled team, reasonable levels of accuracy (98%) and sensitivity (96%) have been achieved [76]. However, unlike breast cancer and other cancers, the purpose of SLNB in colorectal cancer is to achieve a refined staging rather that to change the surgical procedure. Since all the collected lymph nodes are being examined, a false-negative sentinel node will never lead to undertreatment.

The prognostic information obtained from SLNB can be clinically significant, leading to possible upstaging in up to 15% of patients, a value that is even greater if we include also patients with positive aberrant sentinel nodes. Large prospective studies are needed to establish the prognostic significance of upstaging and the consequences of adjuvant therapy. These studies should focus on patients with stage I to II colorectal cancer, since stage III and IV already meet the criteria for adjuvant chemotherapy, so their treatment is not affected by the outcome of the SLNB.

Experience with SLNB in rectal cancer is still limited. The results show a lower sensitivity rate than in colon cancer, probably due to differences of the lymphatic drainage and neoadjuvant irradiation leading to disruption of the native lymphatic vessels, which can potentially hinder the identification of the proper sentinel node.

In conclusion, up-to-date data on SLNB in colorectal cancer suggest that, despite the improved detection rate and the reduced false-negative rate, the sensitivity of this method remains low to support a clinical guideline. Thereafter, this procedure is currently used only to help the pathologist detect in a more precise way the first nodes that drain the tumor. However, further studies are needed in order to assess the feasibility of SLNB in specific colorectal cancer subgroups, in particular stage I and II patients.

# References

[1] Ferlay J., Soerjomataram I., Ervik M., Dikshit R., Eser S., Mathers C., et al. *GLOBOCAN 2012 v1.0, Cancer Incidence and Mortality Worldwide: IARC CancerBase No. 11* [Internet]. Lyon, France: International Agency for Research on Cancer. Available from: http://globocan.iarc.fr, accessed on 27/03/2018.

[2] American College of Surgeons. *AJCC Cancer Staging Manual (Eighth Edition).* Springer. 2017.

[3] Benson A. B., Venook A. P., Cederquist L., Chan E., Chen Y. J., Cooper H. S., et al. Colon Cancer, Version 1.2017, NCCN Clinical Practice Guidelines in Oncology. *J Natl Compr Canc Netw. 2017*;15:370–398.

[4] Vogel J. D., Eskicioglu C., Weiser M. R., Feingold D. L., Steele S. R. The American Society of Colon and Rectal Surgeons Clinical Practice Guidelines for the Treatment of Colon Cancer. *Dis Colon Rectum. 2017*;60:999–1017. doi: 10.1097/DCR.0000000000000926.

[5] Tournigand C., André T., Bonnetain F., Chibaudel B., Lledo G., Hickish T., et al. Adjuvant therapy with fluorouracil and oxaliplatin in stage II and elderly patients (between ages 70 and 75 years) with colon cancer: subgroup analyses of the Multicenter International Study of Oxaliplatin, Fluorouracil, and Leucovorin in the Adjuvant Treatment of Colon Cancer trial. *J Clin Oncol. 2012*;30:3353–3360. doi: 10.1200/JCO.2012.42.5645.

[6] Wilkinson N. W., Yothers G., Lopa S., Costantino J. P., Petrelli N. J., Wolmark N. Long-term survival results of surgery alone versus surgery plus 5-fluorouracil and leucovorin for stage II and stage III colon cancer: pooled analysis of NSABP C-01 through C-05. A baseline from which to compare modern adjuvant trials. *Ann Surg Oncol. 2010*;17:959–966. doi:10.1245/s10434-009-0881-y.

[7] Niedzwiecki D., Bertagnolli M. M., Warren R. S., Compton C. C., Kemeny N. E., Benson A. B., et al. Documenting the natural history of patients with resected stage II adenocarcinoma of the colon after random assignment to adjuvant treatment with edrecolomab or observation: results from CALGB 9581. *J Clin Oncol. 2011*; 29:3146–3152. doi:10.1200/JCO.2010.32.5357.

[8] American Cancer Society. *Colorectal Cancer Facts & Figures 2017-2019.* Atlanta, Ga: American Cancer Society 2017. Available from: https://www.cancer.org/cancer/colon-rectal-cancer.html, accessed on 27/03/2018.

[9] Kumar A., Kennecke H. F., Renouf D. J., Lim H. J., Gill S., Woods R., et al. Adjuvant chemotherapy use and outcomes of patients with high-risk versus low-risk stage II colon cancer. *Cancer. 2015*;121:527–534. doi:10.1002/cncr.29072.

[10] Figueredo A., Coombes M. E., Mukherjee S. Adjuvant therapy for completely resected stage II colon cancer. *Cochrane Database Syst Rev. 2008*;CD005390. doi: 10.1002/14651858.CD005390.pub2.

[11] van der Zaag E. S., Bouma W. H., Tanis P. J., Ubbink D. T., Bemelman W. A., Buskens C. J. Systematic review of sentinel lymph node mapping procedure in colorectal cancer. *Ann Surg Oncol. 2012*;19:3449–3459. doi:10.1245/s10434-012-2417-0.

[12] Benson A. B., Schrag D., Somerfield M. R., Cohen A M., Figueredo A. T., Flynn P. J., et al. American Society of Clinical Oncology recommendations on adjuvant chemotherapy for stage II colon cancer. *J Clin Oncol. 2004*;22:3408–3419. doi: 10.1200/JCO.2004.05.063.

[13] Stojanoski S., Manevska N., Antovic S., Pop-Gjorcheva D., Vaskova O., Miladinova D., et al. Sentinel Lymph Node Detection in Colorectal Cancer - First Experience. *Open Access Maced J Med Sci. 2017*;5:744–750. doi:10.3889/oamjms.2017.166.

[14] Chen S. L., Bilchik A. J. More extensive nodal dissection improves survival for stages I to III of colon cancer: a population-based study. *Annals of surgery. 2006*; 244:602–610. doi:10.1097/01.sla.0000237655.11717.50.

[15] Sfeclan M. C., Vilcea I. D., Barisic G., Mogoanta S. S., Moraru E., Ciorbagiu M. C., et al. The sentinel lymph node (SLN) significance in colorectal cancer: methods and results. General report. *Rom J Morphol Embryol. 2015*;56:943–947.

[16] National Cancer Institute, DCCPS. *Surveillance, Epidemiology, and End Results (SEER) Program Research Data (1973-2014)* [released April 2017]. available from: www.seer.cancer.gov, accessed 27/03/2018.

[17] Saha S., Dan A. G., Beutler T., Wiese D., Schochet E., Badin J., et al. Sentinel lymph node mapping technique in colon cancer. *Semin Oncol. 2004*;31:374–381.

[18] Emile S.H., Elfeki H., Shalaby M., Sakr A., Sileri P., Laurberg S., et al. Sensitivity and specificity of indocyanine green near-infrared fluorescence imaging in detection of metastatic lymph nodes in colorectal cancer: Systematic review and meta-analysis. *J Surg Oncol. 2017*;116:730–740. doi:10.1002/jso.24701.

[19] Saha S., Wiese D., Badin J., Beutler T., Nora D., Ganatra B. K., et al. Technical details of sentinel lymph node mapping in colorectal cancer and its impact on staging. *Ann Surg Oncol. 2000*;7:120–124.

[20] Cancer Research UK. *Bowel cancer survival statistics 2016.* Available from: http://www.cancerresearchuk.org/health-professional/cancer-statistics/statistics-by-cancer-type/bowel-cancer/survival, accessed 27/03/2018.

[21] Liefers G. J., Cleton-Jansen A. M., van de Velde C. J., Hermans J., van Krieken J. H., Cornelisse CJ, et al. Micrometastases and survival in stage II colorectal cancer. *N Engl J Med. 1998*;339:223–228. doi:10.1056/NEJM199807233390403.

[22] Nelson H., Petrelli N., Carlin A., Couture J., Fleshman J, Guillem J., et al. Guidelines 2000 for colon and rectal cancer surgery. *J Natl Cancer Inst. 2001*;93:583–596.

[23] Wells K. O., Hawkins A. T., Krishnamurthy D. M., Dharmarajan S., Glasgow S. C, Hunt S. R., et al. Omission of Adjuvant Chemotherapy Is Associated With Increased Mortality in Patients With T3N0 Colon Cancer With Inadequate Lymph Node Harvest. *Dis Colon Rectum. 2017*;60:15–21. doi:10.1097/DCR.0000000000000729.

[24] Smith J., Hwang H., Wiseman K. W., Filipenko D., Phang P. T. Ex vivo sentinel lymph node mapping in colon cancer: improving the accuracy of pathologic staging? *Am J Surg. 2006*;191:665–668. doi:10.1016/j.amjsurg.2006.01.045.

[25] Mitchell P. J., Ravi S., Grifftiths B., Reid F., Speake D., Midgley C., et al. Multicentre review of lymph node harvest in colorectal cancer: are we understaging colorectal cancer patients? *Int J Colorectal Dis. 2009*;24:915–921. doi:10.1007/s00384-009-0697-z.

[26] van der Pas M. H., Meijer S., Hoekstra O. S., Riphagen I. I., de Vet H. C. W., Knol D. L., et al. Sentinel-lymph-node procedure in colon and rectal cancer: a systematic review and meta-analysis. *Lancet Oncol. 2011*;12:540–550. doi:10.1016/S1470-2045(11)70075-4.

[27] Bilchik A., Nissan A., Wainberg Z., Shen P., McCarter M., Protic M., et al. Surgical quality and nodal ultrastaging is associated with long-term disease-free survival in early colorectal cancer: an analysis of 2 international multicenter prospective trials. *Annals of surgery. 2010*;252:467–74; discussion 474–6. doi: 10.1097/SLA.0b013e3181f19767.

[28] Bilchik A. J., Hoon D. S. B., Saha S., Turner R. R., Wiese D., DiNome M., et al. Prognostic impact of micrometastases in colon cancer: interim results of a prospective multicenter trial. *Ann Surg. 2007*;246:568–75; discussion 575–7. doi: 10.1097/SLA.0b013e318155a9c7.

[29] Rosenberg R., Hoos A., Mueller J., Baier P., Stricker D., Werner M., et al. Prognostic significance of cytokeratin-20 reverse transcriptase polymerase chain reaction in lymph nodes of node-negative colorectal cancer patients. *J Clin Oncol. 2002*; 20:1049–1055. doi:10.1200/JCO.2002.20.4.1049.

[30] Koyanagi K., Bilchik A. J., Saha S., Turner R. R., Wiese D., McCarter M., et al. Prognostic relevance of occult nodal micrometastases and circulating tumor cells in colorectal cancer in a prospective multicenter trial. *Clin Cancer Res. 2008*;14:7391–7396. doi:10.1158/1078-0432.CCR-08-0290.

[31] Iddings D., Ahmad A., Elashoff D., Bilchik A., The prognostic effect of micrometastases in previously staged lymph node negative (N0) colorectal carcinoma: a meta-analysis. *Ann Surg Oncol. 2006*;13:1386–1392. doi:10.1245/s10434-006-9120-y.

[32] Sloothaak D. A. M., Sahami S., van der Zaag-Loonen H. J., van der Zaag E. S., Tanis P. J., Bemelman W. A., et al. The prognostic value of micrometastases and isolated

tumour cells in histologically negative lymph nodes of patients with colorectal cancer: a systematic review and meta-analysis. *Eur J Surg Oncol. 2014*;40:263–269. doi:10.1016/j.ejso.2013.12.002.

[33] Messerini L., Cianchi F., Cortesini C., Comin C. E. Incidence and prognostic significance of occult tumor cells in lymph nodes from patients with stage IIA colorectal carcinoma. *Hum Pathol. 2006*;37:1259–1267. doi:10.1016/j.humpath.2006.04.023.

[34] Bukholm I. R. K., Bondi J., Wiik P., Nesland J. M., Andersen S. N., Bakka A., et al. Presence of isolated tumour cells in mesenteric lymph nodes predicts poor prognosis in patients with stage II colon cancer. *Eur J Surg Oncol. 2003*;29:862–866.

[35] Rahbari N. N., Bork U., Motschall E., Thorlund K., Büchler M. W., Koch M., et al. Molecular detection of tumor cells in regional lymph nodes is associated with disease recurrence and poor survival in node-negative colorectal cancer: a systematic review and meta-analysis. *J Clin Oncol. 2012*;30:60–70. doi:10.1200/JCO.2011.36.9504.

[36] Joosten J. J., Strobbe L. J., Wauters C. A., Pruszczynski M., Wobbes T., Ruers T. J., Intraoperative lymphatic mapping and the sentinel node concept in colorectal carcinoma. *Br J Surg. 1999*;86:482–486. doi:10.1046/j.1365-2168.1999.01051.x.

[37] Paramo J. C., Summerall J., Wilson C., Cabral A., Willis I., Wodnicki H., et al. Intraoperative sentinel lymph node mapping in patients with colon cancer. *Am J Surg. 2001*;182:40–43.

[38] Tuech J. J., Pessaux P., Regenet N., Bergamaschi R., Colson A. Sentinel lymph node mapping in colon cancer. *Surg Endosc. 2004*;18:1721–1729. doi:10.1007/s00464-004-9031-6.

[39] Redston M., Compton C. C., Miedema B. W., Niedzwiecki D., Dowell J. M., Jewell S. D., et al. Analysis of micrometastatic disease in sentinel lymph nodes from resectable colon cancer: results of Cancer and Leukemia Group B Trial 80001. *J Clin Oncol. 2006*;24:878–883. doi:10.1200/JCO.2005.03.6038.

[40] Bertagnolli M., Miedema B., Redston M., Dowell J., Niedzwiecki D., Fleshman J., et al. Sentinel node staging of resectable colon cancer: results of a multicenter study. *Ann Surg. 2004*;240:624–8; discussion 628–30.

[41] Wood T. F., Nora D. T., Morton D. L., Turner R. R., Rangel D., Hutchinson W., et al. One hundred consecutive cases of sentinel lymph node mapping in early colorectal carcinoma: detection of missed micrometastases. *J Gastrointest Surg. 2002*;6:322–9; discussion 229–30.

[42] Bembenek A., String A., Gretschel S., Schlag P. M. Technique and clinical consequences of sentinel lymph node biopsy in colorectal cancer. *Surg Oncol. 2008*; 17:183–193. doi:10.1016/j.suronc.2008.05.003.

[43] Stojadinovic A., Nissan A., Protic M., Adair C. F., Prus D., Usaj S., et al. Prospective randomized study comparing sentinel lymph node evaluation with standard pathologic evaluation for the staging of colon carcinoma: results from the United States

Military Cancer Institute Clinical Trials Group Study GI-01. *Annals of surgery. 2007*; 245:846–857. doi:10.1097/01.sla.0000256390.13550.26.

[44] van der Zaag E. S., Bouma W. H., Peters H. M., Bemelman W. A., Buskens C. J., Implications of sentinel lymph node mapping on nodal staging and prognosis in colorectal cancer. *Colorectal Dis. 2012*;14:684–690. doi:10.1111/j.1463-1318.2012.02949.x.

[45] Wong J. H., Steineman S., Calderia C., Bowles J., Namiki T. Ex vivo sentinel node mapping in carcinoma of the colon and rectum. *Ann Surg. 2001*;233:515–521.

[46] Tuech J. J., Pessaux P., Di Fiore F., Nitu V., Lefebure B., Colson A., et al. Sentinel node mapping in colon carcinoma: in-vivo versus ex-vivo approach. *Eur J Surg Oncol. 2006*;32:158–161. doi:10.1016/j.ejso.2005.11.004.

[47] Bilchik A. J., Saha S., Tsioulias G. J., Wood T. F., Morton D. L., Aberrant drainage and missed micrometastases: the value of lymphatic mapping and focused analysis of sentinel lymph nodes in gastrointestinal neoplasms. *Ann Surg Oncol. 2001*;8:82S–85S.

[48] Paramo J. C., Summerall J., Poppiti R., Mesko T. W., Validation of sentinel node mapping in patients with colon cancer. *Ann Surg Oncol. 2002*;9:550–554.

[49] Saha S., Monson K. M., Bilchik A., Beutler T., Dan A. G., Schochet E., et al. Comparative analysis of nodal upstaging between colon and rectal cancers by sentinel lymph node mapping: a prospective trial. *Dis Colon Rectum. 2004*;47:1767–1772.

[50] Wakeman C., Yu V., Chandra R., Staples M., Wale R., McLean C., et al. Lymph node yield following injection of patent blue V dye into colorectal cancer specimens. *Colorectal Dis. 2011*;13:e266–e269. doi:10.1111/j.1463-1318.2011.02673.x.

[51] de Haas R. J., Wicherts D. A., Hobbelink M. G. G., van Diest P. J., Vleggaar F. P., Borel Rinkes I. H. M., et al. Sentinel lymph node mapping in colon cancer using radiocolloid as a single tracer: a feasibility study. *Nucl Med Commun. 2012*;33:832–837. doi:10.1097/MNM.0b013e328353bc0c.

[52] Xiong L., Gazyakan E., Yang W., Engel H., Hünerbein M., Kneser U., et al. Indocyanine green fluorescence-guided sentinel node biopsy: a meta-analysis on detection rate and diagnostic performance. *Eur J Surg Oncol. 2014*;40:843–849. doi: 10.1016/j.ejso.2014.02.228.

[53] de Haas R. J., Wicherts D. A., Hobbelink M. G. G., Borel Rinkes I. H. M., Schipper M. E. I., van der Zee J. A., et al. Sentinel lymph node mapping in colon cancer: current status. *Ann Surg Oncol. 2007*;14:1070–1080. doi:10.1245/s10434-006-9258-7.

[54] Saha S. Selective lymph node mapping in colorectal cancer–a prospective study for impact on staging, limitations and pitfalls. *Cancer Treat Res. 2002*;111:109–116.

[55] Hirche C., Mohr Z., Kneif S., Doniga S., Murawa D., Strik M., et al. Ultrastaging of colon cancer by sentinel node biopsy using fluorescence navigation with indocyanine green. *Int J Colorectal Dis. 2012*;27:319–324. doi:10.1007/s00384-011-1306-5.

[56] Vîlcea I. D., Vasile I., Mirea C. S., Mesina C., Enache S. D., Tenovici M., et al. Sentinel lymph node study in colorectal cancer using serial sectioning and Hematoxylin-Eosin staining: importance and limitations. *Rom J Morphol Embryol. 2011*;52:379–383.

[57] Ceranic M. S., Kecmanovic D. M., Pavlov M. J., Nale D. P., Micev M. T., Kovacevic P. A., et al. Validation and feasibility of ex vivo sentinel lymph node "mapping" by methylene blue in colorectal cancer. *Hepatogastroenterology. 2010*;57:1113–1118.

[58] Retter S. M., Herrmann G., Schiedeck T. H. K., Clinical value of sentinel node mapping in carcinoma of the colon. *Colorectal Dis. 2011*;13:855–859. doi: 10.1111/j.1463-1318.2010.02293.x.

[59] Sommariva A., Donisi P. M., Gnocato B., Vianello R., Stracca Pansa V., Zaninotto G. Factors affecting false-negative rates on ex vivo sentinel lymph node mapping in colorectal cancer. *Eur J Surg Oncol. 2010*;36:130–134. doi:10.1016/j.ejso.2009.06.007.

[60] Finan K. R., Lewis J. S., Winslow E., Mutch M. G., Birnbaum E. H., Fleshman J. W. Ex vivo sentinel lymph node mapping in patients undergoing proctectomy for rectal cancer. *Dis Colon Rectum. 2010*;53:243–250. doi: 10.1007/DCR.0b013e3181c3822b.

[61] Ivanov K., Kolev N., Ignatov V., Madjov R., Intraoperative sentinel lymph node mapping in patients with colorectal cancer. *Hepatogastroenterology. 2009*;56:99–105.

[62] Nordgård O., Oltedal S., Kørner H., Aasprong O. G., Tjensvoll K., Gilje B., et al. Quantitative RT-PCR detection of tumor cells in sentinel lymph nodes isolated from colon cancer patients with an ex vivo approach. *Ann Surg. 2009*;249:602–607. doi: 10.1097/SLA.0b013e31819ec923.

[63] Park J. S., Chang I. T., Park S. J., Kim B. G., Choi Y. S., Cha S. J., et al. Comparison of ex vivo and in vivo injection of blue dye in sentinel lymph node mapping for colorectal cancer. *World J Surg. 2009*;33:539–546. doi:10.1007/s00268-008-9872-6.

[64] van der Zaag E. S., Buskens C. J., Kooij N., Akol H., Peters H. M., Bouma W. H., et al. Improving staging accuracy in colon and rectal cancer by sentinel lymph node mapping: a comparative study. *Eur J Surg Oncol. 2009*;35:1065–1070. doi: 10.1016/j.ejso.2009.02.001.

[65] Dragan R., Nebojsa M., Dejan S., Ivan P., Dragos S., Damir J., et al. Clinical application of sentinel lymph node biopsy for staging, treatment and prognosis of colon and gastric cancer. *Hepatogastroenterology. 2009*;56:1606–1611.

[66] Chan S. H., Ng C., Looi L. M. Intraoperative methylene blue sentinel lymph node mapping in colorectal cancer. *ANZ J Surg. 2008*;78:775–779. doi:10.1111/j.1445-2197.2008.04648.x.

[67] Faerden A. E., Sjo O. H., Sjo O., Andersen S. N., Hauglann B., Nazir N., et al. Sentinel node mapping does not improve staging of lymph node metastasis in colonic cancer. *Dis Colon Rectum. 2008*;51:891–896. doi:10.1007/s10350-007-9185-0.

[68] Bembenek A. E., Rosenberg R., Wagler E., Gretschel S., Sendler A., Siewert J. R., et al. Sentinel lymph node biopsy in colon cancer: a prospective multicenter trial. *Ann Surg. 2007*;245:858–863. doi:10.1097/01.sla.0000250428.46656.7e.

[69] Bianchi P. P., Ceriani C., Rottoli M., Torzilli G., Roncalli M., Spinelli A., et al. Laparoscopic lymphatic mapping and sentinel lymph node detection in colon cancer: technical aspects and preliminary results. *Surg Endosc. 2007*;21:1567–1571. doi: 10.1007/s00464-006-9152-1.

[70] Kelder W., Braat A. E., Karrenbeld A., Grond J. A. K., De Vries J. E., Oosterhuis J. W. A., et al. The sentinel node procedure in colon carcinoma: a multi-centre study in The Netherlands. *Int J Colorectal Dis. 2007*;22:1509. doi:10.1007/s00384-007-0351-6.

[71] Liberale G., Lasser P., Sabourin J. C., Malka D., Duvillard P., Elias D., et al. Sentinel lymph nodes of colorectal carcinoma: reappraisal of 123 cases. *Gastroenterol Clin Biol. 2007*;31:281–285.

[72] Matter M., Winckler M., Aellen S., Bouzourene H. Detection of metastatic disease with sentinel lymph node dissection in colorectal carcinoma patients. *Eur J Surg Oncol. 2007*;33:1183–1190. doi:10.1016/j.ejso.2007.03.019.

[73] Tiffet O., Kaczmarek D., Chambonnière M. L., Guillan T., Baccot S., Prévot N., et al. Combining radioisotopic and blue-dye technique does not improve the false-negative rate in sentinel lymph node mapping for colorectal cancer. *Dis Colon Rectum. 2007*; 50:962–970. doi:10.1007/s10350-007-0236-3.

[74] van Schaik P. M., van der Linden J. C., Ernst M. F., Gelderman W. A. H., Bosscha K. Ex vivo sentinel lymph node "mapping" in colorectal cancer. *Eur J Surg Oncol. 2007*;33:1177–1182. doi:10.1016/j.ejso.2007.03.006.

[75] Yagci G., Unlu A., Kurt B., Can M. F., Kaymakcioglu N., Cetiner S., et al. Detection of micrometastases and skip metastases with ex vivo sentinel node mapping in carcinoma of the colon and rectum. *Int J Colorectal Dis. 2007*;22:167–173. doi: 10.1007/s00384-006-0132-7.

[76] Saha S., Sehgal R., Seghal R., Patel M., Doan K., Dan A., et al. A multicenter trial of sentinel lymph node mapping in colorectal cancer: prognostic implications for nodal staging and recurrence. *Am J Surg. 2006*;191:305–310. doi: 10.1016/j.amjsurg.2005.10.028.

[77] Thomas K. A., Lechner J., Shen P., Waters G. S., Geisinger K. R., Levine E. A. Use of sentinel node mapping for cancer of the colon: 'to map or not to map". *Am Surg. 2006*;72:606–11; discussion 611–2.

[78] Bell S. W., Mourra N., Fléjou J. F., Parc R., Tiret E. Ex Vivo Sentinel Lymph Node Mapping in Colorectal Cancer. *Dis Colon Rectum. 2005*;48:74–79. doi: 10.1007/s10350-004-0782-x.

[79] Braat A. E., Oosterhuis J. W. A., Moll F. C. P., de Vries J. E., Wiggers T. Sentinel node detection after preoperative short-course radiotherapy in rectal carcinoma is not reliable. *Br J Surg. 2005*;92:1533–1538. doi:10.1002/bjs.5169.

[80] Khafagy W., El-Dawoody A., El-Ghawalby N., El-Shobaky M., Atwan N. Ultrastaging of Rectal Cancer Based on Identification of Micrometastases in Sentinel Lymph Node. *Coloproctol. 2005*;27:153–160. doi:10.1007/s00053-005-5164-x.

[81] Bertoglio S., Sandrucci S., Percivale P., Goss M., Gipponi M., Moresco L., et al. Prognostic value of sentinel lymph node biopsy in the pathologic staging of colorectal cancer patients. *J Surg Oncol. 2004*;85:166–170. doi:10.1002/jso.20030.

[82] Broderick-Villa G., Amr D., Haigh P. I., O'Connell T. X., Danial T., Difronzo L. A. Ex vivo lymphatic mapping: a technique to improve pathologic staging in colorectal cancer. *Am Surg. 2004*;70:937–941.

[83] Patten L. C., Berger D. H., Rodriguez-Bigas M., Mansfield P., Delpassand E., Cleary K. R., et al. A prospective evaluation of radiocolloid and immunohistochemical staining in colon carcinoma lymphatic mapping. *Cancer. 2004*;100:2104–2109. doi: 10.1002/cncr.20233.

[84] Wong J. H., Johnson D. S., Namiki T., Tauchi-Nishi P. Validation of ex vivo lymphatic mapping in hematoxylin-eosin node-negative carcinoma of the colon and rectum. *Ann Surg Oncol. 2004*;11:772–777. doi:10.1245/ASO.2004.11.026.

[85] Viehl C. T., Hamel C. T., Marti W. R., Guller U., Eisner L., Stammberger U., et al. Identification of sentinel lymph nodes in colon cancer depends on the amount of dye injected relative to tumor size. *World J Surg. 2003*;27:1285–1290. doi: 10.1007/s00268-003-7086-5.

[86] Bendavid Y., Latulippe J. F., Younan R. J., Leclerc Y. E., Dube S., Heyen F., et al. Phase I study on sentinel lymph node mapping in colon cancer: a preliminary report. *J Surg Oncol. 2002*;79:81–4; discussion 85.

[87] Cox E. D., Kellicut D., Adair C., Marley K., Otchy D. P., Peoples G. E. Sentinel lymph node evaluation is technically feasible and may improve staging in colorectal cancer. *Curr Surg. 2002*;59:301–306.

[88] Fitzgerald T. L., Khalifa M. A., Al Zahrani M., Law C. H. L., Smith A. J. Ex vivo sentinel lymph node biopsy in colorectal cancer: a feasibility study. *J Surg Oncol. 2002*;80:27–32; discussion 33. doi:10.1002/jso.10091.

[89] Gandy C. P., Biddlestone L. R., Roe A. M., O'Leary D. P. Intra-operative injection of Patent Blue V dye to facilitate nodal staging in colorectal cancer. *Colorectal Dis. 2002*;4:447–449.

[90] Esser S., Reilly W. T., Riley L. B., Eyvazzadeh C., Arcona S. The role of sentinel lymph node mapping in staging of colon and rectal cancer. *Dis Colon Rectum. 2001*; 44:850–4; discussion 854–6.

[91] Covarelli P., Cristofani R., Boselli C., Servoli A., Burattini M. F., Badolato M., et al. Preliminary study on radioguided sentinel node identification in colon cancer. *Am Surg. 2007*;73:222–226.

[92] Dahl K., Westlin J., Kraaz W., Winqvist O., Bergkvist L., Thörn M. Identification of sentinel nodes in patients with colon cancer. *Eur J Surg Oncol. 2005*;31:381–385. doi:10.1016/j.ejso.2004.12.015.

[93] Lim S. J., Feig B. W., Wang H., Hunt K. K., Rodriguez-Bigas M. A., Skibber J. M., et al. Sentinel lymph node evaluation does not improve staging accuracy in colon cancer. *Ann Surg Oncol. 2008*;15:46–51. doi:10.1245/s10434-007-9629-8.

[94] Merrie A. E., van Rij A. M., Phillips L. V., Rossaak J. I., Yun K., Mccall J. L. Diagnostic use of the sentinel node in colon cancer. *Dis Colon Rectum. 2001*;44:410–417.

[95] Quadros C. A., Lopes A., Araujo I., Fregnani J. H., Fahel F. Upstaging benefits and accuracy of sentinel lymph node mapping in colorectal adenocarcinoma nodal staging. *J Surg Oncol. 2008*;98:324–330. doi:10.1002/jso.21112.

[96] Sandrucci S., Mussa B., Goss M., Mistrangelo M., Satolli M. A., Sapino A., et al. Lymphoscintigraphic localization of sentinel node in early colorectal cancer: results of a monocentric study. *J Surg Oncol. 2007*;96:464–469. doi:10.1002/jso.20848.

[97] Terwisscha Van Scheltinga S. E. J., Den Boer F. C., Pijpers R., Meyer G. A., Engel A. F., Silvis R., et al. Sentinel node staging in colon carcinoma: value of sentinel lymph node biopsy with radiocolloid and blue staining. *Scand J Gastroenterol Suppl. 2006*;153–157. doi:10.1080/00365520600664524.

[98] Bembenek A., Rau B., Moesta T., Markwardt J., Ulmer C., Gretschel S., et al. Sentinel lymph node biopsy in rectal cancer–not yet ready for routine clinical use. *Surgery. 2004*;135:498–505; discussion 506–7. doi:10.1016/j.surg.2003.10.004.

[99] Hladík P., Vizd'a J., Hadzi Nikolov D., Dvorák J., Voboril Z. Radio-guided sentinel node detection during the surgical treatment of rectal cancer. *Nucl Med Commun. 2005*;26:977–982.

[100] Kitagawa Y., Watanabe M., Hasegawa H., Yamamoto S., Fujii H., Yamamoto K., et al. Sentinel node mapping for colorectal cancer with radioactive tracer. *Dis Colon Rectum. 2002*;45:1476–1480. doi:10.1097/01.DCR.0000029592.14749.74.

[101] Kusano M., Tajima Y., Yamazaki K., Kato M., Watanabe M., Miwa M. Sentinel node mapping guided by indocyanine green fluorescence imaging: a new method for sentinel node navigation surgery in gastrointestinal cancer. *Dig Surg. 2008*;25:103–108. doi:10.1159/000121905.

[102] Liberale G., Vankerckhove S., Galdon M. G., Donckier V., Larsimont D., Bourgeois P. Fluorescence imaging after intraoperative intravenous injection of indocyanine green for detection of lymph node metastases in colorectal cancer. *Eur J Surg Oncol. 2015*;41:1256–1260. doi:10.1016/j.ejso.2015.05.011.

[103] Handgraaf H. J. M., Boogerd L. S. F., Verbeek F. P. R., Tummers Q. R. J. G., Hardwick J. C. H., Baeten C. I. M., et al. Intraoperative fluorescence imaging to localize tumors and sentinel lymph nodes in rectal cancer. *Minim Invasive Ther Allied Technol. 2016*;25:48–53. doi:10.3109/13645706.2015.1042389.

[104] Nishigori N., Koyama F., Nakagawa T., Nakamura S., Ueda T., Inoue T., et al. Visualization of Lymph/Blood Flow in Laparoscopic Colorectal Cancer Surgery by ICG Fluorescence Imaging (Lap-IGFI). *Ann Surg Oncol. 2016*;23 Suppl 2:S266–S274. doi:10.1245/s10434-015-4509-0.

[105] Noura S., Ohue M., Seki Y., Tanaka K., Motoori M., Kishi K., et al. Feasibility of a lateral region sentinel node biopsy of lower rectal cancer guided by indocyanine green using a near-infrared camera system. *Ann Surg Oncol. 2010*;17:144–151. doi: 10.1245/s10434-009-0711-2.

[106] Cahill R. A., Anderson M., Wang L. M., Lindsey I., Cunningham C., Mortensen N. J. Near-infrared (NIR) laparoscopy for intraoperative lymphatic road-mapping and sentinel node identification during definitive surgical resection of early-stage colorectal neoplasia. *Surg Endosc. 2012*;26:197–204. doi:10.1007/s00464-011-1854-3.

[107] Viehl C. T., Guller U., Langer I., Laffer U., Oertli D., Zuber M. Factors influencing the success of in vivo sentinel lymph node procedure in colon cancer patients: Swiss prospective, multicenter study sentinel lymph node procedure in colon cancer. *World J Surg. 2013*;37:873–877. doi:10.1007/s00268-013-1910-3.

[108] Cahill R. A., Bembenek A., Sirop S., Waterhouse D. F., Schneider W., Leroy J., et al. Sentinel node biopsy for the individualization of surgical strategy for cure of early-stage colon cancer. *Ann Surg Oncol. 2009*;16:2170–2180. doi:10.1245/s10434-009-0510-9.

[109] Trocha S. D., Nora D. T., Saha S. S., Morton D. L., Wiese D., Bilchik A. J. Combination probe and dye-directed lymphatic mapping detects micrometastases in early colorectal cancer. *J Gastrointest Surg. 2003*;7:340–5; discussion 345–6.

[110] Nagata K., Endo S., Hidaka E., Tanaka J. I., Kudo S. E., Shiokawa A. Laparoscopic sentinel node mapping for colorectal cancer using infrared ray laparoscopy. *Anticancer Res. 2006*;26:2307–2311.

[111] Watanabe J., Ota M., Suwa Y., Ishibe A., Masui H., Nagahori K. Evaluation of lymph flow patterns in splenic flexural colon cancers using laparoscopic real-time indocyanine green fluorescence imaging. *Int J Colorectal Dis. 2017*;32:201–207. doi:10.1007/s00384-016-2669-4.

[112] Liberale G., Vankerckhove S., Caldon M. G., Ahmed B., Moreau M., Nakadi I. E., et al. Fluorescence Imaging After Indocyanine Green Injection for Detection of Peritoneal Metastases in Patients Undergoing Cytoreductive Surgery for Peritoneal Carcinomatosis From Colorectal Cancer: A Pilot Study. *Ann Surg. 2016*;264:1110–1115. doi:10.1097/SLA.0000000000001618.

[113] Viehl C. T., Guller U., Cecini R., Langer I., Ochsner A., Terracciano L., et al. Sentinel lymph node procedure leads to upstaging of patients with resectable colon cancer: results of the Swiss prospective, multicenter study sentinel lymph node procedure in colon cancer. *Ann Surg Oncol. 2012*;19:1959–1965. doi:10.1245/s10434-012-2233-6.

[114] Cahill R. A. What's wrong with sentinel node mapping in colon cancer? *World J Gastroenterol. 2007*;13:6291–6294.

In: The Sentinel Lymph Node
Editors: A. Londero, S. Bertozzi and C. Cedolini
ISBN: 978-1-53614-557-1


*Chapter 16*

# LIVER LYMPHATICS, SENTINEL NODE MAPPING AND POSSIBLE CLINICAL APPLICATIONS OF SENTINEL LYMPH NODE BIOPSY IN LIVER SURGERY

***Luca Roncati**, Massimo Lupi, Chiara Cavatorta and Antonio Manenti***
From the Departments of Pathology and Surgery,
University Hospital of Modena, Modena (MO), Italy

**Abstract**

A great amount of lymph is produced daily by a normal liver, thanks to the high porosity of the hepatic sinusoids, which allows an easy passage of fluids and other plasma components into the Disse's spaces. The proximity to the distal lymphatic capillaries induces a lymph flow that is conveyed to the Glissonian sheath and, subsequently, outside the liver parenchyma, to different lymph nodal stations located in the perihepatic region. In the case of liver diseases, mainly cirrhosis, this basic mechanism is subverted by the "capillarization" of the hepatic sinusoids, which no longer retain their proper permeability. In addition, the absence of proper valves in the lymphatic vessels of the portal pedicle allowing a double current flow and extended interconnections between different lymph nodal stations explain the onset of "skip" metastases. These features oppose the routine implementation of the sentinel lymph node biopsy in tumors of the liver, hepatic hilum and hepatic pedicle.

**Keywords:** sentinel lymph node, liver, hepatic pedicle, skip metastases, cirrhosis, liver tumor, podoplanin, tertiary lymphatic organs

## 1. Introduction

The practical value and perspectives of sentinel lymph node biopsy (SLNB) in liver and biliary tract diseases, as in many other organs, are directly correlated with the pathophysiological aspects of the respective lymphatic apparatus and drainage. The absence of an

*Corresponding Author E-mail: emailmedical@gmail.com.

already implemented and well-tested policy of SLNB procedure in diseases of the liver and biliary system reflects the particular anatomo-functional conditions of this district.

## 2. Anatomopathological Aspects of Liver Lymphatics and District Lymph Circulation

It is well-known that a large amount of lymph is produced daily by liver thanks to the high degree of permeability of its sinusoids, allowing the hepatocytes to metabolize many substances absorbed by the intestinal apparatus [1]. At the periphery of the hepatic lobule, in the Mall's space, the sinusoids come in contact with the lymphatic capillaries, enabling a process of nutrient absorption and lymph production [1]. Within the entire liver parenchyma, most lymphatic capillaries converge toward the Glissonian sheath, while others flow into larger peripheral pre-collectors and, subsequently, into collector channels, located inside the vasculo-biliary sheaths above and also within the liver hilum, where proper lymph nodes are also found [2, 3]. Therefore, the lymphatic system of the liver parenchyma can be distinguished into three interconnecting sectors: a first peripheral one, located below the liver surface; a second central one located in the "hepatic core", which has a predominant size and drains most of the liver; and a third one just above the hilar region [4, 5, 6]. Outside the Glissonian sheath of the liver, the lymphatic vessels run through the liver ligaments to the corresponding extra-hepatic lymph nodes, located at the hepatic hilum, in the hepatic pedicle, in the neighbouring districts of the upper abdomen and also in the mediastinum [2, 3]. The latter are placed along the internal thoracic arteries, the oesophagus and the tracheo-bronchial tree. Other posterior intra-hepatic lymphatic vessels drain directly into the lymph nodes located around the intra-thoracic inferior vena cava.

The central hepatic and supra-hilar lymphatics are connected with the lymph nodes of the hepatic hilum, the hepatic pedicle and with those located along the proper hepatic artery, the common hepatic artery, the celiac trunk, and with those around the pancreatic head [7, 1].

It is noteworthy that in the lymphatic vessels at the hepatic hilum or the hepatic pedicle, no proper valves can be found with light microscopy [3]. This explains a possible double direction of the lymph flow from and towards the hepatic hilum, depending on the different pathophysiological conditions, and under the action of different forces, such as positive intra-abdominal pressure, diaphragm movements, tension within the lymphatic channels, etc. [3, 8]. All these characteristics outline the hepatic lymphatic network as a widely open system with multiple interconnections, equipped with absorbent lymphatics and collectors as in other organs [9, 10]. In oncology, considering the possible passage of neoplastic cells into the lymphatic flow through the capillary walls, the onset of distant and unexpected metastases can be easily explained [9]. Additionally, in the case of obstructive jaundice, part of the conjugated bilirubin passes abnormally from the hepatocytes into the Disse's spaces and, subsequently, into the lymphatic capillaries at the periphery of the hepatic lobules; thus, the hepatic lymphatic system acts as a collateral drainage for conjugated bilirubin from the liver to the systemic circulation [11].

Hepatic cirrhosis induces the "capillarization" of the hepatic sinusoids, which lose their particular fenestration and acquire a basal membrane. Their internal pressure increases proportionally to the portal hypertension, whilst their permeability, compared to that of the normal hepatic sinusoids, is greatly reduced, due to the interchanges with the hepatocytes [12, 13, 14, 15]. Therefore, as in several other organs, the lymphatic production process originates from an absorption mechanism of the interstitial fluid, ultra-filtrated from the capillaries in quantities proportional to the hepato-portal vein gradient, typically increased in cirrhosis [16]. In addition, the abnormal architecture of the cirrhotic parenchyma also involves the lymphatic system, with an absolute scarcity of lymphatic capillaries at the periphery of the neo-lobules [17]. As a result, the ultra-filtrated capillary fluid flows in the interstitial spaces outside any vascular structure, before being absorbed by the lymphatic capillaries, which are mainly present at the periphery of the liver parenchyma (Figures 1 and 2), where they appear overcharged due to the abnormally reduced number of other draining lymphatic structures, such as the pre-collector and collector pre-lymph nodal vessels. This condition can be followed by the onset of lymphatic pools inside the Glissonian sheath, visible as white to translucent spots protruding on the liver surface [18]. Based on our experience, they can spill lymph directly into the peritoneum [16].

In addition, the progressive surcharge of the lymphatic stations at the periphery of the cirrhotic liver, correlated with the grade of parenchymal fibrosis and portal hypertension, has a corresponding impact on the lymphatic structures, collector channels and lymph nodes of the liver hilum and hepatic pedicle. This is also reflected in other lymphatic structures located in the adjacent peritoneal or retroperitoneal districts, where a volumetric enlargement and fibrosis of the corresponding lymph nodes can be observed. This lymph dynamic condition aggravates the overfilling of the splanchnic micro-circulation, already present in hepatic cirrhosis, thus favouring the onset or increase of ascites, sometimes even chylous [19, 20].

In oncology, the presence of lymphatic capillaries also in the submucosa of the common bile duct explains the possible precocious lymphatic diffusion of cholangiocarcinoma, and the consequent policy of extending the margins of surgical resection beyond 1 cm (Figure 3). In addition, the lymphatic collectors of the hepatic pedicle, connected to other abdominal stations and completely devoid of valvular structures (Figure 4), justify the onset of "skip" metastatic lymph nodal lesions, often unexpected [21]. With the same mechanism, metastases, even from distant organs, may be able to involve and infiltrate the lymph nodes of the hepatic pedicle with its obstruction and subsequent cholestatic jaundice [22].

All these particular morpho-functional features of the lymphatic circulation of the liver, under normal and pathological conditions, are in contrast with the practice of SLNB, which is based on a constant and topographically regular flow of lymph from each individual organ or part of it to a single nodal station.

## 3. Anatomical Levels of Liver Lymph Nodes

A clear and universally accepted systematization of the different lymph nodal stations related to the lymphatics of the liver or hepatic pedicle has not yet been implemented, which is essential before validating any SLNB procedure [23].

On the basis of a simple topographic criterion, we propose to consider as first-level the lymph nodes at the hepatic hilum, placed above or around the portal bifurcation, just below the hilar plate together with the corresponding arterial, venous and biliary branches.

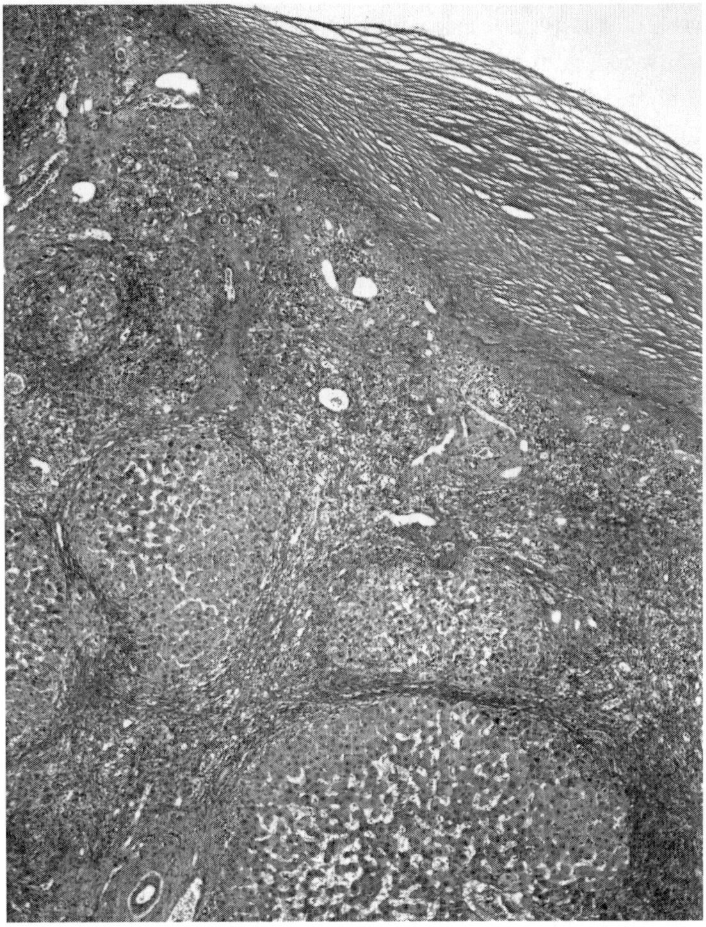

Figure 1. Cirrhotic liver with clearly visible regenerative nodules and ectasic lymphatic spaces, optically empty, just beneath Glisson's fibrous capsule (PAS diastase stain; objective: 4x).

Similarly, the lymph nodes along the falciform ligament can be ascribed to the same first-level. Conversely, the lymph nodes present in the hepatic pedicle and wrapped by the fine peritoneal sheath of the hepato-duodenal ligament can be classified as second-level. The other lymph nodal stations, which accompany the common hepatic, the celiac, the pyloric, the gastro-duodenal and the pancreato-duodenal arteries, represent third-level stations, such as those located around the abdominal oesophagus and cardias.

The lymph nodes of the right renal vein, the lumbo-aortic ones and those around the inferior vena cava or abdominal aorta are considered distant lymphatic stations, being located in the retroperitoneum and directly connected with the main lymphatic outflow pathways from the abdomen. Their secondary neoplastic involvement can be referred to distant metastases.

In any case, the current interest in SLNB in oncological surgery of the liver and biliary tract is justified by the good results obtained in the corresponding diseases of other organs, such as breast and skin [24, 25, 26, 27, 28], where lymphadenectomy has definite

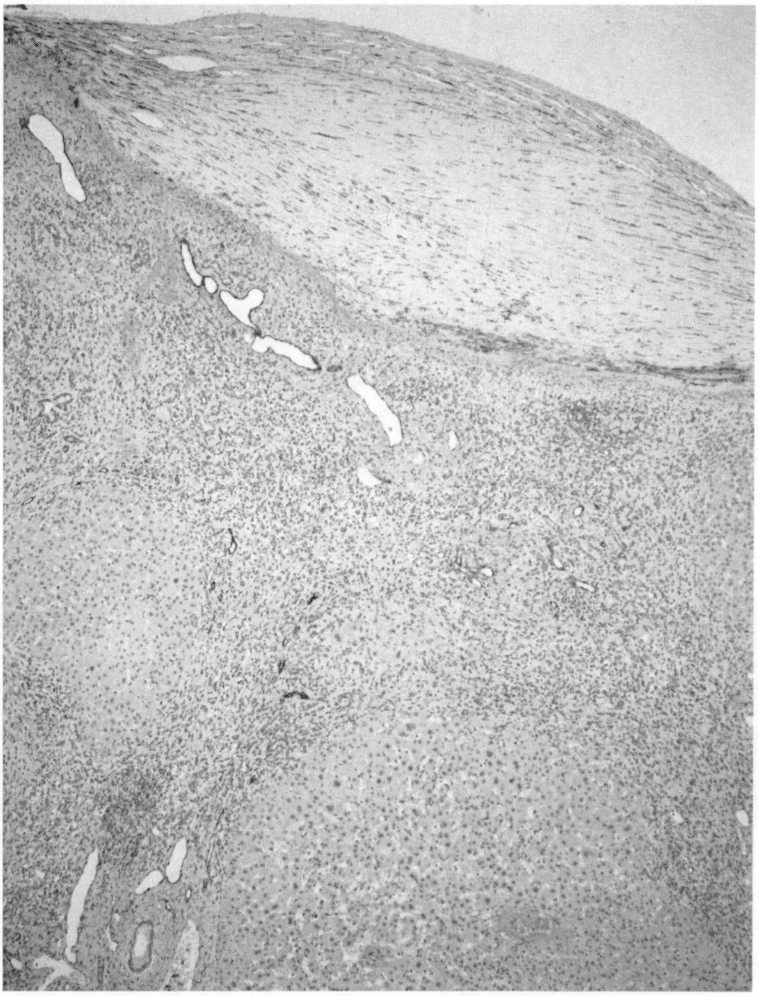

Figure 2. Same photographic field of Figure 1: the ectasic lymphatics are brown-stained by immunohistochemistry for the transmembrane mucoprotein podoplanin, expressed selectively in the lymphatic endothelium (clone: D2-40 Ventana; chromogen: 3,3' diaminobenzidine tetrahydrochloride hydrate; objective: 4x).

indications and can be performed according to precise anatomical criteria. All this leads to a better staging of each neoplastic disease and avoids unnecessary surgical dissections.

This is not the case of many abdominal and intra-thoracic surgical procedures, where there are multiple ways of lymph drainage, which avoid the danger of congestion of the upstream lymphatic pathways [29]. The chylous thorax, a specific complication of mediastinal lymphadenectomy, is rare and, usually, secondary to the injury of the main thoracic duct, rather than to an extended lymphadenectomy. In abdominal surgery, the corresponding complication is represented by chylous ascites, which is usually self-limiting and often followed by spontaneous resolution.

However, it is generally accepted that lymphadenectomy of the hepatic pedicle allows a better staging of tumors of the liver or its hilum [30]. On the contrary, its therapeutic

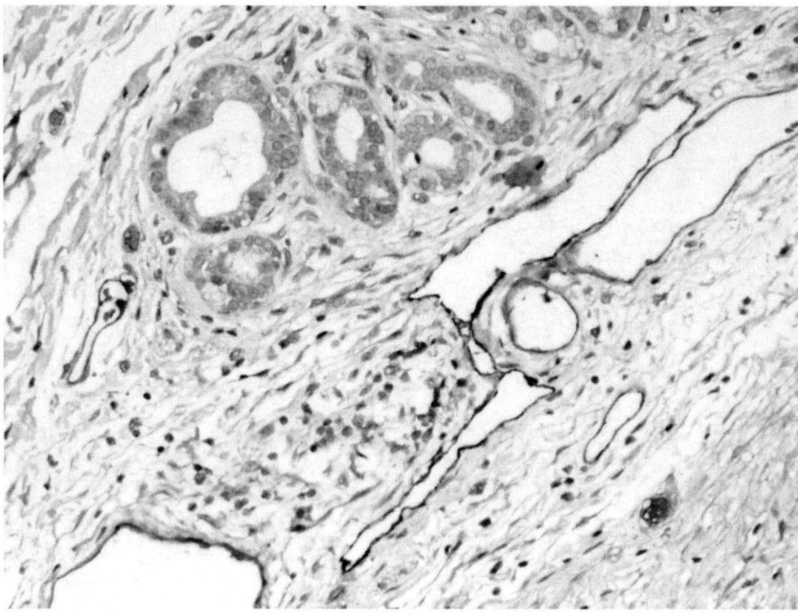

Figure 3. Dilated lymphatics capillary not containing erythrocytes in the submucosa of the common bile duct, brown-stained by immunohistochemistry for podoplanin (clone: D2-40 Ventana; chromogen: 3,3' diaminobenzidine tetrahydrochloride hydrate; objective: 20x), near adjacent to blood capillaries fuchsia-stained by immunohistochemistry for CD31, the well-known specific marker of hematic endothelia (clone: JC70 Ventana; chromogen: new fuchsin; objective: 20x).

advantage has not yet been proven, according to most authors [31, 32, 33, 34, 35, 36, 37, 38, 39]. Moreover, it is difficult to achieve a radical "en bloc" resection of the hilar lymphatic structures [40], due to the absence of a proper sheath, other than the thin peritoneal layer of the hepatic pedicle, the multiple interconnections with proximal lymph node stations and the proximity to vital structures, such as the portal vein, the proper hepatic artery and the common bile duct.

## 4. Ways of Diffusion of District Lymphatic Metastases

In addition to a rigid topographic classification, other characteristics of lymphatic metastases can be considered as indicative tool for better staging liver or hepatic pedicle tumors. It is important to outline that there is a remarkable difference between a limited localization of neoplastic cells within the parenchyma of a lymph node from its extensive invasion, mainly with the involvement of its capsule, of the adjacent areolar tissue or, even, the surrounding peritoneal sheath. Furthermore, the discovery of aggregates of neoplastic cells inside the lymphatic vessels, capillaries, pre-collectors and collectors indicates their great lymphatic tropism in a system devoid of proper valves and with multiple and unexpected ways of diffusion. We must also consider, as for other important lymphatic districts, the development of new "tertiary" lymphatic organs under the action of different neoplastic or

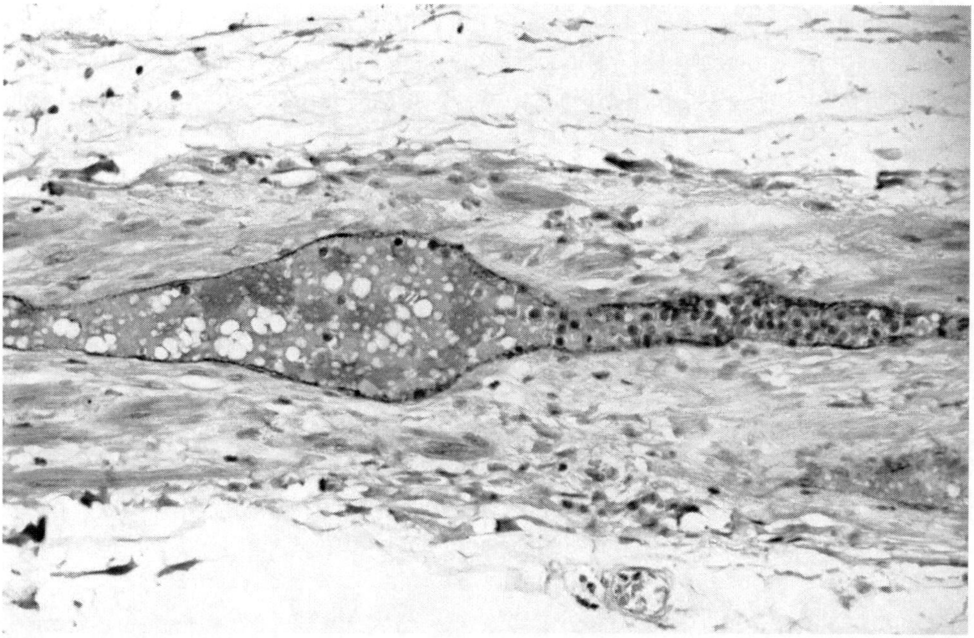

Figure 4. A collector lymphatic of the hepatic pedicle, brown-stained by immunohistochemistry for podoplanin, completely devoid of valvular structures (clone: D2-40 Ventana; chromogen: 3,3' diaminobenzidine tetrahydrochloride hydrate; objective: 40x).

inflammatory stimuli [41, 42, 43].

They are little-known lymphatic structures, typically containing a much lower number of lymphocytes imported from blood and lymph, which can be found theoretically in any abdominal or extra-abdominal site; within the peritoneal cavity, especially in the greater omentum, they have been described by the figurative term of "milky spots" [44]. The aforementioned anatomical and pathophysiological observations outline the real limits to the SLNB procedure in tumors of the liver and its hilum. On the other hand, they explain the possible onset of "skip" or "micro-skip" metastases, the detection of "in-transit" aggregates of neoplastic cells in the lymphatic capillaries and the involvement of "tertiary" lymphatic organs.

## 5. Sentinel Node Mapping and Possible Clinical Applications of Sentinel Node Biopsy in Liver Surgery

Clearly, the technique of SLNB should usefully precede any lymphadenectomy procedure and complete any surgical exploration. However, a negative result does not absolutely exclude the possible presence of distant or unexpected lymphatic metastases. In any case, the dissection of the first-level stations, if anatomically easily performed, can be considered a precautionary measure.

In practice, in the case of a hepatic tumor, the preferred site of injection may correspond to the space surrounding the tumor, where open lymphatic channels can be found.

This manoeuvre can be performed directly or under ultrasound control, using methylene or isosulfan blue dye as tracers [45]. The stained lymph node is excised and subjected to an intraoperative pathological examination in order to assess any subsequent surgical steps.

## Conclusion

The SLNB procedure is based on an adequate lymphatic network, capable of absorbing tracer into or around the tumor, a valid system of collecting vessels relative to the lymph nodes belonging to a single or, alternatively, two contiguous stations. In the case of liver tumors, especially those associated with cirrhosis, or hepatic pedicle tumors, these conditions are not encountered.

A fortiori, we advise surgeons to perform a detailed diagnostic study and staging of each hepato-biliary tumour, nowadays facilitated by cross-sectional imaging. Therefore, it is to be considered the specific pros and cons of any surgical step, including the SLNB procedure, also based on the surgical anatomy of each case. Even today, in hepato-biliary diseases, the SLNB procedure requires further basic and clinical researches.

## References

[1] Ohtani O., Ohtani Y., Lymph circulation in the liver. *Anat Rec (Hoboken). 2008*; 291:643–652. doi:10.1002/ar.20681.

[2] Roncati L., Manenti A., Zizzo M., Farinetti A. Re: Anatomy of hepatic lymphatics and its implications in hepatic malignancies. *ANZ J Surg. 2017*;87:103–104. doi: 10.1111/ans.13829.

[3] Manenti A., Roncati L., Barbolini G., Rivasi F. Lymphatic network of the common bile duct. *Webmed Central Pathology. 2012*;3:WMC002983. doi: 10.9754/journal.wmc.2012.002983.

[4] Manenti A., Roncati L., Farinetti A., Zizzo M. The "Hepatic Core": How to Reach It. *J Am Coll Surg. 2016*;223:542. doi:10.1016/j.jamcollsurg.2016.05.016.

[5] Roncati L., Manenti A., Simonini E. Image-Guided Proper Liver Segmentectomy. *World J Surg. 2018*;42:1857–1859. doi:10.1007/s00268-017-4397-5.

[6] Manenti A., Roncati L., Simonini E., Farinetti A. HCC chemoembolization: Still a challenge. *Clin Res Hepatol Gastroenterol. 2017*;41:e14–e16. doi: 10.1016/j.clinre.2016.07.003.

[7] Akishima Y., Ito K., Zhang L., Ishikawa Y., Orikasa H., Kiguchi H., et al. Immunohistochemical detection of human small lymphatic vessels under normal and pathological conditions using the LYVE-1 antibody. *Virchows Arch. 2004*;444:153–157. doi:10.1007/s00428-003-0950-8.

[8] Breslin J. W. Mechanical forces and lymphatic transport. *Microvasc Res. 2014*;96:46–54. doi:10.1016/j.mvr.2014.07.013.

[9] Azzali G. Tumor cell transendothelial passage in the absorbing lymphatic vessel of transgenic adenocarcinoma mouse prostate. *Am J Pathol. 2007*;170:334–346. doi: 10.2353/ajpath.2007.060447.

[10] Roncati L., Barbolini G., Pusiol T., Piscioli F., Maiorana A. New advances on placental hydrops and related villous lymphatics. *Lymphology. 2015*;48:28–37.

[11] Szabó G., Magyar Z., Szentirmai A., Jakab F., Mihaly K. Bile constituents in blood and lymph during biliary obstruction. II. The absorption and transport of bile acids and bilirubin. *Lymphology. 1975*;8:36–42.

[12] Iwakiri Y. The lymphatic system: A new frontier in hepatology. *Hepatology. 2016*; 64:706–707. doi:10.1002/hep.28650.

[13] Poisson J., Lemoinne S., Boulanger C., Durand F., Moreau R., Valla D., et al. Liver sinusoidal endothelial cells: Physiology and role in liver diseases. *J Hepatol. 2017*; 66:212–227. doi:10.1016/j.jhep.2016.07.009.

[14] Brunt E. M., Gouw A. S. H., Hubscher S. G., Tiniakos D. G., Bedossa P., Burt A. D., et al. Pathology of the liver sinusoids. *Histopathology. 2014*;64:907–920. doi: 10.1111/his.12364.

[15] Greuter T., Shah V. H. Hepatic sinusoids in liver injury, inflammation, and fibrosis: new pathophysiological insights. *J Gastroenterol. 2016*;51:511–519. doi: 10.1007/s00535-016-1190-4.

[16] Manenti A., Roncati L., Barbolini G. The role of lymphatics in portal biliopathy. *J Visc Surg. 2016*;153:81. doi:10.1016/j.jviscsurg.2015.10.009.

[17] Ekataksin W., Kaneda K. Liver microvascular architecture: an insight into the pathophysiology of portal hypertension. *Semin Liver Dis. 1999*;19:359–382. doi:10.1055/s-2007-1007126.

[18] Weickert U., Siegel E., Schilling D., Eickhoff A., Jakobs R., Bohrer M. H., et al. [The diagnosis of liver cirrhosis: a comparative evaluation of standard laparoscopy, mini-laparoscopy and histology]. *Z Gastroenterol. 2005*;43:17–21. doi:10.1055/s-2004-813874.

[19] Chung C., Iwakiri Y. The lymphatic vascular system in liver diseases: its role in ascites formation. *Clin Mol Hepatol. 2013*;19:99–104. doi:10.3350/cmh.2013.19.2.99.

[20] Steinemann D. C., Dindo D., Clavien P. A., Nocito A. Atraumatic chylous ascites: systematic review on symptoms and causes. *J Am Coll Surg. 2011*;212:899–905.e1–4. doi:10.1016/j.jamcollsurg.2011.01.010.

[21] Bonetti L. R., Manenti A., Domati F., Farinetti A. Mesocolic micro-skip metastasis. *Clin Res Hepatol Gastroenterol. 2017*;41:341–343. doi:10.1016/j.clinre.2017.01.007.

[22] Manenti A. [Secondary neoplastic involvement of the hepatic pedicle (author's transl)]. *Sem Hop. 1982*;58:1627–1629.

[23] Miyazaki M., Ohtsuka M., Miyakawa S., Nagino M., Yamamoto M., Kokudo N., et al. Classification of biliary tract cancers established by the Japanese Society of Hepato-Biliary-Pancreatic Surgery: 3(rd) English edition. *J Hepatobiliary Pancreat Sci. 2015*; 22:181–196. doi:10.1002/jhbp.211.

[24] Roncati L., Barbolini G., Piacentini F., Piscioli F., Pusiol T., Maiorana A. Prognostic Factors for Breast Cancer: an Immunomorphological Update. *Pathol Oncol Res. 2016*; 22:449–452. doi:10.1007/s12253-015-0024-7.

[25] Piscioli F., Pusiol T., Roncati L. Higher predictive value of sentinel lymph node biopsy in patients with histological subcategorization of thin melanoma. *Int J Dermatol. 2017*;56:e93–e94. doi:10.1111/ijd.13548.

[26] Piscioli F., Pusiol T., Roncati L. Wisely choosing thin melanomas for sentinel lymph node biopsy. *J Am Acad Dermatol. 2017*;76:e25. doi:10.1016/j.jaad.2016.08.069.

[27] Roncati L., Piscioli F., Pusiol T. Current controversies on sentinel node biopsy in thin and thick cutaneous melanoma. *Eur J Surg Oncol. 2017*;43:506–507. doi: 10.1016/j.ejso.2016.09.014.

[28] Roncati L., Piscioli F., Pusiol T. Sentinel Lymph Node in Thin and Thick Melanoma. *Klin Onkol. 2016*;29:393–394.

[29] Roncati L., Manenti A., Sighinolfi P. Immunohistochemical improvement in the analysis of the lymphatic metastases from lung carcinoma. *Ann Thorac Surg. 2014*;97:380–381. doi:10.1016/j.athoracsur.2013.06.072.

[30] Roncati L., Manenti A., Pavesi E., Piscioli F., Farinetti A., Pusiol T. Surgicopathologic correlations regarding lymphatics in hilar cholangiocarcinoma. *Surgery. 2016*; 159:1483. doi:10.1016/j.surg.2016.01.006.

[31] Nakayama T., Tsuchikawa T., Shichinohe T., Nakamura T., Ebihara Y., Hirano S. Pathological confirmation of para-aortic lymph node status as a potential criterion for the selection of intrahepatic cholangiocarcinoma patients for radical resection with regional lymph node dissection. *World J Surg. 2014*;38:1763–1768. doi: 10.1007/s00268-013-2433-7.

[32] Kambakamba P., Linecker M., Slankamenac K., DeOliveira M. L. Lymph node dissection in resectable perihilar cholangiocarcinoma: a systematic review. *Am J Surg. 2015*;210:694–701. doi:10.1016/j.amjsurg.2015.05.015.

[33] Manenti A., Pavesi E., Farinetti A., Roncati L. For a clearer comprehension of the lymphatic system in perihilar cholangiocarcinoma. *Am J Surg. 2016*;211:493. doi: 10.1016/j.amjsurg.2015.07.014.

[34] Deoliveira M. L., Schulick R. D., Nimura Y., Rosen C., Gores G., Neuhaus P., et al. New staging system and a registry for perihilar cholangiocarcinoma. *Hepatology. 2011*;53:1363–1371. doi:10.1002/hep.24227.

[35] Bradatsch A., Kornprat P., Bacher H., Cerwenka H., Haybaeck J., Mischinger H. J. The Value of Lymph Node Dissection in the Surgery of Colorectal Cancer Liver Metastases. *Anticancer Res. 2016*;36:2993–2997.

[36] Amini N., Ejaz A., Spolverato G., Maithel S. K., Kim Y., Pawlik T. M. Management of lymph nodes during resection of hepatocellular carcinoma and intrahepatic cholangiocarcinoma: a systematic review. *J Gastrointest Surg. 2014*;18:2136–2148. doi:10.1007/s11605-014-2667-1.

[37] Adachi T., Eguchi S. Lymph node dissection for intrahepatic cholangiocarcinoma: a critical review of the literature to date. *J Hepatobiliary Pancreat Sci. 2014*;21:162–168. doi:10.1002/jhbp.30.

[38] Morine Y., Shimada M. The value of systematic lymph node dissection for intrahepatic cholangiocarcinoma from the viewpoint of liver lymphatics. *J Gastroenterol. 2015*;50:913–927. doi:10.1007/s00535-015-1071-2.

[39] Guglielmi A., Ruzzenente A., Campagnaro T., Valdegamberi A., Bagante F., Bertuzzo F., et al. Patterns and prognostic significance of lymph node dissection for surgical treatment of perihilar and intrahepatic cholangiocarcinoma. *J Gastrointest Surg. 2013*; 17:1917–1928. doi:10.1007/s11605-013-2331-1.

[40] Roncati L., Barbolini G., Scacchetti A. T., Busani S., Maiorana A. Unexpected death: anaphylactic intraoperative death due to Thymoglobulin carbohydrate excipient. *Forensic Sci Int. 2013*;228:e28–e32. doi:10.1016/j.forsciint.2013.02.036.

[41] Ruddle N. H. Lymphatic vessels and tertiary lymphoid organs. *J Clin Invest. 2014*; 124:953–959. doi:10.1172/JCI71611.

[42] Ruddle N. H. High Endothelial Venules and Lymphatic Vessels in Tertiary Lymphoid Organs: Characteristics, Functions, and Regulation. *Front Immunol. 2016*;7:491. doi: 10.3389/fimmu.2016.00491.

[43] Pitzalis C., Jones G. W., Bombardieri M., Jones S. A. Ectopic lymphoid-like structures in infection, cancer and autoimmunity. *Nat Rev Immunol. 2014*;14:447–462. doi: 10.1038/nri3700.

[44] Roncati L., Manenti A. Tertiary lymphatic organs of the female pelvis: not negligible structures. *Clin Exp Obstet Gynecol. 2018*;[in press].

[45] Wada H., Hyun H., Vargas C., Genega E. M., Gravier J., Gioux S., et al. Sentinel Lymph Node Mapping of Liver. *Ann Surg Oncol. 2015*;22 Suppl 3:S1147–S1155. doi:10.1245/s10434-015-4601-5.

In: The Sentinel Lymph Node
Editors: A. Londero, S. Bertozzi and C. Cedolini
ISBN: 978-1-53614-557-1


*Chapter 17*

# LESS COMMON APPLICATIONS OF THE SENTINEL LYMPH NODE BIOPSY

***Serena Bertozzi[1]*, Carla Cedolini[1], Luca Seriau[1], Roberta Di Vora[1], Ambrogio P. Londero[2] and Andrea Risaliti[1]***
[1]Breast Unit, Clinic of Surgery, DAME,
University of Udine, University Hospital of Udine, Udine, Italy
[2]Clinic of Obstetrics and Gynecology,
University Hospital of Udine, Udine, Italy

**Abstract**

Sentinel lymph node biopsy is currently indicated in many solid tumors, representing a standard of care in early-stage melanoma, breast, anus, cervix, vulva, endometrium and thyroid cancer, with a relevant impact on prognosis and therapeutic management. In other cancers such as colorectal carcinoma, Sentinel lymph node biopsy may help the pathologist evaluate the first lymph node involved by the lymphatic drainage from the tumor, but it does not prevent complete lymph node dissection. However, many other indications for sentinel lymph node biopsy have been proposed in the literature, including gastric, ovarian and various urological cancers. The main aim of the procedure in these clinical cases is to determine the prognosis and the therapeutic management, while sparing patients from complete lymphadenectomy and its consequent high rate of complications. The techniques used to identify and analyze the sentinel nodes are the same as for other solid tumors. In particular, the combination of technetium-99 and blue dye significantly improves the detection rate, and indocyanine green appears to be very promising either alone, combined or even hybridized with other techniques. The main challenge in solid tumors, described in this chapter, is probably sentinel node localization, due to the high variability of lymphatic drainage patterns in certain intra-abdominal districts. However, the results in terms of detection rate and accuracy are very promising, especially thanks to the constant technical evolution that we are witnessing.

**Keywords:** urologic cancer, gastric cancer, ovarian cancer, sentinel lymph node biopsy

*Corresponding Author E-mail: dr.bertozzi@gmail.com.

# 1. Introduction

First introduced in the 1950s [1, 2, 3, 4], sentinel lymph node biopsy (SLNB) became part of the clinical practice in the 1990s, only following the development of a dynamic intraoperative lymphatic mapping technique for the treatment of melanoma [5]. Subsequently, it has been shown to be a safe and effective technique, and has become a standard of care in certain neoplastic diseases such as breast cancer [5, 6, 7].

Currently, SLNB is indicated in many solid tumors, representing a standard of care in early-stage melanoma, breast, anus, cervix, vulva, endometrium and thyroid cancer [8, 9, 10, 11, 12, 13, 14], with a significant impact on prognosis and therapeutic management. In other cancers such as colorectal carcinoma, SLNB may help the pathologist assess the first lymph node involved by the lymphatic drainage from the tumor, but does not prevent complete lymph node dissection [15].

However, many other indications have been proposed for SLNB in the literature, including gastric, ovarian and various urological cancers. Therefore, in this chapter we will discuss these less common SLNB applications, their technical aspects and clinical implications.

# 2. Gastric Cancer

Many patients with early gastric cancer are currently treated with advanced laparoscopic gastrectomy procedures, such as laparoscopy-assisted distal gastrectomy and laparoscopy-assisted total gastrectomy [16, 17, 18, 19]. These types of intervention contribute to improving aesthetic results, early postoperative recovery, reducing perioperative complications and improving patients' quality of life.

Since the lymph node status is one of the most important factors to consider when deciding on resection and determining the clinical outcome of patients with gastric cancer, the lymph node evaluation method has become a crucial issue [20]. However, any minimally invasive procedure should be considered carefully, because stomach drainage is much more complicated and skip metastases appear to be more common, especially in the second or third compartment of regional lymph nodes [21]. To overcome this issue, the concept of SLNB has been proposed as a novel diagnostic tool for the identification of clinically undetectable lymph node metastases in patients with early gastric cancer [5, 22, 23]. Moreover, given the unsatisfactory accuracy of preoperative imaging for the detection of nodal metastases, intraoperative SLNB may be a useful additional method not only for predicting nodal metastases, but also for determining the extent of nodal dissection required [24, 25].

Single institutional results from a recent multicenter trial of SLNB for early gastric cancer demonstrated an acceptable sentinel node detection rate and great accuracy in determining lymph node status [26, 27, 28]. In particular, Takeuchi and colleagues submitted to SLNB patients with clinical T1-2 (less than 4 cm in diameter) and clinically node-negative tumors. The authors chose a dual-tracer method involving radioactive colloids and blue dyes injected submucosally through endoscopy [26].

The combination of radiotracer and vital dye was found to be the most reliable method for the detection of sentinel nodes in patients with early gastric cancer [28, 29]. In fact, the accumulation of radioactive colloids facilitates the ex vivo detection of the sentinel node in excised specimens, while the blue dye allows the intraoperative lymphatic flow identification. The radioactive tracers of choice used in gastric surgery are technetium-99 tin colloid, technetium-99 sulfur colloid and technetium-99 antimony sulfur colloid. On the other hand, the most commonly used vital dyes are isosulfan blue, patent blue and indocyanine green.

The first step in the detection of sentinel nodes during laparoscopy is the division of the gastrocolic ligament for the laparoscopic visualization of all the possible directions of the lymphatic flow from its primary site in the stomach [29, 30]. In this perspective, the use of vital dyes enables a real-time observation of the lymphatic flow. Based on the main arteries of the stomach, the gastric lymphatic basins may be divided into five groups: left gastric artery area, right gastric artery area, left gastroepiploic artery area, right gastroepiploic artery area and posterior gastric artery area [31].

Blue-stained or radioactive lymph nodes identified both intraoperatively or in the resected specimens are then sent for intraoperative pathological examination. After gastrectomy, the absence of residual radioactivity in the upper abdominal cavity is confirmed by the gamma probe, which is inserted into the abdominal cavity from a trocar port or small abdominal wound. In any case, SLNB is recommended to include a sort of focused lymph node dissection involving both hot and blue nodes [28, 29].

Other authors tested also the clinical utility of intraoperative indocyanine green, which successfully improves the visualization of sentinel nodes even in the adipose tissue [32, 33, 34, 35]. Also other authors suggested indocyanine green fluorescence imaging for SLNB in laparoscopic surgery for early gastric cancer to be feasible, but a limitation of this technique is the subjectivity of bright node evaluation [36].

Single-institutional studies have demonstrated a high sentinel node detection rate for SLNB in gastric surgery of about 90-100%, as well as a high accuracy in determining the lymph node status of about 85-100%, and thus comparable to that of melanoma or breast surgery [29]. In any case, the clinical application of SLNB for early gastric cancer remains highly controversial, due to its wide sensitivity ranging from 50% to 100% [37, 38].

A meta-analysis of Wang and colleagues on 38 studies including 2128 patients who underwent SLNB for gastric cancer demonstrated that the sentinel node detection rate and the accuracy of prediction of lymph node metastases based on the sentinel node status were 94% and 92%, respectively [39], concluding that SLNB for gastric cancer is technically feasible, especially in T1 tumors with the use of combined tracers and submucosal injection methods during SLNB procedures. Another Japanese multicenter prospective trial on SLNB performed between 2004 and 2008 on approximately 400 patients with cT12N0M0 single tumors without any previous treatments, using a dual-tracer method with radioactive colloid and blue dye, described a sentinel node detection rate of 98% and an accuracy of 99% [28].

## 3. Ovarian Cancer

Because accurate surgical staging in ovarian cancer is associated with better prognosis, pelvic and para-aortic lymphadenectomy currently represents a mandatory part of surgical care in early-stage ovarian cancer, although its therapeutic value and impact on survival are under discussion [40]. The prevalence of nodal metastases among patients with a suspected early-stage ovarian cancer is 20% [41]. In order to provide adequate information on the lymph node status in early-stage ovarian cancer, a number of specific retroperitoneal sites should be explored including: para-aortic and para-caval nodes between the inferior mesenteric artery and the renal vein, superficial iliac nodes, and obturator fossa nodes [42].

Although at least 10 nodes should be evaluated from the different aforementioned sites, a higher number of nodes removed reduces the false-negative rate [43] but not without any additional risks. In fact, an increasing extent of lymphadenectomy intuitively correlates with a higher rate of complications, such as increased blood loss and transfusion need, increased operative time and hospital stay [42, 44].

Although the sentinel node concept has been adopted for early-stage vulvar, cervical, and endometrial cancer [45, 12, 13, 14], in early-stage ovarian cancer it remains controversial because of the laborious choice of intra-abdominal injection site, the likely slow uptake of common tracers and the potential spillage of neoplastic cells through injection. A first attempt of SLNB in ovarian cancer was performed by Nyberg and colleagues in 2011 using intraoperative combined injection of blue dye and technetium-99 into the normal postmenopausal ovaries of women at high risk of uterine cancer [46]. All sentinel nodes were located in the para-aortic region and were correctly detected in 94% of cases. Subsequently, the technique was tested on women with ovarian cancer and systematically followed by traditional lymphadenectomy, with a sentinel node detection rate of 100% after combined injection of blue dye and technetium-99 into the ovarian ligaments [47].

A recent study recruited 20 premenopausal women operated on for unilateral or bilateral ovarian masses to perform on the intraoperative combined injection of blue dye and technetium-99 into the mesovarium outside the area suspicious for malignancy to prevent any potential neoplastic dissemination [48]. A median of 2 sentinel nodes were found in every region explored, and a third of sentinel nodes were located in the para-aortic region. With a detection rate of 100%, these results confirm that SLNB for early-stage ovarian cancer is feasible and that blue dye and radioisotope are quickly transported from the mesovarium to the regional lymph nodes.

A review of more than 1200 early-stage ovarian cancer cases confirmed a predictable distribution of sentinel node sites. In particular, para-aortic metastases alone were found in 50% of patients, both para-aortic and pelvic metastases in 30% of patients, and pelvic metastases alone in 20% of patients. Moreover, in the case of a unilateral tumor, 56% of the metastases were ipsilateral, 21% contralateral and 41% bilateral [43].

A recent article describing a considerable number of lymphatic vessels in the mesovarium along the entire length of the ovary found no connections between right and left ovarian drainage and distinguished 3 lymphatic drainage pathways from the ovaries. The two main pathways drained the ovaries via the suspensory ligament to the para-aortic and para-caval regions and via the proper ligament of the ovaries to the obturator fossa and the internal iliac artery, while the third less common pathway drained them via the round ligament to the inguinal lymph nodes [47, 49].

## 4. Penile Cancer

The application of the sentinel node concept has also been attempted in various urological malignancies, with different injection techniques and lymphatic drainage patterns. For example, lymphatic drainage in penile cancer is mainly superficial to the groin, whereas in prostate cancer and other urological tumors it is usually deep along the iliac vessels and in other intra-abdominal complex regions [50].

Penile cancer is a relatively rare disease with a usual lymphatic spread to the inguinal regions. Therefore, lymph node involvement is the single most important prognostic factor for penile cancer-specific mortality [51]. To date, surgery remains the only adequate staging method, as the available non-invasive staging techniques are not enough accurate and reliable enough for nodal staging. However, only 20-25% of clinically node-negative patients have occult nodal metastases after complete lymphadenectomy, which therefore represents an unnecessary overtreatment in most cases and is associated with recognized substantial morbidity [52].

SLNB for penile cancer was first introduced in 1977 by Ramon Cabaas [2], who nevertheless did not take into account the likely individual variability in lymphatic drainage patterns and sentinel node location, which was recognized about 15 years later by Morton and colleagues by performing the SLNB in melanoma patients [5]. Thanks to the technical evolution of the SLNB, which determined its safety and reliability as a staging technique [53, 54, 55], the SLNB procedure for penile cancer was reintroduced in 1994 by Horenblas and colleagues [56], and joined the European Association of Urology guidelines in 2009 as the standard staging tool for clinically node-negative patients (defined by ultrasound-guided fine needle cytology) with at least T1G2 tumors [57].

There is a reasonable consensus on the preoperative lymphatic mapping procedure, based on an intradermal injection of 0.2 - 0.4 cc technetium-99 nanocolloid into three sites within 1 cm proximally from the tumor and the subsequent lymphoscintigraphy and intervention on the same day of the injection [55, 58, 59]. The sentinel node visualization rate with blue dye alone is between 55% and 70% [60, 61] but, as with other primary tumors, the combination of blue dye and technetium-99 appears to be the most effective technique. Moreover, additional information on sentinel node location may be provided by single photon emission computed tomography (SPECT) [62, 63, 64, 65].

Another interesting tracer introduced in recent years is indocyanine green, which enables the visualization of the lymphatic pathways using near-infrared imaging systems, but is limited by its rapid migration through the lymphatic ducts [66, 67]. Therefore, a hybrid tracer molecule has recently been introduced in the SLNB for penile cancer, consisting in fluorescent dye indocyanine green covalently attached to technetium-99 nanocolloid, which combines the properties of both detection methods, and allows an intraoperative detection rate of up to 96.8% [68, 69, 60].

Performed in specialized centers, the technique has been proven to be safe and effective even after a previous excision of the primary tumor [70] and after tumor recurrence [71], with a detection rate of 93-97% and an acceptable false-negative rate of about 7% [70, 72, 65]. The lymphatic drainage pattern is bilateral to both groins in 80% of cases [73]. SLNB sensitivity has been improved by histopathological analysis after serial sectioning of the collected sentinel nodes, preoperative ultrasound of cN0 groins with fine needle aspiration cytology of suspicious lymph nodes and groin exploration in the case of non-visualization during lymphoscintigraphy, including intraoperative palpation of the wound to identify suspicious lymph nodes that potentially failed to pick up any radiocolloid due to tumor blockage [65].

Current guidelines recommend additional inguinal node dissection in the presence of sentinel node metastases [57]. A recent comparative study of the 5-year survival rate before and after the introduction of SLNB has demonstrated the significant impact of SLNB in reducing mortality in patients with penile cancer, mainly due to the prompt detection of the microscopic disease and the consequent lymphadenectomy in node-positive patients [74].

## 5. Prostate Cancer

Prostate cancer is the most frequent urogenital malignancy with a prevalent tendency to lymphatic metastasization, therefore lymph node staging is fundamental to its prognosis and management [75, 76]. In fact, the presence of metastatic lymph nodes may influence the choice between local treatment or systemic hormonal therapy in intermediate-risk patients. In the absence of any reliable and non-invasive diagnostic imaging modality, the current European guidelines recommend the use of nomograms to define the indication for nodal dissection (intermediate- and high-risk patients with a risk ¿5% of nodal metastases) [77, 78, 79, 80].

An extended pelvic lymph node dissection (common iliac, external iliac, obturator, internal iliac and presacral regions) is demonstrated to improve both staging accuracy and prognosis in node-positive prostate cancer patients. In particular, the number of nodes removed is correlated with longer survival but also with higher complication rates [81]. However, there is a false-negative rate of 12.5% also in the case of extended lymphadenectomy and in 5-25% of cases sentinel nodes are not included in the extended lymphadenectomy itself. This is due to the fact that, unlike other malignancies, in prostate cancer the tracer distribution may show considerable variation depending on which part of the organ the metastatic spread originates from [82]. Therefore, SLNB has emerged as a valuable technique to improve metastases detection and reduce complications, also in combination with subsequent traditional extended lymphadenectomy to prevent the potential failure of detection of relevant nodes residing outside the extended dissection field [83, 84, 85, 86, 87].

The most widely used tracer for sentinel node detection is also in this case technetium-99, which allows preoperative identification through lymphoscintigraphy and the potential execution of SPECT, which is recognized to significantly increase the sentinel node detection rate up to 98% [88, 89]. In recent years, fluorescent dyes have been increasingly used for sentinel node detection, as they allow real-time visualization of the sentinel nodes and their afferent lymphatic vessels and are not affected by the localization of the sentinel nodes near the tumor due to the relatively high resolution of fluorescence imaging systems. However, they do not allow for preoperative SPECT and, as a consequence, alternative lymph draining patterns may be missed due to the low penetrance of their near-infrared signal [90, 91, 92].

Methodologically, the tracer may be injected transrectally or transperineally, preoperatively or intraoperatively, usually ultrasound-guided, in both lobes of the peripheral zone, where the most prostate cancers develop [93, 94, 95]. With the introduction of MRI-guided injection techniques, ongoing studies should reveal whether the intratumoral injection is superior to several tracer depots within the entire prostate [96]. The advent of minimally invasive (laparoscopic and robot-assisted) approaches has progressively replaced the traditional open surgery setting for the intraoperative identification of the sentinel nodes [87, 97, 98].

The SLNB procedure for prostate cancer was first introduced by the Augsburg group in 1999 [99]. After the initial feasibility report, the effectiveness of SLNB was demonstrated with an overall sensitivity of 97% [100] and a false-negative rate ranging between 1% and 5.5% [84, 85, 93, 88, 99, 101, 102, 103, 104, 105, 106, 107]. SLNB is very sensitive in intermediate- and low-risk patients, in whom it is able to identify about 20% and 10% of metastases, respectively [86], while its sensitivity drops to 76% among high-risk patients [108, 109, 110]. The median number of excised sentinel node is 6 (range 2 - 26), and they are most frequently located in the internal iliac region (32%), the external iliac region (29%) and the obturator fossa (26%). Sentinel node detection rates range from 76% to 100% [85, 93, 95, 111, 101, 112, 113, 102, 103, 104, 105, 106, 107]. A recent meta-analysis reported a pooled detection rate of 94% (89 - 96.6%) and a pooled sensitivity rate of 95% (92 - 97%) [108].

## 6. Bladder Cancer

In bladder cancer, lymph node metastases are common in patients with muscle invasion and strongly associated with survival [114, 115]. As with other urological malignancies, extended lymphadenectomy plays a key role in the staging, planning of therapeutic management and prognosis of bladder cancer [114, 116, 117]. Although hot nodes are generally found in the external iliac (30%), obturator fossa (25%), internal iliac (26%), common iliac (15%) and para-aortic/para-caval regions (4%), there is disagreement on the extent of lymphadenectomy and the minimum number of nodes to remove, as also in this case single nodal metastases can be found even outside of the traditional lymphadenectomy field [118, 119, 120, 121, 122].

SLNB was first introduced in bladder cancer in 2011, providing a minimally invasive technique with the ability to identify metastatic nodes outside of the field of extended lymphadenectomy and to select hot nodes to be submitted to molecular tools (i.e. ultrastaging, immunohistochemistry or reverse transcriptase PCR) to improve micrometastases detection [123, 124, 125, 126, 127, 128]. With regard to the tracer injection, the transurethral approach into four sites of the detrusor muscle adjacent to the primary tumor is preferred [129], but also cystoscopic injection with bladder distension seems to be an optimal option [130]. The most commonly used tracer is radiocolloid, which also allows for preoperative SPECT [120, 128, 131, 132]. Intraoperative sentinel node detection can be carried out by open surgery but a minimally invasive (laparoscopic and robot-assisted) approach is currently preferred [104, 133, 130, 134].

The sentinel node detection rate varies between 81% and 92% and the false-negative rate is about 19% [131]. This relatively high false-negative rate, together with the complexity of the injection and the additional need for an extended nodal dissection, may explain the still limited use of this procedure for bladder cancer.

## 7. Renal Cell Cancer

The management of early-stage renal cell cancer is primarily surgical, even in the presence of metastases [135, 136, 137]. The general assumption is that the first nodes draining renal cell cancers are located in the hilar region, branching off into the para-caval, inter-aortocaval or para-aortic retroperitoneal lymph nodes, but the truth is that the lymphatic drainage pattern of this type of tumor is generally unpredictable. For this reason, the role of lymph node dissection remains very controversial [138]. On the other hand, SLNB could have both prognostic and therapeutic value in identifying and removing nodal disease, but it also gives the possibility to harvest T-lymphocytes from within the sentinel nodes for preparation and reinjection as part of the novel approach of autologous adoptive immunotherapy [139].

The feasibility of SLNB in renal cell cancer was first established in 2010 by injecting technetium-99 percutaneously into the renal tumor, guided by ultrasound or CT and followed by lymphoscintigraphy and SPECT [140, 141]. The sentinel node detection rate ranged between 70% and 90% and in about 30% of patients no lymphatic drainage was found on imaging, likely due to radiocolloid drainage failure or direct drainage into the thoracic duct [139, 142]. Therefore, the potential clinical application of this technique must be validated by further prospective randomized trials.

## 8. Testicular Cancer

Since occult metastases are present in less than 20% of patients, the management of locoregional lymph nodes in stage I testicular cancer (which is the most frequent stage at diagnosis) generally consists in postoperative surveillance. SLNB may then potentially select patients with lymph node metastases to be treated at an early stage, while sparing node-negative patients from unnecessary treatments. SLNB was fist applied to testicular cancer in 2002, using preoperative injection of radiocolloid followed by lymphoscintigraphy and SPECT [143, 144]. Funicular tracer injection showed only inguinal lymph node uptake, while intratesticular injection allowed the visualization of the retroperitoneal sentinel nodes to the areas along the aorta and vena cava, in accordance with the known drainage patterns.

The sentinel node detection rate was observed at 95% [145]. Although SLNB for testicular cancer has been shown to be feasible, given the high cancer-specific survival of testicular cancer from advances in chemo- and radiotherapy, large-scale prospective randomized trials must be planned to demonstrate the added benefit of this procedure in clinical practice.

## Conclusion

To date, SLNB has been tested in many gastro-intestinal, gynecological and urological malignancies with varying success. For instance, in penile cancer the role of this procedure is well-established, while in prostate, gastric and ovarian cancer its potential value requires confirmation by further prospective randomized clinical trials. Moreover, despite its feasibility for bladder, renal and testicular cancer, only a few studies have been published and there are still concerns about its high false-negative rates.

The major issue in the case of aforementioned tumors is their usually unpredictable and highly variable intra-abdominal lymphatic drainage pattern, which makes sentinel node identification more challenging. On the other hand, this minimally invasive procedure helps to identify the sentinel nodes that may be located outside of the traditional lymphadenectomy regions. In this perspective, recent technological advances such as hybrid tracers and novel intraoperative detection tools will hopefully determine the potential of SLNB as part of the clinical practice in many solid tumors.

## References


[1] Gould E. A., Winship T., Philbin P. H., Kerr H. H. Observations on a "sentinel node" in cancer of the parotid. *Cancer. 1960*;13:77–78.

[2] Cabanas R. M. An approach for the treatment of penile carcinoma. *Cancer. 1977*; 39:456–466.

[3] Chiappa S., Uslenghi C., Bonadonna G., Marano P., Ravasi G., Combined testicular and foot lymphangiography in testicular carcinomas. *Surg Gynecol Obstet. 1966*; 123:10–14.

[4] Weissbach L., Boedefeld E. A. Localization of solitary and multiple metastases in stage II nonseminomatous testis tumor as basis for a modified staging lymph node dissection in stage I. *J Urol. 1987*;138:77–82.

[5] Morton D. L., Wen D. R., Wong J. H., Economou J. S., Cagle L. A., Storm F. K., et al. Technical details of intraoperative lymphatic mapping for early stage melanoma. *Arch Surg. 1992*;127:392–399.

[6] Levenback C., Burke T. W., Gershenson D. M., Morris M., Malpica A., Ross M. I. Intraoperative lymphatic mapping for vulvar cancer. *Obstet Gynecol. 1994*;84:163–167.

[7] Giuliano A. E. Mapping a pathway for axillary staging: a personal perspective on the current status of sentinel lymph node dissection for breast cancer. *Arch Surg. 1999*; 134:195–199.

[8] Di Vora R., Cedolini C., Bulligan C., De Biasio F., Parodi P. C., Bertozzi S. *The Sentinel Lymph Node: Detection, Procedures and Clinical Implications*, chapter "Sentinel lymph node biopsy in melanoma", 81–102. Nova Science Publishers, 2019 .

[9] Bertozzi S., Cedolini C., Londero A. P. *The Sentinel Lymph Node: Detection, Procedures and Clinical Implications*, chapter "Sentinel lymph node biopsy in breast cancer", 39–62. Nova Science Publishers, 2019.

[10] Terrosu G., Cedolini C., Scarpa E, Londero A. P., Bertozzi S. *The Sentinel Lymph Node: Detection, Procedures and Clinical Implications*, chapter "Sentinel lymph node biopsy in anal carcinoma", 243–257. Nova Science Publishers, 2019.

[11] Portinari M., Carcoforo P. *The Sentinel Lymph Node: Detection, Procedures and Clinical Implications*, chapter "Sentinel lymph node biopsy in thyroid cancer", 119–127. Nova Science Publishers, 2019.

[12] Londero A. P., Wilhelmer E., Bertozzi S., Fruscalzo A., Lellé R. J. *The Sentinel Lymph Node: Detection, Procedures and Clinical Implications*, chapter "Sentinel lymph node biopsy in vulvar cancer", 129–149. Nova Science Publishers, 2019.

[13] Biasioli A., Trombetta G., Londero A. P., Cagnacci A. *The Sentinel Lymph Node: Detection, Procedures and Clinical Implications*, chapter "Sentinel lymph node biopsy for cervical cancer", 151–168. Nova Science Publishers, 2019.

[14] Della Martina M., Venier M., Londero A. P., Cagnacci A. *The Sentinel Lymph Node: Detection, Procedures and Clinical Implications*, chapter "Sentinel lymph node biopsy in endometrial cancer", 187–200. Nova Science Publishers, 2019.

[15] Terrosu G., Scarpa E., Bertozzi S., Londero A. P. *The Sentinel Lymph Node: Detection, Procedures and Clinical Implications*, chapter "Sentinel lymph node biopsy in colorectal cancer", 259–279. Nova Science Publishers, 2019.

[16] Kitano S., Iso Y., Moriyama M., Sugimachi K. Laparoscopy-assisted Billroth I gastrectomy. *Surg Laparosc Endosc. 1994*;4:146–148.

[17] Adachi Y., Shiraishi N., Shiromizu A., Bandoh T., Aramaki M., Kitano S. Laparoscopy-assisted Billroth I gastrectomy compared with conventional open gastrectomy. *Arch Surg. 2000*;135:806–810.

[18] Shinohara T., Kanaya S., Taniguchi K., Fujita T., Yanaga K., Uyama I. Laparoscopic total gastrectomy with D2 lymph node dissection for gastric cancer. *Arch Surg. 2009*; 144:1138–1142. doi:10.1001/archsurg.2009.223.

[19] Hur H., Jeon H. M., Kim W. Laparoscopy-assisted distal gastrectomy with D2 lymphadenectomy for T2b advanced gastric cancers: three years' experience. *J Surg Oncol. 2008*;98:515–519. doi:10.1002/jso.21155.

[20] Gotoda T., Yanagisawa A., Sasako M., Ono H., Nakanishi Y., Shimoda T., et al. Incidence of lymph node metastasis from early gastric cancer: estimation with a large number of cases at two large centers. *Gastric Cancer. 2000*;3:219–225.

[21] Siewert J. R., Sendler A. Potential and futility of sentinel node detection for gastric cancer. *Recent Results Cancer Res. 2000*;157:259–269.

[22] Giuliano A. E., Kirgan D. M., Guenther J. M., Morton D. L. Lymphatic mapping and sentinel lymphadenectomy for breast cancer. *Ann Surg. 1994*;220:391–8; discussion 398–401.

[23] Bilchik A. J., Saha S., Wiese D., Stonecypher J. A., Wood T. F., Sostrin S., et al. Molecular staging of early colon cancer on the basis of sentinel node analysis: a multicenter phase II trial. *J Clin Oncol. 2001*;19:1128–1136. doi: 10.1200/JCO.2001.19.4.1128.

[24] Kwee R. M., Kwee T. C. Imaging in assessing lymph node status in gastric cancer. *Gastric Cancer. 2009*;12:6–22. doi:10.1007/s10120-008-0492-5.

[25] Lee S. E., Lee J. H., Ryu K. W., Cho S. J., Lee J. Y., Kim C. G., et al. Sentinel node mapping and skip metastases in patients with early gastric cancer. *Ann Surg Oncol. 2009*;16:603–608. doi:10.1245/s10434-008-0283-6.

[26] Takeuchi H., Kitagawa Y. Sentinel lymph node biopsy in gastric cancer. *Cancer J. 2015*;21:21–24. doi:10.1097/PPO.0000000000000088.

[27] Kitagawa Y., Fujii H., Mukai M., Kubota T., Ando N., Watanabe M., et al. The role of the sentinel lymph node in gastrointestinal cancer. *Surg Clin North Am. 2000*; 80:1799–1809.

[28] Kitagawa Y., Takeuchi H., Takagi Y., Natsugoe S., Terashima M., Murakami N., et al. Sentinel node mapping for gastric cancer: a prospective multicenter trial in Japan. *J Clin Oncol. 2013*;31:3704–3710. doi:10.1200/JCO.2013.50.3789.

[29] Takeuchi H., Kitagawa Y. New sentinel node mapping technologies for early gastric cancer. *Ann Surg Oncol. 2013*;20:522–532. doi:10.1245/s10434-012-2602-1.

[30] Takeuchi H., Saikawa Y., Kitagawa Y. Laparoscopic sentinel node navigation surgery for early gastric cancer. *Asian Journal of Endoscopic Surgery. 2009*;2:13–17. doi: 10.1111/j.1758-5910.2009.00002.x.

[31] Kinami S., Fujimura T., Ojima E., Fushida S., Ojima T., Funaki H., et al. PTD classification: proposal for a new classification of gastric cancer location based on physiological lymphatic flow. *Int J Clin Oncol. 2008*;13:320–329. doi:10.1007/s10147-007-0755-x.

[32] Tajima Y., Murakami M., Yamazaki K., Masuda Y., Kato M., Sato A., et al. Sentinel node mapping guided by indocyanine green fluorescence imaging during laparoscopic surgery in gastric cancer. *Ann Surg Oncol. 2010*;17:1787–1793. doi: 10.1245/s10434-010-0944-0.

[33] Ishikawa K., Yasuda K., Shiromizu A., Etoh T., Shiraishi N., Kitano S. Laparoscopic sentinel node navigation achieved by infrared ray electronic endoscopy system in patients with gastric cancer. *Surg Endosc. 2007*;21:1131–1134. doi:10.1007/s00464-006-9062-2.

[34] Nimura H., Narimiya N., Mitsumori N., Yamazaki Y., Yanaga K., Urashima M. Infrared ray electronic endoscopy combined with indocyanine green injection for detection of sentinel nodes of patients with gastric cancer. *Br J Surg. 2004*;91:575–579. doi:10.1002/bjs.4470.

[35] Miyashiro I., Miyoshi N., Hiratsuka M., Kishi K., Yamada T., Ohue M., et al. Detection of sentinel node in gastric cancer surgery by indocyanine green fluorescence imaging: comparison with infrared imaging. *Ann Surg Oncol. 2008*;15:1640–1643. doi:10.1245/s10434-008-9872-7.

[36] Kinami S., Oonishi T., Fujita J., Tomita Y., Funaki H., Fujita H., et al. Optimal settings and accuracy of indocyanine green fluorescence imaging for sentinel node biopsy in early gastric cancer. *Oncol Lett. 2016*;11:4055–4062. doi: 10.3892/ol.2016.4492.

[37] Kitagawa Y., Kitano S., Kubota T., Kumai K., Otani Y., Saikawa Y., et al. Minimally invasive surgery for gastric cancer–toward a confluence of two major streams: a review. *Gastric Cancer. 2005*;8:103–110. doi:10.1007/s10120-005-0326-7.

[38] Bembenek A., Gretschel S., Schlag P. M. Sentinel lymph node biopsy for gastrointestinal cancers. *J Surg Oncol. 2007*;96:342–352. doi:10.1002/jso.20863.

[39] Wang Z., Dong Z. Y., Chen J. Q., Liu J. L. Diagnostic value of sentinel lymph node biopsy in gastric cancer: a meta-analysis. *Ann Surg Oncol. 2012*;19:1541–1550. doi:10.1245/s10434-011-2124-2.

[40] Kim H. S., Ju W., Jee B. C., Kim Y. B., Park N. H., Song Y. S., et al. Systematic lymphadenectomy for survival in epithelial ovarian cancer: a meta-analysis. *Int J Gynecol Cancer. 2010*;20:520–528. doi:10.1111/IGC.0b013e3181d6de1d.

[41] Angioli R., Plotti F., Palaia I., Calcagno M., Montera R., Cafà E. V., et al. Update on lymphadenectomy in early and advanced ovarian cancer. *Curr Opin Obstet Gynecol. 2008*;20:34–39. doi:10.1097/GCO.0b013e3282f2fd68.

[42] Trimbos J. B. Lymphadenectomy in ovarian cancer: standard of care or unnecessary risk. *Curr Opin Oncol. 2011*;23:507–511. doi:10.1097/CCO.0b013e32834847e7.

[43] Kleppe M., Wang T., Van Gorp T., Slangen B. F. M., Kruse A. J., Kruitwagen R. F. P. M. Lymph node metastasis in stages I and II ovarian cancer: a review. *Gynecol Oncol. 2011*;123:610–614. doi:10.1016/j.ygyno.2011.09.013.

[44] Maggioni A., Benedetti Panici P., Dell'Anna T., Landoni F., Lissoni A., Pellegrino A., et al. Randomised study of systematic lymphadenectomy in patients with epithelial ovarian cancer macroscopically confined to the pelvis. *Br J Cancer. 2006*; 95:699–704. doi:10.1038/sj.bjc.6603323.

[45] Cibula D., Oonk M. H. M., Abu-Rustum N. R. Sentinel lymph node biopsy in the management of gynecologic cancer. *Curr Opin Obstet Gynecol. 2015*;27:66–72. doi:10.1097/GCO.0000000000000133.

[46] Nyberg R. H., Korkola P., Mäenpää J. Ovarian sentinel node: is it feasible? *Int J Gynecol Cancer. 2011*;21:568–572. doi:10.1097/IGC.0b013e318211ef75.

[47] Kleppe M., Brans B, Van Gorp T., Slangen B. F. M., Kruse A. J., Pooters I. N. A., et al. The detection of sentinel nodes in ovarian cancer: a feasibility study. *J Nucl Med. 2014*;55:1799–1804. doi:10.2967/jnumed.114.144329.

[48] Nyberg R. H., Korkola P., Mäenpää J. U. Sentinel Node and Ovarian Tumors: A Series of 20 Patients. *Int J Gynecol Cancer. 2017*;27:684–689. doi: 10.1097/IGC.0000000000000948.

[49] Kleppe M., Kraima A. C., Kruitwagen R. F. P. M., Van Gorp T., Smit N. N., van Munsteren J. C., et al. Understanding Lymphatic Drainage Pathways of the Ovaries to Predict Sites for Sentinel Nodes in Ovarian Cancer. *Int J Gynecol Cancer. 2015*; 25:1405–1414. doi:10.1097/IGC.0000000000000514.

[50] Brouwer O. R., van der Poel H. G., Bevers R. F., van Gennep E. J., Horenblas S. Beyond penile cancer, is there a role for sentinel node biopsy in urological malignancies? *Clin Transl Imaging. 2016*;4:395–410. doi:10.1007/s40336-016-0189-4.

[51] Horenblas S., van Tinteren H. Squamous cell carcinoma of the penis. IV. Prognostic factors of survival: analysis of tumor, nodes and metastasis classification system. *J Urol. 1994*;151:1239–1243.

[52] Wespes E. The management of regional lymph nodes in patients with penile carcinoma and reliability of sentinel node biopsy. *Eur Urol. 2007*;52:15–6; discussion 20–1. doi:10.1016/j.eururo.2007.02.045.

[53] Leijte J. A. P., Kroon B. K., Valdés Olmos R. A., Nieweg O. E., Horenblas S. Reliability and safety of current dynamic sentinel node biopsy for penile carcinoma. *Eur Urol. 2007*;52:170–177. doi:10.1016/j.eururo.2007.01.107.

[54] Schubert T., Uphoff J., Henke R. P., Wawroschek F., Winter A. Reliability of radioisotope-guided sentinel lymph node biopsy in penile cancer: verification in consideration of the European guidelines. *BMC Urol. 2015*;15:98. doi:10.1186/s12894-015-0093-7.

[55] Dimopoulos P., Christopoulos P., Shilito S., Gall Z., Murby B., Ashworth D., et al. Dynamic sentinel lymph node biopsy for penile cancer: a comparison between 1- and 2-day protocols. *BJU Int. 2016*;117:890–896. doi:10.1111/bju.13389.

[56] Horenblas S., Jansen L., Meinhardt W., Hoefnagel C. A., de Jong D., Nieweg O. E. Detection of occult metastasis in squamous cell carcinoma of the penis using a dynamic sentinel node procedure. *J Urol. 2000*;163:100–104.

[57] Pizzocaro G., Algaba F., Horenblas S., Solsona E., Tana S., Van Der Poel H., et al. EAU penile cancer guidelines 2009. *Eur Urol. 2010*;57:1002–1012. doi: 10.1016/j.eururo.2010.01.039.

[58] Hadway P., Smith Y., Corbishley C., Heenan S., Watkin N. A. Evaluation of dynamic lymphoscintigraphy and sentinel lymph-node biopsy for detecting occult metastases in patients with penile squamous cell carcinoma. *BJU Int. 2007*;100:561–565. doi: 10.1111/j.1464-410X.2007.07013.x.

[59] Horenblas S., Kroon B. K., Olmos R. A. V., Nieweg O. E. Dynamic Sentinel Lymph Node Biopsy in Penile Carcinoma. In: *Radioguided Surgery, 111–119*. Springer New York. 2008;doi:10.1007/978-0-387-38327-9_11.

[60] Brouwer O. R., van den Berg N. S., Mathéron H. M., van der Poel H. G., van Rhijn B. W., Bex A., et al. A hybrid radioactive and fluorescent tracer for sentinel node

biopsy in penile carcinoma as a potential replacement for blue dye. *Eur Urol. 2014*; 65:600–609. doi:10.1016/j.eururo.2013.11.014.

[61] Kroon B. K., Horenblas S., Meinhardt W., van der Poel H. G., Bex A., van Tinteren H., et al. Dynamic sentinel node biopsy in penile carcinoma: evaluation of 10 years experience. *Eur Urol. 2005*;47:601–6; discussion 606. doi: 10.1016/j.eururo.2004.11.018.

[62] Kroon B. K., Valdés Olmos R., Nieweg O. E., Horenblas S. Non-visualization of sentinel lymph nodes in penile carcinoma. *Eur J Nucl Med Mol Imaging. 2005*; 32:1096–1099. doi:10.1007/s00259-005-1822-z.

[63] Vermeeren L., van der Ploeg I. M. C., Olmos R. A. V., Meinhardt W., Klop W. M. C., Kroon B. B. R., et al. SPECT/CT for preoperative sentinel node localization. *J Surg Oncol. 2010*;101:184–190. doi:10.1002/jso.21439.

[64] Leijte J. A. P., Valdés Olmos R. A., Nieweg O. E., Horenblas S. Anatomical mapping of lymphatic drainage in penile carcinoma with SPECT-CT: implications for the extent of inguinal lymph node dissection. *Eur Urol. 2008*;54:885–890. doi: 10.1016/j.eururo.2008.04.094.

[65] Leijte J. A. P., van der Ploeg I. M. C., Valdés Olmos R. A., Nieweg O. E., Horenblas S. Visualization of tumor blockage and rerouting of lymphatic drainage in penile cancer patients by use of SPECT/CT. *J Nucl Med. 2009*;50:364–367. doi: 10.2967/jnumed.108.059733.

[66] Markuszewski M., Polom W, Cytawa W., Czapiewski P., Lass P., Matuszewski M. Comparison of Real-Time Fluorescent Indocyanine Green and (99m)Tc-Nanocolloid Radiotracer Navigation in Sentinel Lymph Node Biopsy of Penile Cancer. *Clin Genitourin Cancer. 2015*;13:574–580. doi:10.1016/j.clgc.2015.06.005.

[67] Buckle T., van Leeuwen A. C., Chin P. T. K., Janssen H., Muller S. H., Jonkers J., et al. A self-assembled multimodal complex for combined pre- and intraoperative imaging of the sentinel lymph node. *Nanotechnology. 2010*;21:355101. doi: 10.1088/0957-4484/21/35/355101.

[68] van Leeuwen A. C., Buckle T., Bendle G., Vermeeren L., Valdés Olmos R., van de Poel H. G., et al. Tracer-cocktail injections for combined pre- and intraoperative multimodal imaging of lymph nodes in a spontaneous mouse prostate tumor model. *J Biomed Opt. 2011*;16:016004. doi:10.1117/1.3528027.

[69] Brouwer O. R., Buckle T., Vermeeren L., Klop W. M. C., Balm A. J. M., van der Poel H. G., et al. Comparing the hybrid fluorescent-radioactive tracer indocyanine green-99mTc-nanocolloid with 99mTc-nanocolloid for sentinel node identification: a validation study using lymphoscintigraphy and SPECT/CT. *J Nucl Med. 2012*; 53:1034–1040. doi:10.2967/jnumed.112.103127.

[70] Graafland N. M., Valdés Olmos R. A., Meinhardt W., Bex A., van der Poel H. G., van Boven H. H., et al. Nodal staging in penile carcinoma by dynamic sentinel node

biopsy after previous therapeutic primary tumour resection. *Eur Urol. 2010*;58:748–751. doi:10.1016/j.eururo.2010.06.036.

[71] Graafland N. M., Leijte J. A. P., Olmos R. A. V., Van Boven H. H., Nieweg O. E., Horenblas S. Repeat dynamic sentinel node biopsy in locally recurrent penile carcinoma. *BJU Int. 2010*;105:1121–1124. doi:10.1111/j.1464-410X.2009.08894.x.

[72] Leijte J. A. P., Hughes B., Graafland N. M., Kroon B. K., Olmos R. A. V., Nieweg O. E., et al. Two-center evaluation of dynamic sentinel node biopsy for squamous cell carcinoma of the penis. *J Clin Oncol. 2009*;27:3325–3329. doi: 10.1200/JCO.2008.20.6870.

[73] Kroon B. K., Valdés Olmos R. A., van Tinteren H., Nieweg O. E., Horenblas S. Reproducibility of lymphoscintigraphy for lymphatic mapping in patients with penile carcinoma. *J Urol. 2005*;174:2214–2217. doi:10.1097/01.ju.0000181813.43631.e5.

[74] Djajadiningrat R. S., Graafland N. M., van Werkhoven E., Meinhardt W., Bex A., van der Poel H. G., et al. Contemporary management of regional nodes in penile cancer-improvement of survival? *J Urol. 2014*;191:68–73. doi: 10.1016/j.juro.2013.07.088.

[75] Heidenreich A., Bastian P. J., Bellmunt J., Bolla M., Joniau S., van der Kwast T., et al. EAU guidelines on prostate cancer. part 1: screening, diagnosis, and local treatment with curative intent-update 2013. *Eur Urol. 2014*;65:124–137. doi: 10.1016/j.eururo.2013.09.046.

[76] Meinhardt W. Sentinel Node Evaluation in Prostate Cancer. *EAU-EBU Update Series. 2007*;5:223–231. doi:10.1016/j.eeus.2007.07.003.

[77] Briganti A., Chun F. K. H., Salonia A., Gallina A., Farina E., Da Pozzo L. F., et al. Validation of a nomogram predicting the probability of lymph node invasion based on the extent of pelvic lymphadenectomy in patients with clinically localized prostate cancer. *BJU Int. 2006*;98:788–793. doi:10.1111/j.1464-410X.2006.06318.x.

[78] Cagiannos I., Karakiewicz P., Eastham J. A., Ohori M., Rabbani F., Gerigk C., et al. A preoperative nomogram identifying decreased risk of positive pelvic lymph nodes in patients with prostate cancer. *J Urol. 2003*;170:1798–1803. doi: 10.1097/01.ju.0000091805.98960.13.

[79] Eifler J. B., Feng Z., Lin B. M., Partin M. T., Humphreys E. B., Han M., et al. An updated prostate cancer staging nomogram (Partin tables) based on cases from 2006 to 2011. *BJU Int. 2013*;111:22–29. doi:10.1111/j.1464-410X.2012.11324.x.

[80] Kattan M. W., Eastham J. A., Stapleton A. M. F., Wheeler T. M., Scardino P. T. A Preoperative Nomogram for Disease Recurrence Following Radical Prostatectomy for Prostate Cancer. *JNCI: Journal of the National Cancer Institute. 1998*;90:766–771. doi:10.1093/jnci/90.10.766.

[81] Abdollah F., Gandaglia G., Suardi N., Capitanio U., Salonia A., Nini A., et al. More extensive pelvic lymph node dissection improves survival in patients with node-positive prostate cancer. *Eur Urol. 2015*;67:212–219. doi: 10.1016/j.eururo.2014.05.011.

[82] Buckle T., Brouwer O. R., Valdés Olmos R. A., van der Poel H. G., van Leeuwen F. W. B. Relationship between intraprostatic tracer deposits and sentinel lymph node mapping in prostate cancer patients. *J Nucl Med. 2012*;53:1026–1033. doi: 10.2967/jnumed.111.098517.

[83] Weckermann D., Wawroschek F., Harzmann R. Is there a need for pelvic lymph node dissection in low risk prostate cancer patients prior to definitive local therapy? *Eur Urol. 2005*;47:45–50; discussion 50–1. doi:10.1016/j.eururo.2004.07.017.

[84] de Bonilla-Damiá A., Roberto Brouwer O., Meinhardt W., Valdés-Olmos R. A. Lymphatic drainage in prostate carcinoma assessed by lymphoscintigraphy and SPECT/CT: its importance for the sentinel node procedure. *Rev Esp Med Nucl Imagen Mol. 2012*;31:66–70. doi:10.1016/j.remn.2011.09.003.

[85] Meinhardt W., van der Poel H. G., Valdés Olmos R. A., Bex A., Brouwer O. R., Horenblas S. Laparoscopic sentinel lymph node biopsy for prostate cancer: the relevance of locations outside the extended dissection area. *Prostate cancer. 2012*; 2012:751753. doi:10.1155/2012/751753.

[86] Acar C., Kleinjan G. H., van den Berg N. S., Wit E. M., van Leeuwen F. W., van der Poel H. G. Advances in sentinel node dissection in prostate cancer from a technical perspective. *Int J Urol. 2015*;22:898–909. doi:10.1111/iju.12863.

[87] Kleinjan G. H., van den Berg N. S., Brouwer O. R., de Jong J., Acar C., Wit E. M., et al. Optimisation of fluorescence guidance during robot-assisted laparoscopic sentinel node biopsy for prostate cancer. *Eur Urol. 2014*;66:991–998. doi: 10.1016/j.eururo.2014.07.014.

[88] Brenot-Rossi I., Bastide C., Garcia S., Dumas S., Esterni B., Pasquier J, et al. Limited pelvic lymphadenectomy using the sentinel lymph node procedure in patients with localised prostate carcinoma: a pilot study. *Eur J Nucl Med Mol Imaging. 2005*; 32:635–640. doi:10.1007/s00259-004-1750-3.

[89] Vermeeren L., Valdés Olmos R. A., Meinhardt W., Bex A., van der Poel H. G., Vogel WV, et al. Value of SPECT/CT for detection and anatomic localization of sentinel lymph nodes before laparoscopic sentinel node lymphadenectomy in prostate carcinoma. *J Nucl Med. 2009*;50:865–870. doi:10.2967/jnumed.108.060673.

[90] van den Berg N. S., van Leeuwen F. W. B., van der Poel H. G. Fluorescence guidance in urologic surgery. *Curr Opin Urol. 2012*;22:109–120. doi: 10.1097/MOU.0b013e3283501869.

[91] Jeschke S., Lusuardi L., Myatt A., Hruby S., Pirich C., Janetschek G. Visualisation of the lymph node pathway in real time by laparoscopic radioisotope- and fluorescence-guided sentinel lymph node dissection in prostate cancer staging. *Urology. 2012*; 80:1080–1086. doi:10.1016/j.urology.2012.05.050.

[92] Nguyen D. P., Huber P. M., Metzger T. A., Genitsch V., Schudel H. H., Thalmann G. N. A Specific Mapping Study Using Fluorescence Sentinel Lymph Node Detection in Patients with Intermediate- and High-risk Prostate Cancer Undergoing Extended Pelvic Lymph Node Dissection. *Eur Urol. 2016*;70:734–737. doi: 10.1016/j.eururo.2016.01.034.

[93] Jeschke S., Beri A., Grüll M., Ziegerhofer J., Prammer P., Leeb K., et al. Laparoscopic radioisotope-guided sentinel lymph node dissection in staging of prostate cancer. *Eur Urol. 2008*;53:126–132. doi:10.1016/j.eururo.2007.03.064.

[94] Meinhardt W., Valdés Olmos R. A., van der Poel H. G., Bex A., Horenblas S. Laparoscopic sentinel node dissection for prostate carcinoma: technical and anatomical observations. *BJU Int. 2008*;102:714–717. doi:10.1111/j.1464-410X.2008.07674.x.

[95] Manny T. B., Patel M., Hemal A. K. Fluorescence-enhanced robotic radical prostatectomy using real-time lymphangiography and tissue marking with percutaneous injection of unconjugated indocyanine green: the initial clinical experience in 50 patients. *Eur Urol. 2014*;65:1162–1168. doi:10.1016/j.eururo.2013.11.017.

[96] Hansen N., Patruno G., Wadhwa K., Gaziev G., Miano R., Barrett T., et al. Magnetic Resonance and Ultrasound Image Fusion Supported Transperineal Prostate Biopsy Using the Ginsburg Protocol: Technique, Learning Points, and Biopsy Results. *Eur Urol. 2016*;70:332–340. doi:10.1016/j.eururo.2016.02.064.

[97] Wawroschek F., Vogt H., Wengenmair H., Weckermann D., Hamm M., Keil M., et al. Prostate lymphoscintigraphy and radio-guided surgery for sentinel lymph node identification in prostate cancer. Technique and results of the first 350 cases. *Urol Int. 2003*;70:303–310. doi:10.1159/000070140.

[98] Jeschke S., Burkhard F. C., Thurairaja R., Dhar N., Studer U. E. Extended lymph node dissection for prostate cancer. *Curr Urol Rep. 2008*;9:237–242.

[99] Wawroschek F., Vogt H., Weckermann D., Wagner T., Harzmann R. The sentinel lymph node concept in prostate cancer - first results of gamma probe-guided sentinel lymph node identification. *Eur Urol. 1999*;36:595–600. doi:10.1159/000020054.

[100] Wawroschek F., Harzmann R., Weckermann D. [Value of sentinel node biopsy for urological tumors]. *Urologe A. 2005*;44:630–634. doi:10.1007/s00120-005-0834-4.

[101] Holl G., Dorn R., Wengenmair H., Weckermann D., Sciuk J. Validation of sentinel lymph node dissection in prostate cancer: experience in more than 2,000 patients. *Eur J Nucl Med Mol Imaging. 2009*;36:1377–1382. doi:10.1007/s00259-009-1157-2.

[102] Winter A., Kneib T., Henke R. P., Wawroschek F. Sentinel lymph node dissection in more than 1200 prostate cancer cases: rate and prediction of lymph node involvement depending on preoperative tumor characteristics. *Int J Urol. 2014*;21:58–63. doi: 10.1111/iju.12184.

[103] Rousseau C., Rousseau T., Campion L., Lacoste J., Aillet G., Potiron E., et al. Laparoscopic sentinel lymph node versus hyperextensive pelvic dissection for staging clinically localized prostate carcinoma: a prospective study of 200 patients. *J Nucl Med. 2014*;55:753–758. doi:10.2967/jnumed.113.129023.

[104] Inoue S., Shiina H., Mitsui Y., Yasumoto H., Matsubara A., Igawa M. Identification of lymphatic pathway involved in the spread of bladder cancer: Evidence obtained from fluorescence navigation with intraoperatively injected indocyanine green. *Can Urol Assoc J. 2013*;7:E322–E328. doi:10.5489/cuaj.12096.

[105] Häcker A., Jeschke S., Leeb K., Prammer K., Ziegerhofer J., Sega W., et al. Detection of pelvic lymph node metastases in patients with clinically localized prostate cancer: comparison of [18F]fluorocholine positron emission tomography-computerized tomography and laparoscopic radioisotope guided sentinel lymph node dissection. *J Urol. 2006*;176:2014–8; discussion 2018–9. doi:10.1016/j.juro.2006.07.037.

[106] Corvin S., Schilling D., Eichhorn K., Hundt I., Hennenlotter J., Anastasiadis A. G., et al. Laparoscopic sentinel lymph node dissection–a novel technique for the staging of prostate cancer. *Eur Urol. 2006*;49:280–285. doi:10.1016/j.eururo.2005.08.021.

[107] van der Poel H. G., Buckle T., Brouwer O. R., Valdés Olmos R. A., van Leeuwen F. W. B. Intraoperative laparoscopic fluorescence guidance to the sentinel lymph node in prostate cancer patients: clinical proof of concept of an integrated functional imaging approach using a multimodal tracer. *Eur Urol. 2011*;60:826–833. doi:10.1016/j.eururo.2011.03.024.

[108] Sadeghi R., Tabasi K. T., Bazaz S. M. M., Kakhki V. R. D., Massoom A. F., Gholami H., et al. Sentinel node mapping in the prostate cancer. Meta-analysis. *Nuklearmedizin. 2011*;50:107–115. doi:10.3413/nukmed-0339-10-07.

[109] van der Poel H. G., Leijte J. A. P., Horenblas S. Radioguided Sentinel Lymph Node Biopsy and Lymphatic Mapping in Urogenital Malignancies. In: *Radioguided Surgery*, 227–247. Springer International Publishing. 2016;doi:10.1007/978-3-319-26051-8_15.

[110] Van den Bergh L., Joniau S., Haustermans K., Deroose C. M., Isebaert S., Oyen R., et al. Reliability of sentinel node procedure for lymph node staging in prostate cancer patients at high risk for lymph node involvement. *Acta Oncol. 2015*;54:896–902. doi:10.3109/0284186X.2014.987354.

[111] Weckermann D., Dorn R., Trefz M., Wagner T., Wawroschek F., Harzmann R. Sentinel lymph node dissection for prostate cancer: experience with more than 1,000 patients. *J Urol. 2007*;177:916–920. doi:10.1016/j.juro.2006.10.074.

[112] Jakobsen J. K. Sentinel node biopsy in uro-oncology: a history of the development of a promising concept. *Urol Oncol. 2015*;33:486–493. doi: 10.1016/j.urolonc.2015.08.010.

[113] Brenot-Rossi I., Rossi D., Esterni B., Brunelle S., Chuto G., Bastide C. Radioguided sentinel lymph node dissection in patients with localised prostate carcinoma: influence of the dose of radiolabelled colloid to avoid failure of the procedure. *Eur J Nucl Med Mol Imaging. 2008*;35:32–38. doi:10.1007/s00259-007-0516-0.

[114] Herr H. W., Donat S. M. Outcome of patients with grossly node positive bladder cancer after pelvic lymph node dissection and radical cystectomy. *J Urol. 2001*; 165:62–4; discussion 64. doi:10.1097/00005392-200101000-00015.

[115] Stenzl A., Cowan N. C., De Santis M., Kuczyk M. A., Merseburger A. S., Ribal M. J., et al. Treatment of muscle-invasive and metastatic bladder cancer: update of the EAU guidelines. *Eur Urol. 2011*;59:1009–1018. doi:10.1016/j.eururo.2011.03.023.

[116] Jensen J. B., Ulhøi B. P., Jensen K. M. E. Extended versus limited lymph node dissection in radical cystectomy: impact on recurrence pattern and survival. *Int J Urol. 2012*;19:39–47. doi:10.1111/j.1442-2042.2011.02887.x.

[117] Wosnitzer M. S., Hruby G. W., Murphy A. M., Barlow L. J., Cordon-Cardo C., Mansukhani M., et al. A comparison of the outcomes of neoadjuvant and adjuvant chemotherapy for clinical T2-T4aN0-N2M0 bladder cancer. *Cancer. 2012*;118:358–364. doi:10.1002/cncr.26278.

[118] Sharir S., Fleshner N. E.. Lymph node assessment and lymphadenectomy in bladder cancer. *J Surg Oncol. 2009*;99:225–231. doi:10.1002/jso.21253.

[119] Hurle R., Naspro R. Pelvic lymphadenectomy during radical cystectomy: a review of the literature. *Surg Oncol. 2010*;19:208–220. doi:10.1016/j.suronc.2009.05.004.

[120] Roth B., Wissmeyer M. P., Zehnder P., Birkhäuser F. D., Thalmann G. N., Krause T. M., et al. A new multimodality technique accurately maps the primary lymphatic landing sites of the bladder. *Eur Urol. 2010*;57:205–211. doi: 10.1016/j.eururo.2009.10.026.

[121] Leissner J., Ghoneim M. A., Abol-Enein H., Thüroff J. W., Franzaring L., Fisch M., et al. Extended radical lymphadenectomy in patients with urothelial bladder cancer: results of a prospective multicenter study. *J Urol. 2004*;171:139–144. doi: 10.1097/01.ju.0000102302.26806.fb.

[122] Triantafyllou M., Studer U. E., Birkhäuser F. D., Fleischmann A., Bains L. J., Petralia G., et al. Ultrasmall superparamagnetic particles of iron oxide allow for the detection of metastases in normal sized pelvic lymph nodes of patients with bladder and/or prostate cancer. *Eur J Cancer. 2013*;49:616–624. doi:10.1016/j.ejca.2012.09.034.

[123] Retz M., Lehmann J., Szysnik C., Zwank S., Venzke T., Röder C., et al. Detection of occult tumor cells in lymph nodes from bladder cancer patients by MUC7 nested RT-PCR. *Eur Urol. 2004*;45:314–319. doi:10.1016/j.eururo.2003.10.011.

[124] Copp H. L., Chin J. L., Conaway M., Theodorescu D. Prospective evaluation of the prognostic relevance of molecular staging for urothelial carcinoma. *Cancer. 2006*; 107:60–66. doi:10.1002/cncr.21953.

[125] Kiss B., Thoeny H. C., Studer U. E. Current Status of Lymph Node Imaging in Bladder and Prostate Cancer. *Urology. 2016*;96:1–7. doi:10.1016/j.urology.2016.02.014.

[126] van der Pas M. H., Meijer S., Hoekstra O. S., Riphagen I. I., de Vet H. C. W., Knol D. L., et al. Sentinel-lymph-node procedure in colon and rectal cancer: a systematic review and meta-analysis. *Lancet Oncol. 2011*;12:540–550. doi:10.1016/S1470-2045(11)70075-4.

[127] Gazquez C., Ribal M. J., Marín-Aguilera M., Kayed H., Fernández P. L., Mengual L., et al. Biomarkers vs conventional histological analysis to detect lymph node micrometastases in bladder cancer: a real improvement? *BJU Int. 2012*;110:1310–1316. doi:10.1111/j.1464-410X.2012.11025.x.

[128] Sherif A., De La Torre M., Malmström P. U., Thörn M. Lymphatic mapping and detection of sentinel nodes in patients with bladder cancer. *J Urol. 2001*;166:812–815.

[129] International Atomic Energy Agency IAEA. Guided Intraoperative Scintigraphic Tumour Targeting (Gostt); Implementing Advanced Hybrid Molecular Imaging And Non-Imaging Probes For Advanced Cancer Management: IAEA Human Health Series No. 29. *International Atomic Energy Agency. 2015.*

[130] Schaafsma B. E., Verbeek F. P. R., Elzevier H. W., Tummers Q. R. J. G., van der Vorst J. R., Frangioni J. V., et al. Optimization of sentinel lymph node mapping in bladder cancer using near-infrared fluorescence imaging. *J Surg Oncol. 2014*;110:845–850. doi:10.1002/jso.23740.

[131] Liedberg F., Chebil G., Davidsson T., Gudjonsson S., Mansson W. Intraoperative sentinel node detection improves nodal staging in invasive bladder cancer. *J Urol. 2006*;175:84–8; discussion 88–9. doi:10.1016/S0022-5347(05)00066-2.

[132] Sherif A., Garske U., de la Torre M., Thörn M. Hybrid SPECT-CT: an additional technique for sentinel node detection of patients with invasive bladder cancer. *Eur Urol. 2006*;50:83–91. doi:10.1016/j.eururo.2006.03.002.

[133] Vermeeren L., Valdés Olmos R. A., Meinhardt W., Bex A., van der Poel H. G., Vogel W. V., et al. Intraoperative radioguidance with a portable gamma camera: a novel technique for laparoscopic sentinel node localisation in urological malignancies. *Eur J Nucl Med Mol Imaging. 2009*;36:1029–1036. doi:10.1007/s00259-009-1100-6.

[134] Manny T. B., Hemal A. K. Fluorescence-enhanced robotic radical cystectomy using unconjugated indocyanine green for pelvic lymphangiography, tumor marking, and mesenteric angiography: the initial clinical experience. *Urology. 2014*;83:824–829. doi:10.1016/j.urology.2013.11.042.

[135] Ljungberg B., Cowan N. C., Hanbury D. C., Hora M., Kuczyk M. A., Merseburger A. S., et al. EAU guidelines on renal cell carcinoma: the 2010 update. *Eur Urol. 2010*;58:398–406. doi:10.1016/j.eururo.2010.06.032.

[136] Alt A. L., Boorjian S. A., Lohse C. M., Costello B. A., Leibovich B. C., Blute M. L.. Survival after complete surgical resection of multiple metastases from renal cell carcinoma. *Cancer. 2011*;117:2873–2882. doi:10.1002/cncr.25836.

[137] Aben K. K. H., Heskamp S., Janssen-Heijnen M. L., Koldewijn E. L., van Herpen C. M., Kiemeney L. A., et al. Better survival in patients with metastasised kidney cancer after nephrectomy: a population-based study in the Netherlands. *Eur J Cancer. 2011*; 47:2023–2032. doi:10.1016/j.ejca.2011.03.002.

[138] Blom J. H. M., van Poppel H., Maréchal J. M., Jacqmin D., Schröder F. H., de Prijck L., et al. Radical nephrectomy with and without lymph-node dissection: final results of European Organization for Research and Treatment of Cancer (EORTC) randomized phase 3 trial 30881. *Eur Urol. 2009*;55:28–34. doi: 10.1016/j.eururo.2008.09.052.

[139] Sherif A. M., Eriksson E., Thörn M., Vasko J., Riklund K., Ohberg L., et al. Sentinel node detection in renal cell carcinoma. A feasibility study for detection of tumour-draining lymph nodes. *BJU Int. 2012*;109:1134–1139. doi:10.1111/j.1464-410X.2011.10444.x.

[140] Bernie J. E., Zupkas P., Monga M. Intraoperative mapping of renal lymphatic drainage: technique and application in a porcine model. *J Endourol. 2003*;17:235–237. doi:10.1089/089277903765444375.

[141] Bex A., Vermeeren L., de Windt G., Prevoo W., Horenblas S., Olmos R. A. V. Feasibility of sentinel node detection in renal cell carcinoma: a pilot study. *Eur J Nucl Med Mol Imaging. 2010*;37:1117–1123. doi:10.1007/s00259-009-1359-7.

[142] Bex A., Vermeeren L., Meinhardt W., Prevoo W., Horenblas S., Valdés Olmos R. A. Intraoperative sentinel node identification and sampling in clinically node-negative renal cell carcinoma: initial experience in 20 patients. *World J Urol. 2011*;29:793–799. doi:10.1007/s00345-010-0615-6.

[143] Tanis P. J., Horenblas S., Valdés Olmos R. A., Hoefnagel C. A., Nieweg O. E. Feasibility of sentinel node lymphoscintigraphy in stage I testicular cancer. *Eur J Nucl Med Mol Imaging. 2002*;29:670–673. doi:10.1007/s00259-001-0751-8.

[144] Brouwer O. R., Valdés Olmos R. A., Vermeeren L., Hoefnagel C. A., Nieweg O. E., Horenblas S. SPECT/CT and a portable gamma-camera for image-guided laparoscopic sentinel node biopsy in testicular cancer. *J Nucl Med. 2011*;52:551–554. doi:10.2967/jnumed.110.086660.

[145] Satoh M., Ito A., Kaiho Y., Nakagawa H., Saito S., Endo M., et al. Intraoperative, radio-guided sentinel lymph node mapping in laparoscopic lymph node dissection for Stage I testicular carcinoma. *Cancer. 2005*;103:2067–2072. doi:10.1002/cncr.21049.

In: The Sentinel Lymph Node
Editors: A. Londero, S. Bertozzi and C. Cedolini
ISBN: 978-1-53614-557-1


*Chapter 18*

# THE SENTINEL LYMPH NODE BIOPSY FROM THE PAST TO THE FUTURE

***Serena Bertozzi***[1,*]***, Carla Cedolini***[1] ***and Ambrogio P. Londero***[2]
[1]Breast Unit, DAME, University of Udine,
University Hospital of Udine, Udine, Italy
[2]Clinic of Obstetrics and Gynecology,
University Hospital of Udine, Udine, Italy

**Abstract**

The lymphatic system is recognized as one of the major pathways involved in cancer spread. During the second half of the last century, the concept of the sentinel lymph node biopsy evolved from a pioneering hypothesis to a definite standard technique for cancer staging. Sentinel lymph node biopsy is a minimally invasive procedure that consists in the intraoperative detection of the first lymph node draining a certain cancer, and allows adequate lymph node staging while sparing patients from unnecessary complete lymph node dissections and their traditionally associated harmful complications. Sentinel lymph node biopsy was successfully applied to melanoma for the first time in 1989 and subsequently became a standard of care for breast cancer patients in the 1990's. Subsequently, this procedure was introduced for many other solid cancers, such as thyroid cancer, gynecological cancers including endometrial, cervical and vulvar cancer, gastrointestinal cancers including colorectal, anal and gastric cancer, urological cancers including penile and prostate cancer, with varying rates of success. The current trend towards increased surgical conservatism is intended to spare patients from the sentinel lymph node biopsy itself in the future, when clinicians will be able to preoperatively evaluate lymph nodes through increasingly accurate imaging techniques.

**Keywords:** sentinel node biopsy, conservative surgery, sentinal node mapping, solid tumors

## 1. Introduction

The existence of the lymphatic vessels had already been recognized in the Greco-Roman world. However, the knowledge of these structures was extremely limited, as evidenced

*Corresponding Author E-mail: dr.bertozzi@gmail.com.

by the Hippocratic theory that the liquid in the intestinal lymphatic vessels was a sort of mother's milk en route to the breasts [1]. Later in history, Thomas Bartholin (1653) classified and named the structures of the lymphatic system, which were thereafter detailed by Thomas Wharton (1656) and Marcello Malpighi (1666) [1].

Nowadays, the lymphatic system is recognized as one of the major pathways involved in cancer spread [2]. Over the second half of the last century, the concept of the sentinel lymph node biopsy (SLNB) has evolved from a pioneering hypothesis to be supported to a definite standard cancer staging technique. This has been done thanks to promising clinical studies first and to numerous epidemiological and clinical experimental studies later, which have validated the current SLNB technique.

## 2. The Rationale of Sentinel Lymph Node Biopsy

The SLNB is a minimally invasive procedure that consists in the intraoperative detection of the first lymph node draining a certain cancer. The purpose of this technique is to allow adequate lymph node staging while sparing patients from unnecessary complete lymph node dissections and the traditional harmful complications associated with them. In fact, a greater number of lymph nodes removed is correlated with a higher incidence of early and late postoperative complications in each body district.

Among the early lymphatic complications, the most frequent is lymphocele, a lymph collection within the operated field that usually reabsorbs spontaneously within a few weeks, but which can also be drained by a syringe. On the other hand, the most dreadful late complication is lymphedema, which consists in lymph retention in the affected upper or lower limb with a consequent increase in the limb diameter, a reduction in motility and an increase in locoregional infection incidence. Lymphedema usually occurs within a few months of lymph node surgery, but may be triggered by subsequent predisposing events such as limb trauma, blood sampling, radiotherapy or chemotherapy administration. Lymphedema treatment is heterogeneous, including limb dressing, lymphatic drainage massage and targeted gymnastic, but has a disappointing effectiveness. Clearly, the incidence of lymphedema collapsed with the introduction of SLNB, but it has not been completely eradicated [3, 4].

Although the first attempts at the SLNB were made in the 1950s [5, 6, 7, 8], only the development of a dynamic intraoperative lymphatic mapping technique for the treatment of melanoma in the 1990s by Morton and colleagues [9] led to the acceptance of the SLNB as a feasible technique, and therefore as a standard of care in certain neoplastic pathologies [9, 10, 11].

The concept of the SLNB is based on two cornerstones. The first assumption is the existence of an orderly and predictable sequence of lymph nodes involved in the lymphatic drainage of the regional lymph node basin. The second is the ability of the sentinel node to limit the spread of tumor cells to downstream nodes [12, 2]. This hypothesis of sequential tumor dissemination has been corroborated by several studies using SLNB with confirmatory regional lymph node dissection that show a limited number of false-negative rates [9, 13, 11].

Rather, SLNB appears to reduce the false-negative rate of traditional complete lymph node dissection in certain intra-abdominal cancers. For instance, in the case of gynecological or urological cancers, it has been shown that SLNB finds a non-neglectable percentage of metastases in lymph nodes that are not commonly included in the classical lymphadenectomy. Therefore, in some of these cases, SLNB has become a standard procedure in combination with traditional or extended complete lymphadenectomy in order to guide the pathologist in the more rapid search for the first nodes draining the tumor [14, 15, 4, 16, 17, 18, 19].

The SLNB is a safe and effective procedure for adequately assessing the lymph node status in the case of various types of solid cancer [20, 21, 2, 22, 23, 3, 24, 14, 15, 4, 25, 16, 17, 18, 26, 19, 27]. The safety of this procedure has been extensively studied, and a reduction in perioperative complications has been observed in every lymph node district. In particular, as mentioned before, a very low incidence of lymphedema has been reported after SLNB compared with complete locoregional lymph node dissection, which represents an important achievement in the progressive improvement for the quality of life of oncological patients.

As regards the effectiveness of SLNB, many studies have shown an acceptable false-negative rate. As a result, they have confirmed the adequacy of this procedure in the staging of locoregional nodes in many cancer histotypes. In this perspective, it is important to recall the staging role of lymph node excision in oncological surgery, which has completely replaced the previous curative intent. In fact, cancer prognosis is generally guided by distant metastases and not by locoregional extension, while locoregional involvement is fundamental to guide proper cancer staging and decision-making on subsequent therapeutical options.

## 3. Technical Considerations of Sentinel Lymph Node Biopsy

Over time, many techniques have been tested for both detection and analysis of sentinel nodes. With regard to the intraoperative sentinel node detection, it can be performed using vital dyes (patent, methylene or isosulfan blue dye), radiotracers (technetium-99) or fluorescent tracers (indocyanine green), with a very high detection rate, which can even be improved by the combination of two of these methods. Currently, the most widely used technique in most solid tumor is technetium-99 radiocolloid, but its use is strongly limited by the disposability of a nuclear medicine department in the specific local setting. Technetium-99 can also be combined with blue dye, which however is not free of side effects. In particular, anaphylactic reactions are described and a blue tattoo may remain permanently at the injection site. Indocyanine green is the latest proposed tracer and has many promising advantages, such as the ability to detect real-time lymphatic drainage trough near-infrared fluorescence imaging.

To reduce the comorbidity of complete lymph node dissection, these techniques can be combined to select the lymph nodes draining a certain tumor from those that do not. For example, axillary reverse mapping is a newly introduced technique that distinguishes radioactive lymph nodes that drain the breast (after technetium-99 injection into the breast tumor) from blue lymph nodes that drain the ipsilateral arm (after blue dye injection into the ipsilateral forearm). This technique helps to spare patients from unnecessary excision of lymph nodes that do not drain the breast, thus reducing postoperative lymphatic complications. In the future, it will probably be used also in the case of tumors with inguinal lymphatic drainage to spare lymph nodes selectively draining the lower limb.

Taking into account sentinel node analysis, in addition to traditional hematoxylin-eosin staining, the sentinel lymph node can be analyzed by ultrastaging to improve the detection of minor metastatic disease, or by using new molecular techniques such as the one-step nucleic acid amplification (OSNA) assay to reduce the analysis time and consequently anesthesiological time in the case of cancers that require intraoperative decision-making. For example, ultrastaging has been observed to improve the detection of small amounts of metastatic disease within sentinel nodes in gynecological cancers, while the OSNA method is currently used in breast cancer to allow immediate complete axillary lymph node dissection in women with sentinel node macrometastases, sparing them from a second intervention.

SLNB was successfully applied to melanoma for the first time in 1989 and subsequently became a standard of care for breast cancer patients in the 1990s. Thereafter, this procedure was introduced for many other solid cancers, such as thyroid cancer, gynecological cancers including endometrial, cervical and vulvar cancers, gatrointestinal cancers including colorectal, anal and gastric cancers, urological cancers including penile and prostate cancers [20, 21, 2, 22, 23, 3, 24, 14, 15, 4, 25, 16, 17, 18, 26, 19, 27]. Moreover, SLNB has also been described in other cancers, such as hepatic cancer, which has been less successful, usually because of the unfavorable anatomic condition, such as in the case of non-reproducible lymphatic drainage.

This variability in lymphatic drainage patterns is also the reason why SLNB is not yet a standard of care for many other solid malignancies. For instance, cancers in some odd intra-abdominal organs may have an even distribution of lymphatic drainage, which naturally makes it more difficult to identify sentinel lymph nodes. In these cases, bilateral sentinel node detection is demonstrated to be more effective in reducing the false-negative rate and correctly predicting the prognosis [14, 15, 4, 16, 18, 19, 27].

In each type of cancer, SLNB may have different technical aspects, indications, detection rates and complications. For example, in the case of malignant melanoma, the sentinel lymph node localization is always a challenge, depending on the primary tumor site [23]. In particular, melanomas of the lower limb usually drain into the inguinal lymph node basin while melanomas of the upper limb drain into the axillary lymph node basin and head and neck melanomas tend to drain into the latero-cervical lymph node basins. Unfortunately, many melanomas occur in the truncus, where lymphatic drainage is again difficult to predict, with the possibility of draining both into the inguinal or axillary basins, or potentially even into all four sites. In addition, not all sites present the same surgical difficulties. For instance, the latero-cervical nodes are placed in a very delicate area of the neck, and therefore their excision is correlated with a higher perioperative morbidity.

Also in most gynecological and urological cancers there is no uniform lymphatic drainage pattern. Therefore, SLNB does not replace complete lymphadenectomy, but is useful in helping the surgeon locate lymph nodes basins that may be involved by metastases but are not usually included in either traditional or extended lymph node dissection. Moreover, sentinel node identification can also help the pathologist in the postoperative lymph node evaluation in search of potential metastatic disease [14, 15, 4, 16, 18, 19, 27].

In the case of colorectal cancer, SLNB does not prevent the standard mesenteric lymph node dissection, but it may help the pathologist analyze primarily the sentinel nodes in a district that potentially contains several tens of nodes. In this case, for example, the tracer injection can be performed in vivo, as well as ex vivo after surgical excision of the specimen, only to indicate which are the first nodes potentially involved by metastatic disease. The disadvantages of the in vivo injection are the need for an additional preoperative endoscopy and a very short operative time to avoid the tracer migration to secondary non-sentinel nodes, whereas the limit of the ex vivo injection is the need for a manual massage to stimulate lymph movement through the mesocolon to the sentinel nodes [19].

With regard to sentinel node metastases, over the past decades we have assisted to fundamental changes in their classification and in their predictive and prognostic values. In particular, the metastatic involvement dimension has become of key importance in the decision-making process for many solid tumors. Recently, metastases have been divided by size as follows: macrometastases if above 2 mm, micrometastases if below 2 mm but above 0,2 mm, and isolated tumor cells (ITCs) if below 0,2 mm [28]. As a result, the attitude towards the presence of lymph node metastases also varies among cancers.

As already mentioned, mesenteric dissection for colorectal cancer is performed independently of the result of SLNB. This is because there is no certainty about the predictive role of sentinel node metastases towards the presence of other metastatic non-sentinel nodes, together with the fact that sparing patients from mesocolon resection is not correlated with significantly lower perioperative morbidity, as with skin or breast cancers, conversely.

In the case of melanoma, each metastatic involvement is treated with complete locoregional dissection independently of the size of the metastases. On the other hand, in the case of breast cancer, it is well-established that micrometastases and ITCs do not require additional lymph node dissection. Moreover, studies are underway to potentially avoid complete axillary lymph node dissection even in the presence of a macrometastatic sentinel node, as well as to spare clinically and radiologically node-negative patients from SLNB itself [21].

In these perspective, preoperative lymph node evaluation has evolved to improve metastases detection in an increasingly less invasive way. The most effective imaging technique for lymph node status assessment is the ultrasound, a very easy to learn and cheap technique that does not expose patients to any radiation or other potential toxic sources [22, 16]. If there is any doubt, there is the possibility of performing an ultrasound-guided fine needle aspiration citology or a core needle biopsy to distinguish healthy from metastatic nodes before surgery and subsequently select patients for SLNB or primary complete lymphadenectomy. Moreover, computed tomography may help identify morphologically altered lymph nodes susceptible to preoperative biopsy. Finally, magnetic resonance imaging and positron emission tomography provide a metabolic assessment of lymph nodes, regardless of their altered or normal morphology, and represent the most effective method for detecting lymph node metastases. However, these latter techniques are very expensive and require devices and expertise, that may not be accessible in every single setting.

## Conclusion

In conclusion, in this surgical era when conservative surgery is progressively replacing traditional oncological interventions, SLNB currently represents a milestone, allowing to avoid unnecessary and harmful lymph node dissections in node-negative patients. Moreover, the new technologies might revolutionize the sentinel node mapping procedures in many solid tumors. Finally, this trend towards increased surgical conservatism is likely to spare patients from SLNB itself in the future when clinicians will be able to preoperatively evaluate the lymph node status through increasingly accurate imaging techniques.

## References

[1] O'Dowd M., Philipp E. *The History of Obstetrics and Gynaecology*. CRC Press. 2000. doi:10.1201/b14682.

[2] Seriau L., Bertozzi S., Cedolini C., Londero A. P. *The Sentinel Lymph Node: Detection, Procedures and Clinical Implications*, chapter "Cancer dissemination pathways, conservative surgery, and the rational of the sentinel lymph node biopsy", 9–18. Nova Science Publishers, 2019.

[3] Cedolini C., Bertozzi S., Seriau L., Noce L., Londero A. P. *The Sentinel Lymph Node: Detection, Procedures and Clinical Implications*, chapter "Complications of the sentinel lymph node biopsy for breast cancer and melanoma", 103–117. Nova Science Publishers, 2019.

[4] Biglia N., Bounous V. E., Robba E., Menato G. *The Sentinel Lymph Node: Detection, Procedures and Clinical Implications*, chapter "Complications of lymphadenectomy and sentinel lymph node biopsy in patients with gynecological cancer", 169–189. Nova Science Publishers, 2019.

[5] Gould E., Winship T., Philbin P., Kerr H. Observations on a "sentinel node" in cancer of the parotid. *Cancer. 1960*;13:77–78.

[6] Cabanas R. M. An approach for the treatment of penile carcinoma. *Cancer. 1977*; 39:456–466.

[7] Chiappa S., Uslenghi C., Bonadonna G., Marano P., Ravasi G. Combined testicular and foot lymphangiography in testicular carcinomas. *Surgery, gynecology & obstetrics. 1966*;123:10–14.

[8] Weissbach L., Boedefeld E. A. Localization of solitary and multiple metastases in stage II nonseminomatous testis tumor as basis for a modified staging lymph node dissection in stage I. *The Journal of urology. 1987*;138:77–82.

[9] Morton D. L., Wen D. R., Wong J. H., Economou J. S., Cagle L. A., Storm F. K., et al. Technical details of intraoperative lymphatic mapping for early stage melanoma. *Archives of surgery (Chicago, Ill : 1960). 1992*;127:392–399.

[10] Levenback C., Burke T. W., Gershenson D. M., Morris M., Malpica A., Ross M. I. Intraoperative lymphatic mapping for vulvar cancer. *Obstetrics and gynecology. 1994*;84:163–167.

[11] Giuliano A. E. Mapping a pathway for axillary staging: a personal perspective on the current status of sentinel lymph node dissection for breast cancer. *Archives of surgery (Chicago, Ill : 1960). 1999*;134:195–199.

[12] Tanis P. J., Nieweg O. E., Valdés Olmos R. A., Th Rutgers E. J., Kroon B. B. History of sentinel node and validation of the technique. *Breast cancer research : BCR. 2001*; 3:109–112.

[13] Turner R. R., Ollila D. W., Krasne D. L., Giuliano A. E. Histopathologic validation of the sentinel lymph node hypothesis for breast carcinoma. *Annals of surgery. 1997*; 226:271–6; discussion 276–8.

[14] Londero A. P., Wilhelmer E, Bertozzi S., Fruscalzo A, Lellé RJ. *The Sentinel Lymph Node: Detection, Procedures and Clinical Implications*, chapter "Sentinel lymph node biopsy in vulvar cancer", 129–149. Nova Science Publishers, 2019.

[15] Biasioli A., Trombetta G., Londero A. P., Cagnacci A. *The Sentinel Lymph Node: Detection, Procedures and Clinical Implications*, chapter "Sentinel lymph node biopsy for cervical cancer", 151–168. Nova Science Publishers, 2019.

[16] Xholli A., Cecchini F., Londero A. P., Cagnacci A. *The Sentinel Lymph Node: Detection, Procedures and Clinical Implications*, chapter "Ultrasound nodal staging in cervical and endometrial cancer", 201–219. Nova Science Publishers, 2019.

[17] Terrosu G., Cedolini C., Scarpa E., Londero A. P., Bertozzi S. *The Sentinel Lymph Node: Detection, Procedures and Clinical Implications*, chapter "Sentinel lymph node biopsy in anal carcinoma", 243–257. Nova Science Publishers, 2019.

[18] Della Martina M., Venier M., Londero A. P., Cagnacci A. *The Sentinel Lymph Node: Detection, Procedures and Clinical Implications*, chapter "Sentinel lymph node biopsy in endometrial cancer", 187–200. Nova Science Publishers, 2019.

[19] Terrosu G., Scarpa E., Bertozzi S., Londero A. P. *The Sentinel Lymph Node: Detection, Procedures and Clinical Implications*, chapter "Sentinel lymph node biopsy in colorectal cancer", 259–279. Nova Science Publishers, 2019.

[20] Orsaria M., Bertozzi S., Marzinotto S., Londero A. P., Mariuzzi L. *The Sentinel Lymph Node: Detection, Procedures and Clinical Implications*, chapter "Technical aspects of the sentinel lymph node evaluation", 19–38. Nova Science Publishers, 2019.

[21] Bertozzi S., Cedolini C., Londero A. P. *The Sentinel Lymph Node: Detection, Procedures and Clinical Implications*, chapter "Sentinel lymph node biopsy in breast cancer", 39–62. Nova Science Publishers, 2019.

[22] Viola L., Londero A. P., Bertozzi S., Gatta G. *The Sentinel Lymph Node: Detection, Procedures and Clinical Implications*, chapter "Breast cancer nodal staging", 63–80. Nova Science Publishers, 2019.

[23] Di Vora R., Cedolini C., Bulligan C., De Biasio F., Parodi P. C., Bertozzi S. *The Sentinel Lymph Node: Detection, Procedures and Clinical Implications*, chapter "Sentinel lymph node biopsy in melanoma", 81–102. Nova Science Publishers, 2019.

[24] Portinari M., Carcoforo P. *The Sentinel Lymph Node: Detection, Procedures and Clinical Implications*, chapter "Sentinel lymph node biopsy in thyroid cancer", 119–127. Nova Science Publishers, 2019.

[25] Andretta M., Cedolini C., Bertozzi S., Londero A. P. *The Sentinel Lymph Node: Detection, Procedures and Clinical Implications*, chapter "Sentinel lymph node detection technique", 19–35. Nova Science Publishers, 2019.

[26] Roncati L., Lupi M., Cavatorta C., Manenti A. *The Sentinel Lymph Node: Detection, Procedures and Clinical Implications*, chapter "Liver lymphatics, sentinel node mapping and possible clinical applications of sentinel lymph node biopsy in liver surgery", 281–293. Nova Science Publishers, 2019.

[27] Bertozzi S., Cedolini C., Valotto C., Di Vora R., Londero A. P., Rialiti A. *The Sentinel Lymph Node: Detection, Procedures and Clinical Implications*, chapter "Less common applications of the sentinel lymph node biopsy", 295–314. Nova Science Publishers, 2019.

[28] American College of Surgeons. *AJCC Cancer Staging Manual (Eighth Edition)*. Springer. 2017.

# Editors Contact Information


***Ambrogio Pietro Londero, MD, PhD***

Udine University Hospital, Italy

Email: ambrogio.londero@gmail.com

***Serena Bertozzi, MD***

Udine University Hospital, Italy

Email: dr.bertozzi@gmail.com

***Carla Cedolini***

Udine University Hospital, Italy

Email: Carla.cedolini@asuiud.sanita.fvg.it

# INDEX

## A



## B



## C



## D



## E



## F



## G

## H



## I



## L



## M



## N



## O



## P

## R



## S



## T



## U



## V



## W

## Bladder Cancer: Research Advances and Clinical Challenges

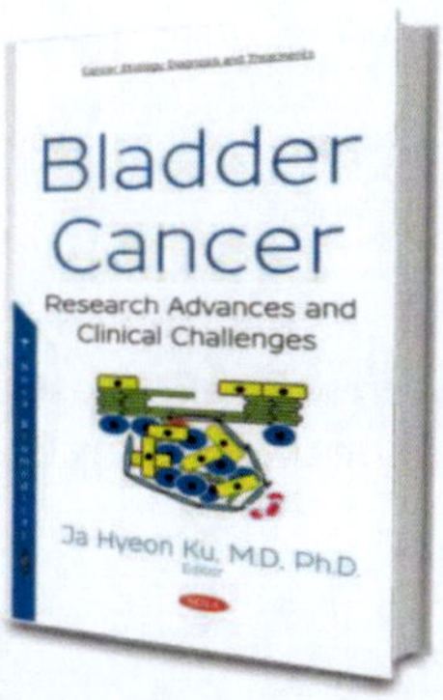


**Editor:** Ja Hyeon Ku, M.D., Ph.D. (Department of Urology, Seoul National University Hospital, Yongon Dong, Jongno Ku, Seoul, Korea)

**Series:** Cancer Etiology, Diagnosis and Treatments

**Book Description:** *Bladder Cancer: Research Advances and Clinical Challenges* is a textbook on bladder cancer written by leading world experts in the field. This new book presents the latest research in this field.

**Hardcover ISBN:** 978-1-53613-354-7
**Retail Price:** $195

## Clinical Oncoproteomics: Proteome-Based Personalized Anti-Cancer Therapy

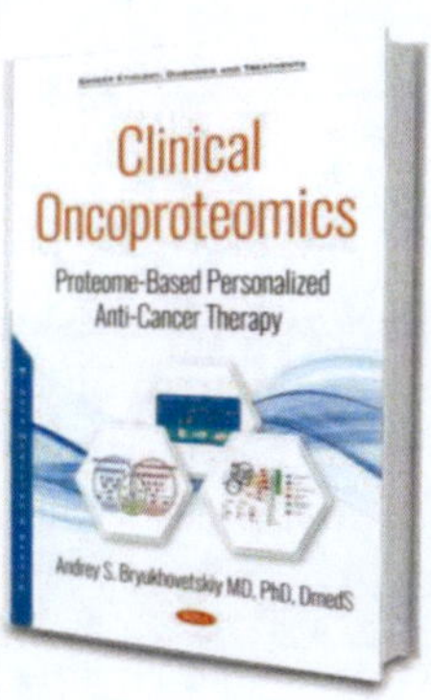


**Author:** Andrey S. Bryukhovetskiy, M.D., Ph.D. (Federal Research Center for Specialized Types of Medical Assistance and Medical Technologies of FMBA of Russia, Moscow, Russia)

**Series:** Cancer Etiology, Diagnosis and Treatments

**Book Description:** This book reviews various academic viewpoints on the informational component and value of the data of clinical oncoproteomics for the diagnostics and treatment of malignant tumors using cellular, genomic and post-genomic technologies.

**Hardcover ISBN:** 978-1-53614-477-2
**Retail Price:** $230